The World Book Health & Medical Annual

1990

World Book, Inc./Chicago • London • Sydney • Toronto

a Scott Fetzer company

Staff

Publisher
William H. Nault

Editor in Chief
Robert O. Zeleny

Executive Editor
A. Richard Harmet

Editorial
Managing Editor
Wayne Wille

Associate Editor
Joan Stephenson

Senior Editors
David L. Dreier
Robin Goldman
Jinger Hoop
Mary A. Krier
Barbara A. Mayes
Jay Myers
Rod Such

Contributing Editors
Sara Dreyfuss
Darlene R. Stille

Cartographic Services
H. George Stoll, Head
Wayne K. Pichler

Editorial Assistant
Ethel Matthews

Art
Art Director
Alfred de Simone

Senior Artist,
Health & Medical Annual
Melanie J. Lawson

Senior Artists
Nikki Conner
Lucy Smith

Photographs
Photography Director
John S. Marshall

Senior Photographs Editor
Sandra M. Ozanick

Photographs Editor
Geralyn Swietek

Research Services
Director
Mary Norton

Product Production
Executive Director
Peter Mollman

Director of Manufacturing
Henry Koval

Manufacturing, Manager
Sandra Van den Broucke

Pre-Press Services
Jerry Stack, Director
Barbara Podczerwinski
Randi Park

Proofreaders
Anne Dillon
Marguerite Hoye
Daniel Marotta

Copyright © 1989
World Book, Inc.
Merchandise Mart Plaza, Chicago, Illinois 60654
All rights reserved

ISBN 0-7166-1190-2
ISSN 0890-4480
Library of Congress Catalog Card Number: 87-648075
Printed in the United States of America

IMPORTANT NOTE: The information contained in *The World Book Health & Medical Annual* is not intended to take the place of the care and attention of a physician or other medical or health-care professional. The information contained in *The World Book Health & Medical Annual* is believed to be accurate, but cannot be warranted. On any matters related to health, always consult a physician or other appropriate health-care professional.

Editorial Advisory Board

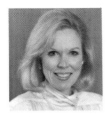
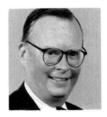
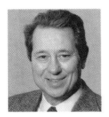
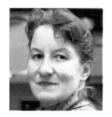
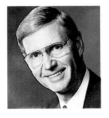

Contents

Special Reports

Fifteen articles present in-depth information about topics of current importance in the fields of health and medicine.

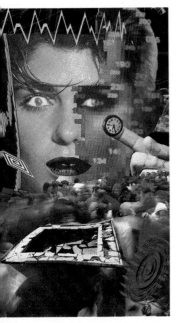

See page 10.

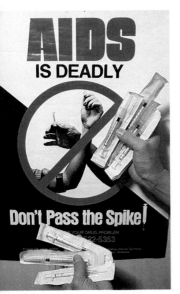

See page 119.

No Need to Panic
by Daniel Goleman
Phobias, panic attacks, and other anxiety disorders are among the most common, most treatable psychiatric problems.   10

Answers to Your Questions About Breast Cancer
by Susan M. Love with Karen Lindsey
A noted cancer surgeon presents a down-to-earth discussion of one of women's most feared diseases.   26

Steroid Abuse: Turning Winners into Losers
by Thomas H. Maugh II
Athletes who hope to gain a winning edge by taking drugs called anabolic steroids risk serious health problems.   42

What Everyone Needs to Know About Stroke
by Beverly Merz
Stroke is the third leading cause of death in the United States. Fortunately, much can be done to prevent it.   56

The Inside Story on Ulcers
by John Schaffner
Forget the old ideas about what causes peptic ulcers.   70

Soviet Medicine: The Promise and the Problems
by Michael Woods
The Soviet Union seeks to reconcile a goal of free health care for all and a reality that falls far short.   82

Make Mine Vegetarian?
by Johanna T. Dwyer
An expert on nutrition takes a look at vegetarian diets.   98

Medical Ethics and the AIDS Epidemic
by Carol Levine
AIDS has raised many troubling questions for society. Bioethicists are helping us find some answers.   112

When a Kiss Can Make You Sick
by Patricia Thomas
The mononucleosis virus touches nearly everyone.   126

The Great White Plague: A History of TB
by William H. Allen
Tuberculosis has long been the subject of myth.   140

The Puzzle of Legionnaires' Disease
by John Camper
What caused the deadly disease that surfaced at a 1976
American Legion convention?   154

The Hidden Dangers of Lead
by Jan Ziegler
The symptoms of lead poisoning are often unrecognized, and its
many sources are not readily apparent.   168

Living with Asthma
by François Haas and Sheila Sperber Haas
With education and medication, asthmatics can take control of
their disease and their lives.   182

Oh, My Aching Back!
by Joseph Wallace
Most Americans will have problems with their backs during
their lives. And the causes and treatments are plentiful.   198

Treating the Severely Burned
by Richard Trubo
Ever-better treatments are saving lives of burn patients.   212

Health & Medical File
Forty-one alphabetically arranged articles, plus six   228
Health & Medical Annual Close-Ups, report on the
year's major developments in health and medicine.

People in Health Care
In *Rescuing Young Lives: Inside a Trauma Center,*   338
writer Alan Doelp presents a dramatic account of
how the special expertise of a children's trauma
center can make the difference between life and
death. *They Fly to Save Sight,* by Mary Krier,
profiles the work of a flying eye hospital and its
mission to fight world blindness.

Health Studies
In *Vaccines and Your Health* by Boyce Rensberger, *The*   366
World Book Health & Medical Annual takes an in-depth
look at vaccines and their importance in our lives.

Index   385

A tear-out page of cross-reference tabs for insertion in
The World Book Encyclopedia appears after page 384.

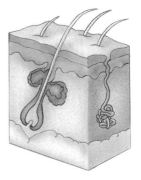

See page 215.

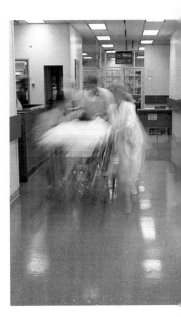

See page 341.

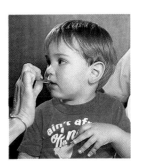

See page 378.

Contributors

Allen, William H., B.S., M.A., M.S.J.
Science Reporter, *St. Louis Post-Dispatch.*
[Special Report, *The Great White Plague: A History of TB; Diabetes; Smoking*]

Balk, Robert A., M.D.
Director of Medical Intensive Care Unit and Director of Respiratory Therapy, Rush-Presbyterian-St. Luke's Medical Center.
[*Respiratory System*]

Barone, Jeanine, M.S.
Nutritionist and Exercise Physiologist,
American Health Foundation.
[*Nutrition and Food*]

Baum, John, M.D.
Professor of Medicine, Pediatrics, and Rehabilitation, University of Rochester School of Medicine.
[*Arthritis and Connective Tissue Disorders*]

Birnbaum, Gary, M.D.
Professor of Neurology, University of Minnesota Medical School.
[*Brain and Nervous System*]

Bower, Bruce, B.A., M.A.
Behavioral Sciences Editor, *Science News.*
[*Child Development; Mental and Behavioral Disorders*]

Camper, John, B.A.
Reporter, *Chicago Tribune.*
[Special Report, *The Puzzle of Legionnaires' Disease*]

Cates, Willard, Jr., M.D., M.P.H.
Director, Division of Sexually Transmitted Diseases, Centers for Disease Control.
[*Sexually Transmitted Diseases*]

Crawford, Michael H., M.D.
Professor of Medicine, University of Texas Health Science Center.
[*Heart and Blood Vessels*]

Doelp, Alan
Free-lance Writer; Author, *In the Blink of an Eye* (1989).
[People in Health Care, *Rescuing Young Lives: Inside a Trauma Center*]

Dover, Jeffrey S., M.D., F.R.C.P. (C)
Dermatologist, Deaconess Hospital, Harvard Medical School.
[*Skin*]

Dwyer, Johanna T., D.Sc., R.D.
Professor of Medicine, Tufts University Medical School.
[Special Report, *Make Mine Vegetarian?*]

Franklin, James L., M.D.
Associate Professor, Rush-Presbyterian-St. Luke's Medical Center.
[*Digestive System*]

Friedman, Emily, B.A.
Contributing Editor, *Hospitals* and *Medical World News.*
[*Financing Health Care; Health Care Facilities*]

Gartland, John J., M.D.
Chairman Emeritus, Department of Orthopaedic Surgery, Jefferson Medical College.
[*Bone Disorders*]

Goleman, Daniel, Ph.D.
Contributing Writer, *The New York Times.*
[Special Report, *No Need to Panic*]

Goldstein, Robert A., M.D., Ph.D.
Acting Director, Division of Allergy, Immunology and Transplantation,
National Institute of Allergy and Infectious Diseases.
[*Allergies and Immunology*]

Haas, François, Ph.D.
Director, Pulmonary Function Laboratory, New York University Medical Center.
[Special Report, *Living with Asthma*]

Haas, Sheila Sperber, Ph.D.
Free-lance Writer.
[Special Report, *Living with Asthma*]

Hamilton, Gayle R., Ph.D.
President, Drug Abuse Training Associates; Adjunct Professor, George Mason University.
[*Alcohol and Drug Abuse*]

Hussar, Daniel A., B.S., M.S., Ph.D.
Remington Professor of Pharmacy,
Philadelphia College of Pharmacy and Science.
[*Drugs*]

Jubiz, William, M.D.
Director, Medical Service, Department of Veterans Affairs.
[*Glands and Hormones*]

Lake, Laura M., B.A., M.A., Ph.D.
Adjunct Assistant Professor of Environmental Science and Engineering, School of Public Health, University of California at Los Angeles.
[*Environmental Health*]

Lane, Thomas J., B.S., D.V.M.
Extension Veterinarian, University of Florida.
[*Veterinary Medicine*]

Levine, Carol, M.A.
Executive Director, Citizens Commission on AIDS.
[Special Report, *Medical Ethics and the AIDS Epidemic*]

Lindsey, Karen, B.A., M.A.
Free-lance Writer.
[Special Report, *Answers to Your Questions About Breast Cancer*]

Love, Susan M., B.S., M.D., Ph.D.
Director, Faulkner Breast Centre.
[Special Report, *Answers to Your Questions About Breast Cancer*]

Maugh, Thomas H., II, Ph.D.
Science Writer,
Los Angeles Times.
[Special Report, *Steroid Abuse: Turning Winners into Losers*]

McInerney, Joseph D., B.S., M.S., M.A.
Director, Biological Sciences Curriculum Study, The Colorado College.
[*Genetics*]

Merz, Beverly, A.B.
Associate Editor,
Journal of the American Medical Association.
[Special Report, *What Everyone Needs to Know About Stroke; Drugs* (Close-Up); *Eye and Vision; Stroke*]

Newman-Horm, Patricia A., B.A.
Chief, Press Office,
National Cancer Institute.
[*Cancer*]

Ovitsky, Margaret Moore, A.M.L.S.
Information Services Librarian, Library of the Health Sciences, University of Illinois at Chicago.
[*Books of Health and Medicine*]

Pessis, Dennis A., B.S., M.D.
Associate Professor,
Rush Medical College.
[*Urology*]

Phillips, Tania J., B.Sc., M.B.B.S., M.R.C.P.
Dermatologist, Boston University School of Medicine.
[*Skin*]

Powers, Robert D., M.D.
Medical Director,
Emergency Medical Services,
University of Virginia Health Sciences Center.
[*Emergency Medicine*]

Rensberger, Boyce, B.S., M.S.
Science Editor, *Washington Post.*
[Health Studies, *Vaccines and Your Health*]

Roodman, G. David, M.D., Ph.D.
Associate Professor,
University of Texas Health Science Center.
[*Blood*]

Schaffner, John, M.D.
Associate Professor of Medicine, Rush Medical College.
[Special Report, *The Inside Story on Ulcers*]

Siegel, Kenneth L., A.B., D.D.S.
Dentist.
[*Dentistry*]

Skinner, James S., Ph.D.
Director, Exercise and Sport Research Institute, and Professor, Department of Health and Physical Education, Arizona State University.
[*Exercise and Fitness* (Close-Up)]

Thomas, Patricia, M.A.
Boston Correspondent,
Medical World News.
[Special Report, *When a Kiss Can Make You Sick; Weight Control; Weight Control* (Close-Up)]

Thompson, Jeffrey R., B.S., M.D.
Assistant Professor of Medicine, University of Texas, Southwestern Medical Center.
[*Kidney*]

Trubo, Richard, B.A., M.A.
Contributing Editor,
Medical World News.
[Special Report, *Treating the Severely Burned; AIDS*]

Tyrer, Louise B., M.D.
Vice President for Medical Affairs, Planned Parenthood Federation of America.
[*Birth Control*]

Wallace, Joseph, B.A.
Free-lance Writer.
[Special Report, *Oh, My Aching Back!*]

Williams, T. Franklin, M.D.
Director, National Institute on Aging.
[*Aging*]

Woods, Michael, B.S.
Science Editor, *Toledo Blade.*
[Special Report, *Soviet Medicine: The Promise and the Problems; Safety.*]

Ziegler, Jan
Free-lance Writer; former Science Editor, United Press International.
[Special Report, *The Hidden Dangers of Lead*]

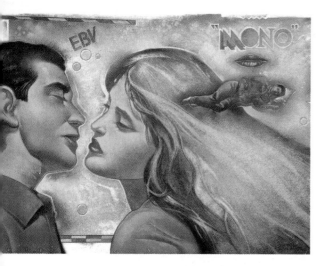

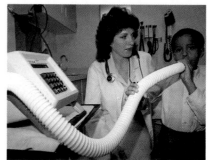

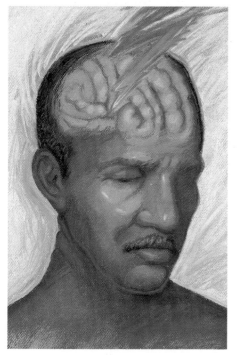

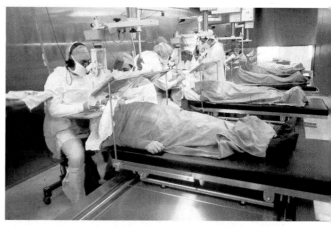

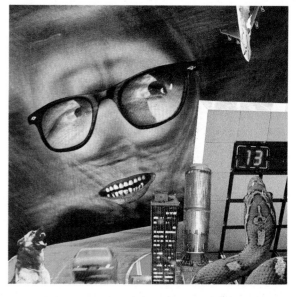

Special Reports

Fifteen Special Reports present in-depth information about topics of current importance in health and medicine.

No Need to Panic
by Daniel Goleman — 10

Answers to Your Questions About Breast Cancer
by Susan M. Love with Karen Lindsey — 26

Steroid Abuse: Turning Winners into Losers
by Thomas H. Maugh II — 42

What Everyone Needs to Know About Stroke
by Beverly Merz — 56

The Inside Story on Ulcers
by John Schaffner — 70

Soviet Medicine: The Promise and the Problems
by Michael Woods — 82

Make Mine Vegetarian?
by Johanna T. Dwyer — 98

Medical Ethics and the AIDS Epidemic
by Carol Levine — 112

When a Kiss Can Make You Sick
by Patricia Thomas — 126

The Great White Plague: A History of TB
by William H. Allen — 140

The Puzzle of Legionnaires' Disease
by John Camper — 154

The Hidden Dangers of Lead
by Jan Ziegler — 168

Living with Asthma
by François Haas and Sheila Sperber Haas — 182

Oh, My Aching Back!
by Joseph Wallace — 198

Treating the Severely Burned
by Richard Trubo — 212

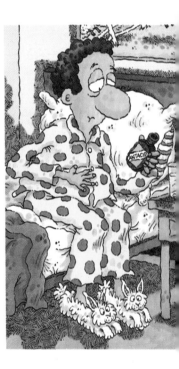

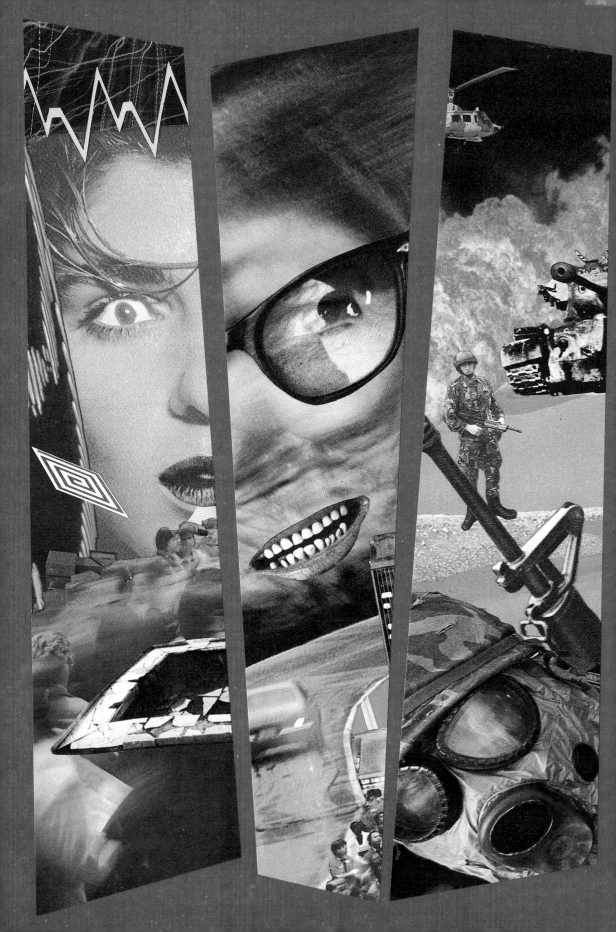

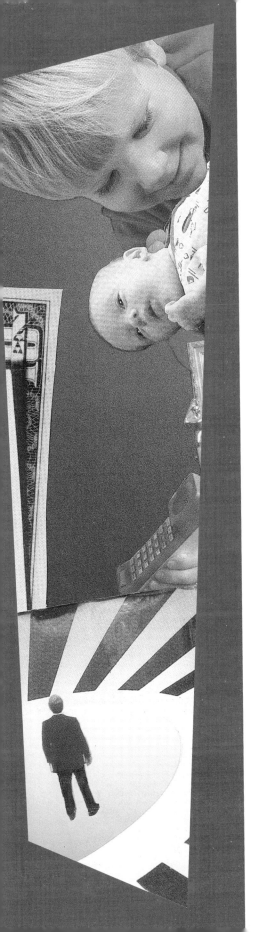

Phobias, panic attacks, and other anxiety disorders are among the most common psychiatric problems of all— and the most easily treated.

No Need to Panic

By Daniel Goleman

*E*llen, a 23-year-old law clerk, was working late doing research for a case. Suddenly she felt flooded with dread that something awful was about to happen. Then she found herself gasping for air. Her whole body felt flushed and tingling; her arms and legs went numb. Then a bolt of pain stabbed across her chest. Ellen was terrified she was dying of a heart attack, all alone in the law firm's library.

Jack, a Vietnam veteran in his 40's, is haunted with memories of the war, decades ago. Often he can't concentrate on his work or even just watch TV. Instead, his mind drifts off to images of the wounded and dead he saw on the battlefield. Many nights he wakes shaking from a vivid nightmare in which an enemy soldier is about to kill him.

Jane, in her 50's, is afraid to drive a car. The fear began more than 10 years ago, when she was driving on a rural two-lane road and

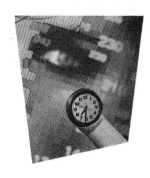

a drunken driver hit her car head-on. After the accident, Jane quit driving—though that meant finding a new job closer to home and depending on friends to take her shopping. Even when someone else is driving, Jane refuses to sit in the front seat. When she tries, she freezes, paralyzed with fear.

We all worry about something—our health, our friends, our grades in school. But for some people anxiety is more than a response to a problem; anxiety *is* the problem.

Ellen, Jack, and Jane suffer from *anxiety disorders*—mental and behavioral problems in which ordinary situations cause extreme anxiety. Ellen's anxiety attacks are the primary sign of *panic disorder.* Jack's problem is *post-traumatic stress disorder* (PTSD), an anxiety disorder linked with a traumatic past event. Jane has a *simple phobia*, an unreasonable fear of a specific situation or thing.

According to a survey of 18,500 people conducted between 1980 and 1984 by the National Institute of Mental Health (NIMH), 14.8 per cent of Americans suffer from an anxiety disorder at some point in their lives. By comparison, the lifetime rate for depression and related disorders is 8.3 per cent. Only drug or alcohol abuse, which occurs among 16.4 per cent of Americans, poses a higher lifetime risk. Among women—who account for twice as many anxiety cases as men—anxiety is the most commonly diagnosed psychiatric problem of all. (Some experts suggest that this reflects more willingness among women to seek help for anxiety disorders.)

Still, anxiety's many sufferers are not doomed to lives of fear and worry. Anxiety disorders are among the easiest to treat of all psychiatric problems. And researchers are working to pinpoint the causes of anxiety disorders and to develop even more effective treatments for them.

Types of anxiety disorders

It is normal to feel anxious on occasion, such as when giving a speech or facing an exam. But anxiety disorders go beyond normal nervousness in two ways. First, people with these disorders are anxious in situations in which most other people are not, or they are anxious to a disproportionate degree. Second, their anxiety is so intense that it interferes with their lives—often because they go out of their way to avoid the situations that spark their fears.

For a long time, psychiatry lumped all anxiety problems together under the terms "phobia" or "anxiety neurosis." But in the last decade, psychiatrists have formally recognized several distinct—though related—anxiety disorders. These include panic disorder and the often-associated *agoraphobia* (fear of public places); simple phobias related to specific situations; *social phobia* (unreasonable shyness); PTSD; and *generalized*

The author:

Daniel Goleman is a contributing writer for *The New York Times* and author of the book *Vital Lies, Simple Truths: The Psychology of Self-Deception* (1986).

anxiety disorder (anxiety unrelated to a particular trigger).

Panic disorder. Perhaps the most frightening of the anxiety disorders is that characterized by attacks such as those that plagued Ellen. Symptoms of panic attacks vary, but they generally include several of the following: dizziness or faintness, heart acceleration or palpitations, numbness or shakiness, profuse sweating, hot flashes or chills, stomach upset, choking or a sense of suffocation, and chest pains.

Attacks typically last only a few minutes, though sometimes they go on for hours. The start is usually marked by a feeling of apprehension, which can turn to outright terror. Victims often feel intense fear—of going crazy, of losing control, or of dying. The physical symptoms lead many victims to believe they are having a heart attack. They also make the disorder hard to diagnose, since patients and physicians usually start by investigating possible physical illnesses.

Panic attacks usually first occur during a person's late 20's, though they can start as early as childhood or as late as middle age. Once the problem begins, the attacks may recur more and more frequently. Sometimes the frequency of attacks wanes after a few weeks or months, but more often they continue on and off for years unless they are treated. After her first panic attack, Ellen started to have them once or twice a week. She never knew when one might strike, and she lived in constant dread of the next episode.

This unpredictability of panic attacks, and the fearful anticipation it creates, may become as much of a problem as the attacks themselves. For some patients, this apprehension develops into another anxiety disorder: agoraphobia.

Agoraphobia occurs most often in people with panic disorder. Although its name (Greek for "fear of the marketplace") implies that the disorder is a type of simple phobia, it is not— that is, the fear does not focus on a specific object or situation. Rather, agoraphobia is a generalized fear of public places, such as stores, theaters, restaurants, or public transportation. People with this disorder avoid these places for fear that in an emergency—such as a panic attack—they will be unable to get help or to escape without embarrassment.

In its mildest forms, agoraphobia may lead people to avoid normal situations, such as shopping or going to work. In the most severe cases, sufferers will leave their homes only with a trusted companion—or won't go out at all.

Simple phobia refers to any fear that focuses on a specific cause—such as spiders, snakes, heights, or flying. People with a simple phobia feel immediate, agonizing anxiety when they are exposed to whatever it is they fear. Someone with a phobia of dogs, for instance, would have anxiety symptoms—such

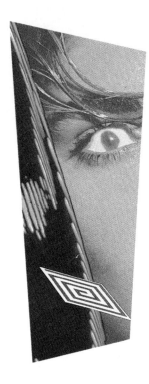

as a racing heart or sweating—upon seeing a dog. The closer the feared object, the worse the anxiety. Jane's fear of driving became more intense if she sat in the front seat.

Even though people with phobias know their fears are exaggerated, they feel powerless to control them. Instead, they go to great lengths to avoid the things they fear. A phobia may matter little if a person rarely encounters the feared situation. For example, a person who lives in the country might face no difficulty from a fear of tall buildings. But for someone who lives in a city, this phobia can make life miserable.

Sometimes the source of a phobia can be traced to a traumatic experience. In Jane's case, that was an auto accident. Being in an airplane that goes through such intense turbulence it seems it may crash might lead to a fear of flying; being attacked by a vicious dog might lead to a phobia of dogs. Most phobias, however, do not seem to stem from an event.

Phobias are by far the most common of anxiety disorders, and they can begin at any point in life. Many children's phobias—such as fears of dogs or the dark—disappear as they grow older. But if such a phobia continues into adulthood, it is likely to remain unless the person receives treatment.

Social phobia is the technical name for extreme shyness. People with social phobia fear that they will do something embarrassing while other people are watching—such as become speechless while giving a lecture, be unable to urinate in a public lavatory, or say something foolish when meeting someone new. The mere prospect of having to meet strangers or speak up in a group can evoke trembling or panic.

People who are merely shy can still endure the social situations that make them uncomfortable, but those with social phobia become so distressed that it interferes with their work and their relationships. For example, ordinary shyness may make a person reluctant to meet a stranger, but social phobia might lead someone to refuse to go to a party for fear of being introduced to a stranger.

As with simple phobia, people with social phobia may realize their fear is unreasonable and limiting, yet feel powerless to do much about it. Often these people fall prey to a cycle in which they worry that someone will notice that they are nervous, and that worry increases their nervousness.

Post-traumatic stress disorder stems from the lingering psychological impact of an intensely frightening experience. The types of events that cause this problem—such as auto accidents, rape, mugging, or war—would be upsetting to almost anyone. But although most people largely recover from such trauma within a month or two, those who develop PTSD feel the emotional impact for six months or longer—often years.

The primary symptom of PTSD is *flashbacks*, episodes in which the person's awareness floods with images or emotions

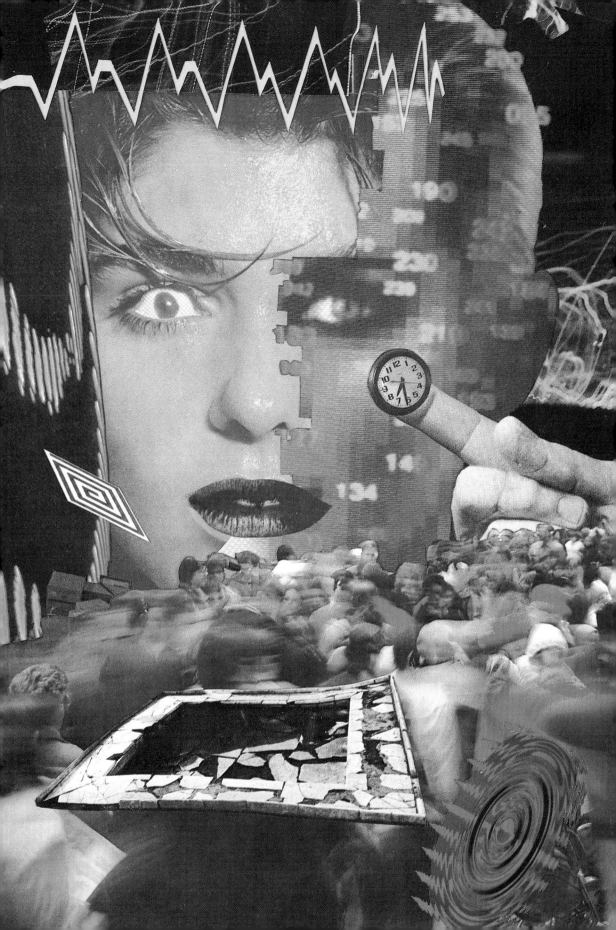

associated with the event. Sometimes the flashbacks are provoked by an encounter that resembles the original event, or by an occasion—such as an anniversary—that revives the memories. In rare instances, the person seems to relive the event as though it were happening at that moment.

This happened to Jack during a business trip. He ran into an old war buddy, and the two men went to a bar and talked over memories of Vietnam. Walking back to his hotel, Jack began to believe that the people he passed were enemy soldiers in disguise. He started shouting at them, threatening to kill them. Someone called the police, and Jack was arrested.

Flashbacks, although the most striking demonstration of PTSD, are not the only symptom. Another hallmark is emotional constriction, or a numbing of responsiveness. Victims may also be overalert and easily startled, as though they were perpetually on guard. Other symptoms may include feelings of guilt, trouble concentrating, nightmares or difficulty with sleeping, or amnesia about all or part of the event.

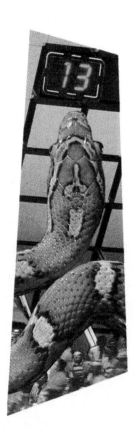

Opposite page: People with *phobias* feel agonizing fear at even the thought of a specific object or situation—such as snakes, heights, or flying. Even though they know their fears are unreasonable, they feel powerless to control them.

The symptoms of PTSD were observed among veterans of World War I, when the syndrome was called "shell shock," and World War II, when it was called "battle fatigue." But it was not until the late 1970's, when the problem was widely noticed among veterans of the Vietnam War, that the disorder was described most fully and given its present name. The disorder is now recognized among people who have survived other deeply traumatic experiences besides combat. Even children may exhibit PTSD after intense events—such as dog bites, rapes, or shootings—or from long-term stressful situations, such as incest, abuse, and war.

Still, Vietnam veterans account for the vast majority of diagnosed cases. A 1988 Veterans Administration study of 3,000 Vietnam veterans found PTSD in nearly 15 per cent of the men and 8.5 per cent of the women. The NIMH survey suggested that PTSD occurred in about 20 per cent of veterans who were wounded in Vietnam, but the proportion dropped to about 3.5 per cent among veterans who were not wounded.

Generalized anxiety disorder. While most anxiety disorders focus on a specific event, object, or situation, generalized anxiety disorder is marked by chronic, unrealistic anxiety about anything or everything. For a student with this disorder, this "free-floating" worry might focus on tests, grades, or friends. Adults might worry continuously about finances, troubles of family members, or the future. Unlike ordinary worries, which may last a few days or weeks, worries associated with this disorder last for six months or longer, during which time they preoccupy the worrier more days than not.

The anxiety manifests itself in many types of symptoms.

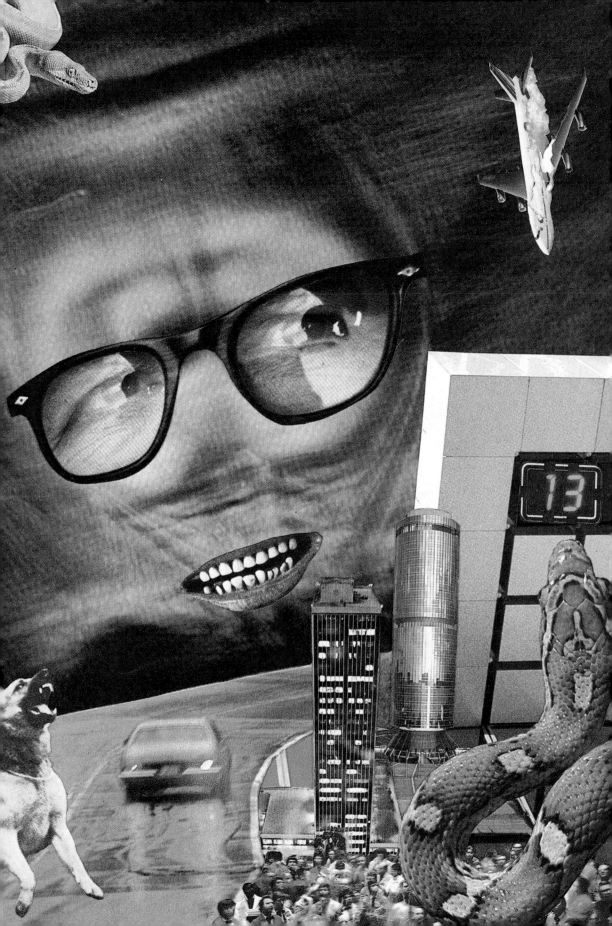

These include various forms of physical tension, such as tiredness, restlessness, trembling, or muscle aches. Another symptom is bodily arousal, the signs of which can include dryness in the mouth, shortness of breath, faintness, nausea or other stomach distress, a lump in the throat, chills or hot flashes, sweating or clamminess, or heart palpitations. Or the anxiety may cause a state of extreme alertness, as expressed in trouble concentrating, irritability, or a tendency to startle easily.

Causes of anxiety disorders

Scientific theories on the causes of anxiety disorders generally fall into two categories: *behavioral theories*, which suggest that anxiety is a learned response to certain objects or situations, and *biological theories*, which propose that a disorder is due to physiological processes in the brain. No single theory explains every kind of anxiety disorder, however. In fact, some scientists believe that individual cases may arise from a combination of both behavioral and biological causes.

Behavioral theories hold that anxiety reactions are learned responses associated with threatening situations. For instance, if a laboratory rat receives an electric shock every time it touches a lever, it will learn to be anxious in response to the lever. By avoiding the lever, it can keep its anxiety under control. Similarly, according to this theory, someone who feels intense anxiety during a turbulent plane flight may then feel the same anxiety later, while taking another plane.

Learning theories seem to explain some anxiety syndromes, such as phobia, which centers on a specific object, or PTSD, which stems from a traumatic experience. But learning theory does not easily explain such problems as panic disorder, in which there is no clear incident that teaches a person to be fearful and no specific situation that triggers the attacks.

Scientists who are pursuing biological theories about anxiety disorders are studying structures and activities of the brain. They believe that people with certain anxiety disorders may have too many of certain kinds of brain cells, or that they produce too much or too little of certain of the large number of brain chemicals that affect these cells.

Some studies are focusing on brain cells that, when stimulated by certain brain chemicals, trigger reactions like those seen during panic attacks—such as a racing heart, trembling, and sweating. Drugs that block the activity of these brain cells are being tested as a means of controlling panic attacks. Other research centers on brain cells that become responsive during stress. In general, brain theories apply most clearly to problems such as panic disorder and generalized anxiety, whose symptoms are not connected to a particular circumstance.

Whether anxiety disorders are caused by psychological factors, physical factors, or both, scientists are finding increasing evidence that some people are more likely than others to develop such disorders. Studies that show anxiety disorders to be unusually common among relatives suggest that some people may inherit an anxiety-prone temperament. For example, in 1983, Norwegian genetic researcher Samuel Torgerson studied 85 pairs of twins in which at least one twin had an anxiety disorder. He found that among identical twins—who have identical genes—both twins had anxiety disorders in 45 per cent of the pairs. But among nonidentical twins—who share fewer of the same genes—both had anxiety disorders only 15 per cent of the time. These results strongly suggest that a tendency toward anxiety disorders has a genetic basis.

Other research suggests that an anxiety-prone temperament is present early in life—perhaps from birth. In a study reported in 1988, Jerome Kagan and J. Steven Reznick, psychologists at Harvard University in Cambridge, Mass., tested 400 2-year-old children from Boston. They found that about 15 per cent of the children were unusually timid, compared with their peers. These shy children also showed more physical signs of stress—such as faster heart rates and greater muscle tension—than did a group of children marked as outgoing.

Kagan and Reznick tested both groups three more times over the next few years. By age 7, about three-fourths of the timid children were still measurably shyer than their peers, and nearly two-thirds of them displayed unusual fears—of, for instance, kidnappers or television shows. The researchers suggested that extreme shyness that can be detected in toddlers is a clue to increased risk of anxiety disorders later.

This study alone, however, did not directly link childhood shyness to anxiety disorders. Seeking such a connection, Jerrold Rosenbaum, a physician at Massachusetts General Hospital in Boston, asked Kagan to evaluate 18 children of patients being treated for panic disorder and agoraphobia. Extreme shyness appeared in 84 per cent of the patients' children. Among a group of children whose parents were not anxiety patients, only the usual 15 per cent were extremely shy.

While these and other studies suggest that anxiety-proneness might be inherited, they do not prove that genetics are solely responsible. For example, instead of passing on anxiety as an inherited trait, anxious parents may simply be teaching their children to react to life with anxiety.

Most experts believe that even if some people are more anxiety-prone than others, specific experiences are necessary to trigger anxiety problems. For example, Kagan found that

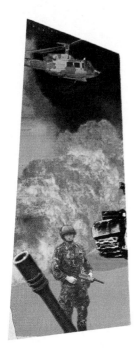

two-thirds of the shy children had older brothers or sisters, while two-thirds of the outgoing children were first-born. This suggests that the stress of living with an older, more dominant sibling may encourage an existing tendency toward shyness.

In fact, stressful events, such as death of a spouse or divorce, often precede the onset of such problems as panic disorder. And some disorders, such as PTSD and phobias, show obvious links to stressful incidents. Still, the same trauma that triggers a disorder in one person will not necessarily do so in another. In all likelihood, the cause of most anxiety disorders lies in a combination of stressful events, learned responses to certain situations, and a biological predisposition.

Treatment of anxiety disorders

Whatever their causes, as many as 4 out of 5 cases of anxiety disorders improve significantly with treatment, according to various studies. In fact, getting patients into treatment may present more of a hurdle than the treatment itself. The Phobia Society of America (a nonprofit organization based in Rockville, Md.) estimates that more than three-fourths of sufferers fail to seek help, and those who do spend an average of eight years before being properly diagnosed and treated.

Treatment for anxiety disorders involves two approaches, which are often used in combination. One is medication to bring the most intense symptoms under control. The other is therapy or counseling to help people overcome their fears and—ideally—eliminate the problem entirely.

Not all anxiety disorders respond equally well to drugs. No medications have been shown to be effective for simple phobia or PTSD. For other disorders, drugs have been used with varying effects.

Benzodiazepines, a class of sedative drugs that includes the tranquilizers Valium and Librium, are often used to control nervousness, especially in people with generalized anxiety disorder. A benzodiazepine derivative called alprazolam has also been shown to work for both nervousness and panic disorder. But these drugs can be addictive, causing withdrawal symptoms unless discontinued gradually. Some also may cause drowsiness. A new drug called buspirone, approved in 1986 as a general antianxiety medication, has been shown to be nonaddictive and less sedative than the benzodiazepines.

Panic attacks and agoraphobia can often be controlled by *antidepressants*, which alter the balance of brain chemicals. These drugs, which include *tricyclics* and *monoamine oxidase inhibitors* (MAOI's), were first developed to treat depression. Antidepressants may produce any of a large range of side effects, including drowsiness, insomnia, dry mouth, constipation, faintness, trembling, blurred vision, or rashes. Patients taking

Opposite page: Memories of war, rape, or other intensely frightening experiences haunt sufferers of *post-traumatic stress disorder*. Victims relive the experience, and the fears associated with it, again and again in their minds.

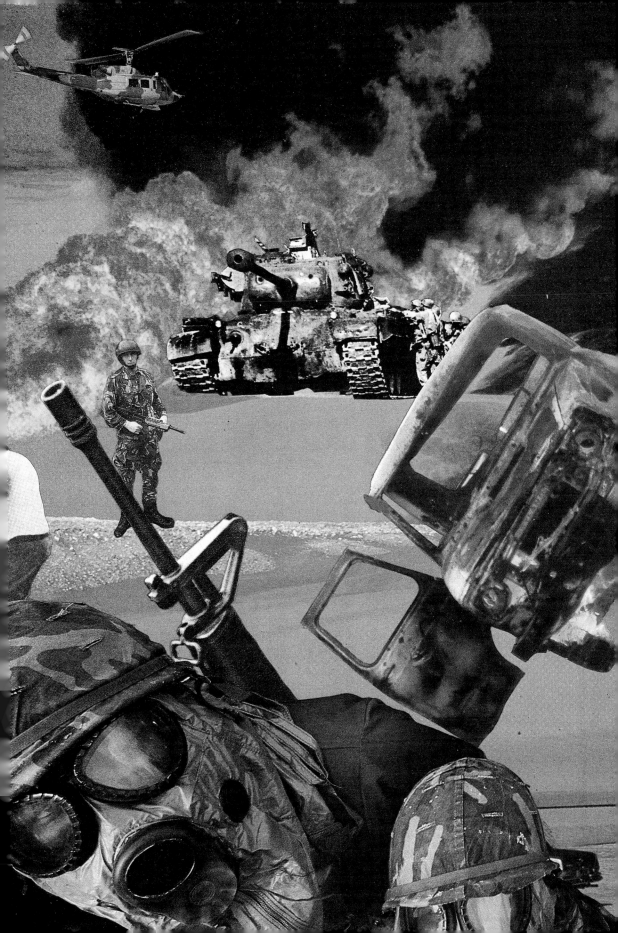

MAOI's must observe some dietary restrictions, because these drugs can interact dangerously with some foods.

Certain MAOI's have shown promise in relieving the fears that underlie social phobia. Researchers are also testing *beta-adrenergic blocking agents*, which are sometimes used by professional performers to counter physical signs of stage fright. These "beta-blockers," by calming the visible symptoms of social phobia—such as a racing heart or tremors—may help break the patient's cycle of increasing nervousness.

The primary drawback of using medication to control anxiety is that drugs only control symptoms temporarily. They do not, in themselves, cure the disorders—and they cannot be used forever. Some patients find that the symptoms come back as soon as they stop taking the drugs. Preventing such recurrence may require therapy or counseling.

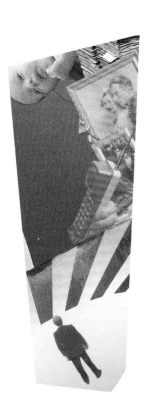

The therapy used most often for anxiety disorders is *cognitive-behavioral therapy*, a combination of two types of psychological techniques. Behavior therapy focuses on correcting the way a person responds. For anxiety problems, this typically involves repeatedly exposing the patients to the things they fear. Cognitive therapy concentrates on the way a person thinks, by helping a person replace unrealistic thoughts with more realistic ones. For anxiety disorders, that means correcting the mistaken beliefs that feed fear and trigger anxiety. Most cognitive-behavioral programs last from 8 to 20 weeks; after completing the program, some patients continue with individual or group therapy to reinforce their treatment.

Jane went to a cognitive-behavioral therapist who helped her plan gradual steps that would lead her, finally, to drive again. One part of Jane's therapy focused on the erroneous beliefs that fed her fears, such as the thought that she was an awful driver or that she was bound to have another accident. Jane learned that when one of these thoughts came to mind, she could talk back to it, telling herself why it was false.

Another part of Jane's therapy put her in the situation she feared most so that she would see that nothing terrible would actually happen to her. Jane went with her therapist to a car, where she sat behind the wheel. As usual, Jane became frightened just sitting there, but with the support of her therapist, she learned to tell herself that the anxiety she felt was just the sensation of fear, not a warning that she was in danger.

After Jane conquered sitting behind the wheel, the next step was to start the engine. At the next session, she drove a few feet. Each week Jane drove a bit more and became more sure of herself. Within three months, Jane was driving normally. She still felt afraid sometimes, but instead of panicking, she could stay behind the wheel until the fears subsided.

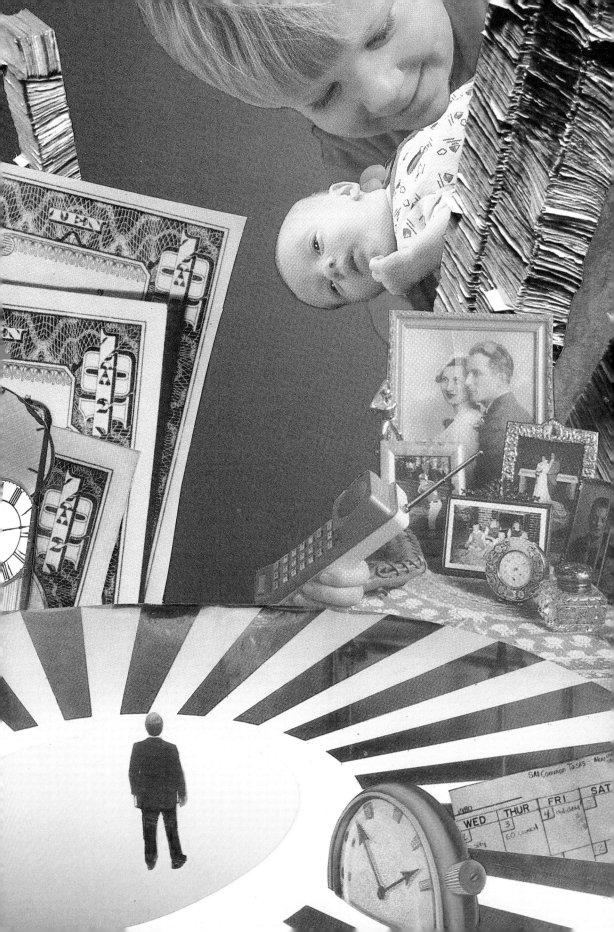

Jane's getting behind the wheel is an example of *in vivo* (real-life) exposure, a behavioral technique in which the patient faces the feared object or situation and stays there until the anxiety lessens. The exposures continue until finally the patient can endure them without fear. This technique is stressful, and some people simply refuse to try it. But studies have found the technique helps up to 75 per cent of patients who do try it—one of the highest rates of improvement for a treatment of a psychological problem.

Other exposure techniques rely on the imagination. In *systematic desensitization*, the patient is put into a state of deep relaxation and then told to visualize an increasingly anxiety-producing series of scenes. Someone with a phobia of snakes, for instance, might first imagine looking at a picture of a snake, and progress to imagining picking up a snake. When anxiety begins, the patient falls back to a relaxation exercise before continuing. In *imaginal flooding*, the patient begins directly with imagining the most frightening scene and maintains that image until the anxiety begins to decrease. This technique, like *in vivo* exposure, is stressful and requires a trained therapist and high motivation on the patient's part.

Treatment for panic attacks takes a different course. When Ellen first went to a psychotherapist, she was having two or three panic attacks a week and living in constant dread of the next one. The first step in her treatment was medication, which got her panic attacks under control. But Ellen realized that medication would only control her problem, not eliminate it. Her therapist began cognitive-behavioral therapy with her.

Because Ellen was so afraid of her panic symptoms, the therapist had her simulate those symptoms purposely during the treatment sessions. She induced the sensation of chest pain, for instance, by tensing her chest and shoulder muscles; for breathlessness, she ran up a flight of stairs. The therapist had Ellen identify which sensations bothered her most.

Then Ellen's therapist helped her to focus on the thoughts that flashed through her mind just as her panic attacks were beginning. Ellen discovered that she was telling herself that something dreadful was going to happen to her—that she was going to die of a heart attack. To her surprise, she saw that those thoughts triggered the panic symptoms—gasping for air, numbness, chest pain, and the like. And this, in her mind, confirmed her fears of heart attack and escalated the panic.

Ellen learned a relaxation method to use when she first felt an attack coming on. By telling herself that the sensations of panic were not a true catastrophe and relaxing when she felt them, Ellen learned to stop her panic attacks.

This approach to treating panic disorder has proven highly

successful. In 1986, David H. Barlow, a psychologist and anxiety specialist at the State University of New York at Albany, reported on the treatment of 32 people with panic disorder using these techniques. After 15 weeks of treatment, 85 per cent of the patients no longer had panic attacks. After 6 to 12 months, 72 per cent were still free of problems.

Agoraphobia can be especially responsive to treatment that involves family or friends. Barlow studied a group of women with agoraphobia whose husbands accompanied them to weekly therapy sessions for three months. The husbands also went along to lend support during practice tasks, which involved placing the women into the situations they feared. Two years later, 82 per cent of the women had overcome many of their fears and were able to function better. In a parallel group of agoraphobic women who were treated without their husbands, only 46 per cent overcame their fears, and those women showed more of a tendency to regress.

PTSD treatments often focus on helping a person come to terms with the trauma and the distressing feelings that it continues to cause. The patient is encouraged to talk about the traumatic event, even if that causes a flood of upsetting emotions. Once those emotions are brought out, then the therapist can help the person deal with them more effectively.

One common approach to treating PTSD is group therapy. After his flashback on the street, Jack joined a therapy group of Vietnam veterans who suffered from PTSD. He was relieved to find others who were haunted by disturbing memories of their war years and who understood his problems.

Under the gentle guidance of the therapist who led the group, Jack was able, for the first time, to talk about the war experience that continued to pain him the most: when his closest buddy was killed by an enemy bomb—an explosion that would have killed Jack if his buddy had not insisted on going first into that unfriendly village.

By talking about feelings that had oppressed him for years, Jack slowly came to be more at peace with his experiences. His nightmares and other symptoms gradually waned. After a year or so, Jack felt he didn't need the group any more—but he decided to keep attending so he could help other veterans come to grips with the psychological legacy of combat.

Because they sought help, Jack, Ellen, and Jane all learned to cope with their anxiety. They discovered that the symptoms of anxiety don't mean that a person is dying or going insane. Rather, anxiety disorders are among the most common and easiest to treat of all psychological problems.

A noted cancer surgeon presents
a down-to-earth discussion of one
of women's most feared diseases.

Answers to Your Questions About Breast Cancer

By Susan M. Love
with Karen Lindsey

At least once a week a frightened woman comes to my office
at the Faulkner Breast Centre in Jamaica Plains, Mass. She's
discovered a lump in her breast, she's sure it's breast cancer,
and she's sure that it will kill her or—at the very least—that
her breast will have to be removed.

And, of course, she's right to be concerned. The incidence
of breast cancer in the United States is rising, affecting 1 out
of 10 women in the nation. Luckily, I'm able to reassure my
patients that most breast lumps are totally harmless.

Sometimes, of course, a breast lump does prove to be cancer, and that is terrifying for any woman. But even then, it
may not be nearly as bad as it sounds. We still tend to think
of the word *cancer* as a death sentence, but in fact, 70 per
cent of women whose breast cancer is discovered before it has
spread beyond the breast survive at least five years.

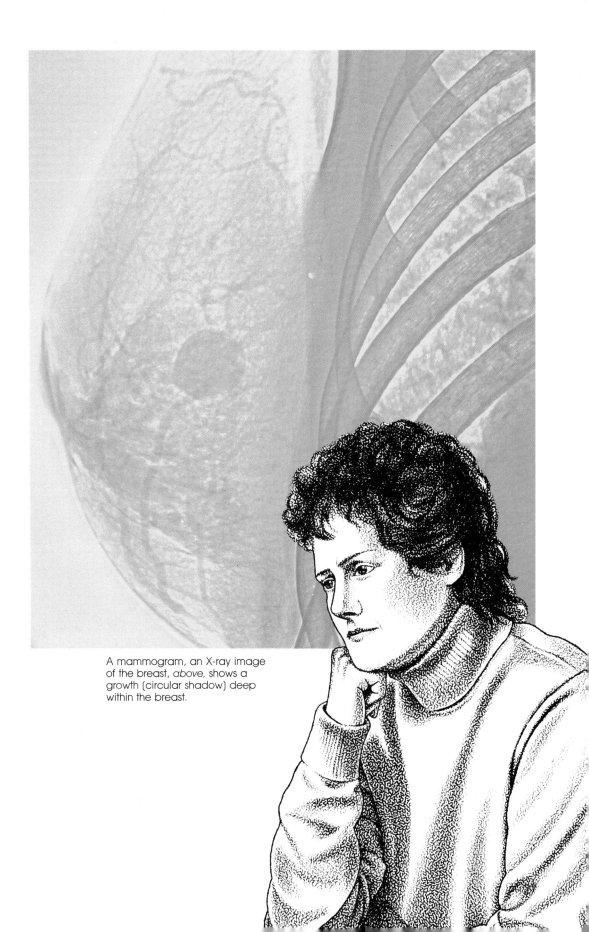

A mammogram, an X-ray image of the breast, *above,* shows a growth (circular shadow) deep within the breast.

What is breast cancer?

Our understanding of all forms of cancer, including breast cancer, is constantly being reexamined. We know that breast cancer often *metastasizes* (spreads throughout the body), going from the breast to the lungs, liver, bones, or brain. Over the years, however, those of us involved in treating breast cancer have refined our perceptions of what breast cancer is and how metastasis occurs.

Experts on cancer once thought that breast cancer started in the breast, rapidly grew into a tumor, and then began sending cancer cells to the rest of the body via the *lymphatic system*, a network of vessels and small masses of tissue called *nodes* that return to the bloodstream the fluid that bathes and nourishes the body's cells. The lymphatic system is vital to the body's disease-fighting immune system because it destroys foreign or harmful matter that enters the bloodstream. Surgeons formerly rushed to remove breast cancer tumors as soon as they were discovered, believing that a delay of even a day or two could give the cancer cells a chance to begin entering the lymphatic system and traveling to other organs.

This course was followed until the late 1970's, when scientists began to realize that, in general, breast cancer tumors grow more slowly than anyone had thought. Most breast cancers require an average of 100 days for a tumor to double in size. It takes about 100 days for the first cell to become two cells, and another 100 days for those two to become four, and for those four to become eight. Thus, by the time there are enough cells to form a detectable lump—about 100 billion cells—the cancer has probably been growing in the breast for 8 to 10 years.

This assumes that all cancers grow at the same rate, which is probably not true. Some may grow rapidly and some extremely slowly. It also assumes that they all grow steadily. In fact, most tumors probably alternate between periods of rest and growth spurts. Nonetheless, it is true that most breast cancer tumors are present a long time before we can detect them through any means. The idea that no cancer cells have entered the bloodstream over such a long period is improbable, and scientific evidence proves that it's likely that some cancer cells leave the breast about three years after the tumor begins growing.

On the basis of this scientific work, Bernard Fisher, a surgeon and researcher at the University of Pittsburgh Medical Center, popularized a new theory about the spread of breast cancer. Because most tumors have sent cells into the bloodstream or lymphatic system before they are detected, Fisher theorized that what is important is not whether cancer cells have escaped, but how successfully the immune system attacked the cells that have probably already escaped. If the

The authors:

Susan M. Love is director of the Faulkner Breast Centre in Boston. She is also assistant clinical professor of surgery at Harvard Medical School and clinical associate in surgical oncology at the Dana Farber Cancer Institute in Boston. Karen Lindsey is a free-lance writer in the Boston area who specializes in women's issues.

28

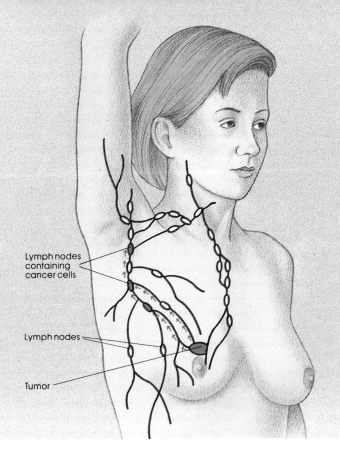

Lymph nodes
containing
cancer cells

Lymph nodes

Tumor

What is breast cancer?

Breast cancer usually starts as a slow-growing tumor in the breast. As it grows, the tumor may send cancer cells to other organs via the bloodstream and the lymphatic system, which destroys foreign or harmful matter in the blood. The presence of cancer cells in some of the lymph nodes near the breast indicates that the cancer has begun to spread throughout the body.

immune system has destroyed all the cells that have traveled beyond the breast, then the woman will be fine; if not, those cells will slowly grow in their new sites until the tumors are big enough to cause harm.

This points up an important fact about breast cancer: Nobody dies of cancer in the breast. You could have a very large lump there and it would not kill you. What kills women with breast cancer is the spread of the cancer to a vital organ, such as the lungs or liver, where the presence of a growing tumor destroys healthy tissue and hinders essential functions.

Interestingly, breast cancer cells that have migrated to other parts of the body are still considered breast cancer. Breast cancer that has spread to the liver, for instance, is not the same thing as liver cancer that originated in liver cells. The escaped breast cancer cells are something like immigrants: If you're an American who moves to France, many essential features of your character remain those of an American, however long you stay in France. Understanding this concept is important because it affects the treatment—in determining which drugs are used to combat the metastasized cancer. It also af-

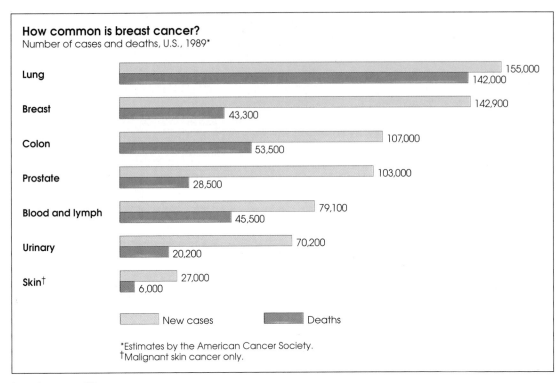

How common is breast cancer?
Number of cases and deaths, U.S., 1989*

Lung	155,000 / 142,000
Breast	142,900 / 43,300
Colon	107,000 / 53,500
Prostate	103,000 / 28,500
Blood and lymph	79,100 / 45,500
Urinary	70,200 / 20,200
Skin†	27,000 / 6,000

New cases   Deaths

*Estimates by the American Cancer Society.
†Malignant skin cancer only.

Breast cancer strikes more American women than any other form of cancer; among the population as a whole (men and women), only lung cancer is more common.

fects the *prognosis*—the forecast of the probable course of a patient's disease—since some forms of cancer are far more aggressive and deadly than others.

Thus, today we look at breast cancer as a disease that affects not just the breast, but the whole body—that is, we view it as a *systemic* illness.

Who is at risk?

It seems as if every week the news media report that something increases your risk of breast cancer. In 1988 and 1989, for example, women were told that two substances commonly used by American women—alcoholic beverages and birth control pills—were linked to the development of breast cancer. Such reports—which remain controversial—panic some women, who immediately try to alter their behavior to eliminate all risk in hopes of avoiding breast cancer altogether. Unfortunately, this is probably not possible. Some women indeed have a much higher risk than average, but the majority of women who get breast cancer have no risk factors at all. In general, the mere fact that we are women is what puts us at risk. (Less than 1 per cent of all breast cancers occur in men. Unfortunately, because many men are unaware that they can get breast cancer, the few who get it tend to ignore their symptoms until the cancer is advanced.)

Nonetheless, the most significant risk factor for breast cancer is family history. If your mother had it, you are slightly more likely to get it than you would be otherwise. But even that is not absolute because there seem to be two levels of risk. In some families, almost every woman in every generation seems to inherit breast cancer. I had one patient whose mother and four sisters had developed breast cancer, and she wanted to have her breasts surgically removed—a procedure known as a *double mastectomy*—as a preventive measure. This woman's family was obviously so predisposed to breast cancer that her desire to have preventive surgery was understandable. Although preventive surgery is rarely warranted, there are a few situations, such as this one, in which it may be considered.

But such cases, where most or all females in a family develop the disease, account for only about 15 per cent of all breast cancer. More common is the situation in which the disease occurs often in a family but not every female gets it. In these families, factors other than genes may be at work. For example, it may be that every woman in the family eats the same diet or begins menstruation early in life or has children late in life—factors that increase a woman's prospects of developing the disease.

For reasons we don't yet understand, the younger a woman is at the onset of menstruation and the older she is when she reaches *menopause* (the time of life when menstruation stops), the more likely she is to get breast cancer. Pregnancy also appears to affect vulnerability to the disease. Women who have never given birth seem to have a higher risk than women who had a child before age 30, but a lower risk than women who had their first child after 30. (Having had a pregnancy before age 30 that was terminated by abortion or miscarriage doesn't seem to affect breast cancer risk.)

Various theories—most of them inconclusive—have been proposed to explain these risk factors, which are linked to the body's production of *sex hormones* (chemicals that regulate body processes involved in puberty and reproduction). It appears that there is a time of vulnerability to cancer-causing agents between the first period and the first pregnancy, which may mean that breast cancer risk is lowered if the onset of menstruation is delayed. One way menstruation is delayed is if girls exercise vigorously during adolescence. And indeed there are some data showing that women who were very athletic in school are less prone to breast cancer than average.

Recently we've learned about a few possible risk factors over which you may have more control. For example, research has suggested that the amount of fat in your diet may affect your vulnerability to breast cancer. Unfortunately, these studies are somewhat contradictory, and they do not make clear whether the danger comes from all fats, fats from animal foods only, or even just the extra calories that you get when you eat a high-fat diet. We do know that the breast cancer rates for women living in countries where people eat low-fat diets, such as Japan, are lower than the rates in countries such as the Netherlands and the United States, where high-fat diets are the norm. Studies suggest that only about 27 per cent of breast cancers are likely to be linked to fat intake, however.

Another possible risk factor is alcohol consumption. Studies published in 1988 suggest that even moderate amounts of alcoholic beverages may increase a woman's susceptibility to breast cancer. Here, too, it seems that the time of greatest danger may be early in life; alcohol consumption after age 30 doesn't appear to affect breast cancer risk as much. Again, the studies are not yet conclusive.

There are a number of other risk factors. Studies have shown some relation between breast cancer risk and high doses of radiation—such as those once given as a treatment for acne—during adolescence. And studies reported in 1989 suggest that a woman who uses birth control pills for more than 10 years before her first childbirth may be at greater risk. Finally, the drug diethylstilbestrol (DES), once given to pregnant women to prevent miscarriage, has been shown to increase risk in the women who took it. In spite of what you may have been told, however, lumpy breasts—a condition sometimes labeled *fibrocystic breast disease*—does not in itself make a woman more vulnerable to breast cancer.

Finally, it's important to put the notion of risk factors into context. When we say that 1 in 10 women will develop breast cancer at some time in her life, we are assuming that all women have the same level of risk and that they will all live to be 110. It may be more helpful to consider the level of risk for women at different ages. Breast cancer is rare in women under 30, and the odds that a woman between 30 and 35 will get breast cancer in any given year are 1 in 5,900. For a woman between 40 and 50, the odds are 1 in 1,200; when she is between 50 and 60, the odds are 1 in 500; and between 70 and 80, they are 1 in 330.

Since these statistics include women at high risk as well as

Do you need a mammogram?

Mammography, a technique for making X rays of the breast using low doses of radiation, is the best method we have for detecting breast cancer at the earliest possible stage. Originally, this procedure was used only to help in diagnosis. If a woman had a suspicious lump, her doctor would order a mammogram before doing a biopsy to see if there were more lumps in the area and to get a sense of the growth's shape.

Mammography is still used diagnostically, but since the 1970's, its usefulness as a way to detect some breast tumors before they are large enough to be felt has become increasingly apparent. A breast cancer tumor typically grows for 10 years before it's large enough to be detectable by feeling, but it may be detectable through mammography a year or two earlier.

The American Cancer Society recommends that every woman have her first mammogram sometime between the ages of 35 and 40. The film should be kept permanently so that it can be used as a reference, or *baseline mammogram,* to compare with the mammograms she will have taken later. Every woman should have mammograms at one- to two-year intervals throughout her 40's, and women at high risk should have them every year. After 50, when breast cancer risk rises, annual mammograms are recommended.

The National Cancer Institute generally agrees with these guidelines and also recommends that women who have had breast cancer receive annual mammograms regardless of age. Aside from those who fall into this category, most women under 40 do not require regular screening mammograms, especially if they have no family history of breast cancer.

Why, if mammography saves lives, shouldn't all women receive them annually? Because, unlike the breast self-examination—which is simple, risk-free, and costs nothing—mammograms cost $50 to $200. Also, the usefulness of mammograms in young women is questionable, since young breasts have a lot of dense breast tissue that X rays can't penetrate. (The older you are, the more fat tissue there is in your breasts, and X rays can, in effect, see through fat tissue.) In addition, any procedure that involves X rays carries a health risk, because large doses of radiation can cause cancer. The amount of radiation used

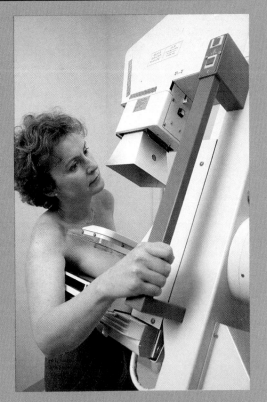

Mammography is a simple process in which the breasts are compressed briefly and X-rayed. Two views of each breast are typically made.

in mammography is very small, but—because the effects of radiation are cumulative—it is best not to begin regular mammograms in most women before age 35.

It's also important to realize that mammography is not 100 per cent accurate. If you have a breast lump, even a normal result on a mammogram should not prevent you from seeking medical evaluation and even a biopsy.

Finally, women who have had their breasts surgically *augmented* (enlarged) with silicone implants may have some difficulty obtaining reliable mammograms, because X rays cannot penetrate the implants. These women should be sure to tell the technician who takes the mammogram about the implants, and they may wish to seek out an expert who specializes in examining augmented breasts.   [S.M.L.]

How is breast cancer treated?

Today, breast cancer patients have more treatment options—and more decisions to make—than ever before. Once cancer is diagnosed, the patient and her doctor, *right,* should discuss what type of surgery should be used to remove the tumor. After surgery, the patient and her doctor must also decide whether drug therapy is needed to kill any cancer cells that have traveled beyond the breast.

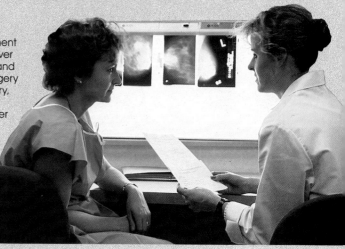

Two surgical options with comparable cure rates

A mastectomy, *below,* (also called a *modified radical mastectomy*) is a surgical procedure in which all the breast tissue is removed along with some lymph nodes. The breast can be reconstructed using plastic surgery techniques.

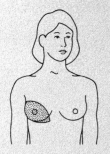

Breast tissue removed

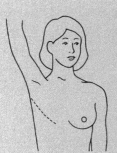

Surgical scar

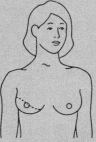

Appearance after reconstruction

A lumpectomy, *below,* involves the removal of only the tumor, some surrounding tissue, and some lymph nodes from under the arm. Follow-up radiation treatments are necessary to ensure that all cancer cells in the breast are destroyed.

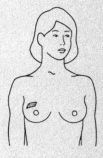

Breast tissue removed

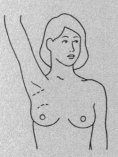

Surgical scars

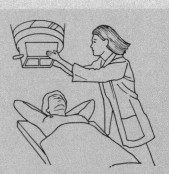

Radiation treatment

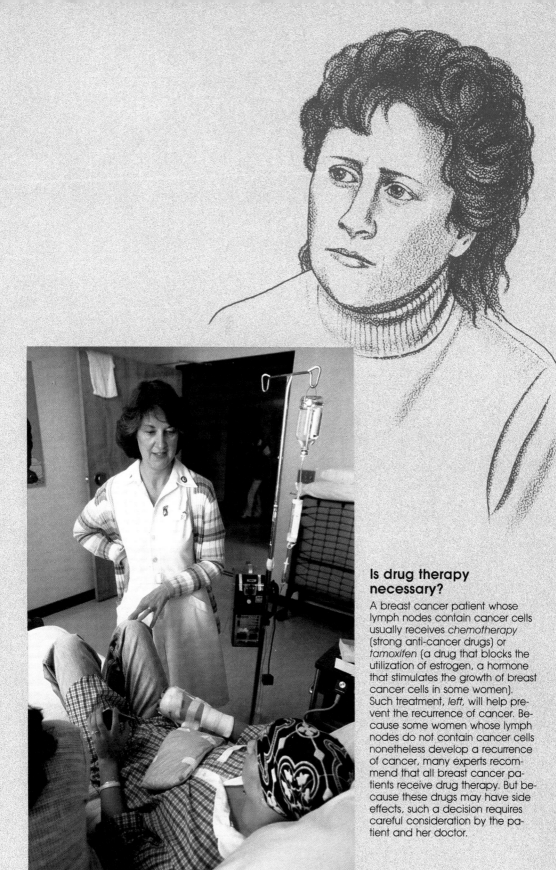

Is drug therapy necessary?

A breast cancer patient whose lymph nodes contain cancer cells usually receives *chemotherapy* (strong anti-cancer drugs) or *tamoxifen* (a drug that blocks the utilization of estrogen, a hormone that stimulates the growth of breast cancer cells in some women). Such treatment, *left,* will help prevent the recurrence of cancer. Because some women whose lymph nodes do not contain cancer cells nonetheless develop a recurrence of cancer, many experts recommend that all breast cancer patients receive drug therapy. But because these drugs may have side effects, such a decision requires careful consideration by the patient and her doctor.

35

women at low risk, they overestimate them for low-risk women and underestimate them for high-risk women. For example, the chances are 1 in 30 that a woman with no risk factors will get breast cancer if she lives 110 years. So if you have a risk factor that doubles your chances of getting breast cancer—if you took birth control pills for 10 years before your first child was born, for example—it may mean that the odds for developing breast cancer by age 110 rise from 1 in 30 to 1 in 15.

How is breast cancer diagnosed?

How do we determine whether someone has breast cancer? The most frequent symptom is a lump in the breast—usually discovered by the woman herself while performing breast self-examination or while washing her breasts in the shower or bath, though sometimes it's found by a doctor during a regular checkup. Sometimes a lump too small to be felt is detected by *mammography*—a special form of X ray that is useful for detecting breast cancer. (See Do you need a mammogram? on page 33 and The breast self-examination on pages 38 and 39 for information on these vitally important procedures.) In rare cases, the first sign that something is wrong may not be a lump in the breast, but another unusual symptom of the breast such as redness, swelling, or dimpling of the skin, bloody discharge from one of the nipples, or flaking of the skin of the nipple.

If the symptom is a lump, chances are good that it is probably one of three harmless varieties—a *cyst*, which is a sac containing fluid, somewhat like an internal blister; a *fibroadenoma*, which is a benign (noncancerous) tumor formed from fibrous and glandular tissue; or a *pseudolump*, which is simply a thickened area of normal breast tissue.

To determine if the lump is a cyst, doctors usually perform a *needle aspiration*. In this procedure, the doctor administers a local anesthetic and inserts a thin needle attached to a syringe into the lump. If the syringe draws out fluid, then we know the lump is a cyst and there is probably nothing to worry about.

If no fluid comes out, the next step is a *biopsy*, performed under local or general anesthetic. Depending on a number of factors, the doctor may use a needle and syringe to get some cells or may cut out either the whole lump or a piece of it. The tissue is then sent to a laboratory to be checked by a pathologist, who examines it under a microscope, looking for cancer cells. If cancer is present, the patient and her doctor should discuss the best way to treat it.

How is breast cancer treated?

In the past, before having a lump in her breast biopsied, it was customary for a woman to sign a consent form saying that if the pathologist found cancer, the surgeon could immediately perform a mastectomy—that is, surgically remove the breast. Nowadays, it's far more common for a woman to have a biopsy, get the pathologist's report from her doctor, and, if the lump is a cancer, discuss treatment options with her doctor and take some time to decide on a course of treatment. Some women still choose to sign a prebiopsy consent form, but I think that urging all women to do so is a mistake. Our best evidence indicates that immediate surgery does not improve the woman's chances for recovery, and it may be hard for a woman to make a reasoned decision about something that is still a hypothetical situation.

The treatment for breast cancer has also changed. Until the mid-1970's, the standard treatment was *radical mastectomy*—surgical removal of the breast, the muscles underneath it, and all the lymph nodes up to the collarbone. The surgery was disfiguring, and the removal of muscle tissue left the arm permanently weakened. Fortunately, we've learned over the years that such extensive surgery is usually unnecessary, and the radical mastectomy is rarely performed nowadays.

Today, there are essentially two surgical options for breast cancer patients. The first is the *modified radical mastectomy*—removal of only the breast, with the underlying muscle left intact. This operation is less disfiguring than the old radical procedure. Many women who have mastectomies also have a plastic-surgery procedure known as *breast reconstruction*, which creates an artificial breast that looks like the one that was removed. The new breast has little or no sensation, and of course it can't be used to breast-feed, but it can be cosmetically pleasing to a woman dismayed by the deformity of a mastectomy.

The other option, which has become more and more popular, is the *lumpectomy*, or partial mastectomy, in which only the cancerous lump and some of the normal tissue surrounding it are removed. The surgery is usually followed by treatment with radiation, which is intended to kill any cancer cells missed by the scalpel. Lumpectomy with radiation is more cosmetically acceptable than mastectomy, and research published by Fisher in 1989 indicates that the survival rate—70 per cent after eight years—is the same for women who have either procedure.

Many women still choose a mastectomy, however, for a

The breast self-examination

Because most breast cancers first appear as lumps that can be felt, it's important to have your doctor look for breast lumps—by visually examining the breasts and then physically examining them and the armpits. Women under 40 should have these clincal breast exams at least once every three years, and after age 40, annual exams are recommended.

It's even more important that you learn to examine your own breasts, and do so every month. If you have not reached menopause, you should examine your breasts just after your menstrual period—a time when the breasts are not swollen. After the menopause, you may want to set a date for a breast self-exam—the first of each month, for example—to help you remember to check your breasts regularly.

Breast self-examination costs nothing and is simple. It's also a habit worth getting into at an early age. The American Cancer Society recommends that you start at age 20. Although breast cancer is rare in women under 30, it's important that every woman learn what her breasts normally look and feel like. Breasts are as individual as faces and figures, and, if you want to be able to detect breast cancer at an early stage, you have to be able to recognize any change.

To begin with, simply look in a mirror at your breasts to see if you notice any obvious changes. It's easiest to visually examine your breasts if you lift your arms to stretch

the tissue out, and then put your hands on your hips and push in, contracting the chest muscles.

In that position, look for visual signs that may indicate cancer, such as a dimpling in one of your breasts that you've never noticed before. Or one of your nipples might suddenly be inverted. In rare cases, you may even be able to see a lump. You might discover some flaking skin on your nipple; this could be a harmless skin disorder, but there's a chance that it is a symptom of a cancer called *Paget's disease*. You might notice some nipple discharge. Or your skin may be an unusual shade of red, or the veins may be unusually prominent. (If you're pregnant, however, the latter symptom is probably one of the normal changes that occur during pregnancy.)

The second part of your self-exam involves *palpation*—feeling your breasts. Some women prefer to do this while they're showering or bathing, because it's easier to detect lumps when the skin is slippery with soap.

If you do it this way, put the hand on the side you want to examine behind your head. This moves the breast tissue that's beneath your armpit to your chest wall. Since the tissue is sandwiched between your skin and your ribcage, this position gives you good access to the breast tissue.

If your breasts are very large, you might find it difficult to examine them while you

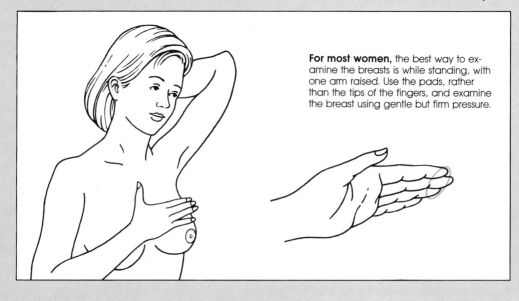

For most women, the best way to examine the breasts is while standing, with one arm raised. Use the pads, rather than the tips of the fingers, and examine the breast using gentle but firm pressure.

are standing or sitting, because even with your arm raised, your breasts hang down. In this case, it's probably better to perform the self-exam while lying on a bed. Follow the same method, putting your hand behind your head.

If your breasts are so large that even in this position they hang over the side of your chest, put a pillow under your shoulder on the side you're examining. This will also help shift the breast tissue toward your chest wall.

Whatever position you use, you should palpate the breast firmly but not roughly. Too soft a touch won't reveal what's in the tissue, while too hard a touch, aside from being uncomfortable, will cause you to feel your ribs rather than breast tissue. Use the pads of your fingers—the fingerprint part—rather than your fingertips. And don't grab the skin; just press down.

You should palpate your breast in a methodical pattern to make sure you feel all the tissue. There are several possible patterns. One is to imagine your breast is a clock, with the nipple as its center, and to feel the breast in the 12 sections that would correspond to hour markings. (This isn't, however, a perfectly round clock. You need to feel the tissue above the breast itself, so be sure to palpate up nearly to your collarbone.)

Another pattern is to palpate the tissue in concentric circles, starting at the nipple and spiraling out and up. A third way is to examine the breast in vertical strips, beginning at the top of your chest and going all the way down the breast, strip by strip. It doesn't matter which pattern you use, as long as you stick with it. You can invent a pattern of your own if you like. All that matters is that you feel the entire breast each time.

While you're feeling the breast, search for fairly large lumps—walnut-sized or larger. If you feel something tiny, like a grain of sand, it's almost never cancer, though your doctor should check the area to confirm this.

And you're also looking for one lump, or at most two or three. If you find dozens of lumps throughout both breasts, they may be fat or normal breast tissue, which in some women is exceptionally thick. Ask your doctor to check these lumps to be sure, however.

When you've finished palpating one breast, reverse the position of your arms and palpate the other breast.

Finally, don't be afraid to see your doctor immediately if you notice anything unusual. After all, seeking medical attention is a no-lose situation. Chances are good that the symptom is harmless, and checking it out with a doctor will put your mind at ease. And if the symptom is an indication of cancer, getting prompt treatment will be the best thing you ever do for yourself. [S.M.L.]

Examine the tissue in each breast methodically, following some pattern that ensures you check every part of the breast. You may want to palpate the breast in vertical strips, or in pie-shaped wedges, or by starting at the nipple and spiraling outward.

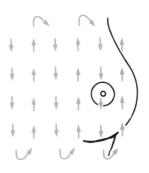 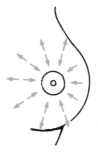 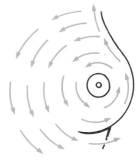

number of reasons. Some do so for peace of mind. With the breast gone, they think they cannot get cancer again—though of course cancer may have already spread to other organs. Some women prefer to avoid radiation treatments, which, though they cause few side effects, typically last for six weeks and can be tiring. One of my patients had saved money all her life to go traveling after she retired, and she decided that keeping her breast was less important to her than immediately embarking on the traveling she'd long dreamed of. Former first lady Nancy Reagan, who had a mastectomy in 1987, told interviewers that her demanding schedule required that her treatment take as little time as possible, and a colleague of mine in a rural area tells me that her patients, who are hard-working farmers, have a similar attitude. Today's availability of breast reconstruction often makes mastectomy even more appealing to these women.

For many women, however, the possibility of keeping their breast by means of a lumpectomy is worth the time and energy necessary for the follow-up radiation therapy, and they realize that scientific studies equate their survival rate with that of women who have mastectomies. So there is no clear right or wrong choice: Each woman knows what the loss of a breast means to her, and what she is willing to do to avoid it.

No matter which surgical procedure a woman elects, it will include the removal of a few lymph nodes in the underarm area. This is crucial, because if the cancer has spread beyond the breast, one sign may be cancer cells in the nodes. (Blood tests and X rays can detect cancer in other organs once tumors have grown large enough.) Because surgery and radiation kill the cancer cells in only the immediate area, the patient will need a systemic treatment if there is any hint that the cancer may have spread. Standard treatment for women who have not yet reached menopause is *chemotherapy* (the use of strong drugs that kill cancer cells) and, for women who have passed menopause, *tamoxifen*. This drug blocks the utilization of estrogen, a sex hormone that appears to stimulate the growth of about 40 per cent of all breast cancers. (Because only some breast cancers are affected by estrogen, a test to determine the effect of the hormone on the tumor is usually performed after the biopsy.)

The current dilemma in the treatment of breast cancer lies in determining whether women who do not have cancer in the lymph nodes should receive systemic treatment—because, unfortunately, in about 20 per cent of these women, the cancer has indeed spread. For this reason, many experts, including those at the National Cancer Institute in Bethesda, Md., now believe that all breast cancer patients should be given systemic therapy.

The problem with this is that 80 per cent of the women without cancer in their lymph nodes do not need further treatment, and chemotherapy can have some very unpleasant side effects—such as nausea, vomiting, and hair loss—and some permanent side effects, such as sterility. Not surprisingly, doctors are sharply divided over whether the risk of giving systemic therapy to all breast cancer patients outweighs the risk of missing a cancer that has spread until it is too late to save the patient's life. Our hope is that we will someday find a more precise method of determining whether breast cancer has metastasized than examining the lymph nodes, and this subject is now being researched.

What's the outlook?

Research into the prevention and treatment of breast cancer is also well underway, and almost daily we learn more about the nature of breast cancer and the ways to cure it. And, truthfully, the picture today is not as grim as it's often painted. Even when breast cancer is found in the lymph nodes, there is a 60 per cent chance of surviving five years. I have many long-term patients who have had no recurrence despite the fact that I discovered cancer cells in their lymph nodes.

Unfortunately, doctors cannot prescribe behaviors guaranteed to keep you from getting breast cancer, though reducing the amount of fats in your diet and cutting down on alcohol may help. But with the continuing refinement of treatment—and with early detection through breast self-examinations and mammography—there is every reason to be optimistic about breast cancer's cure.

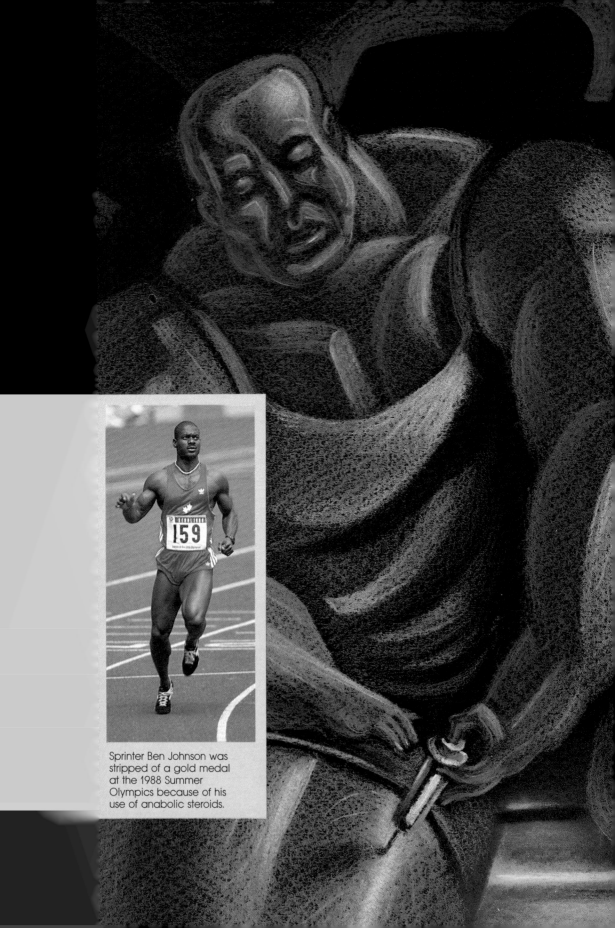

Sprinter Ben Johnson was stripped of a gold medal at the 1988 Summer Olympics because of his use of anabolic steroids.

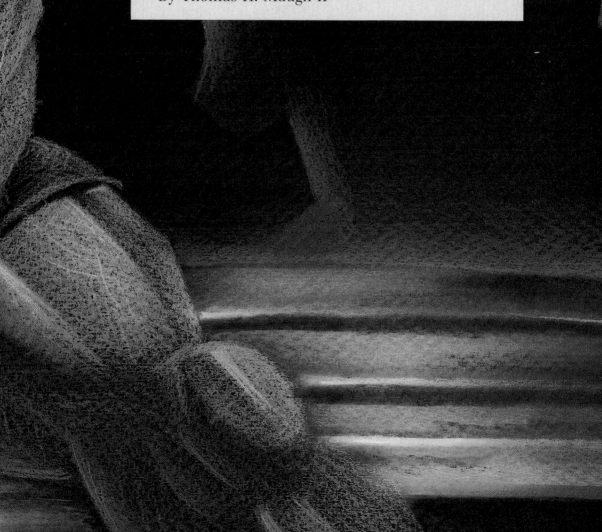

Athletes who hope to gain a winning
edge by taking drugs called anabolic
steroids may acquire something more
ominous: serious health problems.

Steroid Abuse: Turning Winners into Losers

By Thomas H. Maugh II

The story of Ben Johnson's fall from glory into disgrace is by now familiar to nearly everyone. On September 24 in the 1988 Olympic Summer Games in Seoul, the Jamaican-born sprinter, running for Canada, captured a gold medal in the 100-meter dash with the world record time of 9.79 seconds. Three days later, however, Johnson was stripped of both his gold medal and the world record. He was also barred from international competition for two years and banned from the Canadian team for life.

The reason for the sudden reversal of Johnson's fortune was simple: He was caught cheating. Traces of a drug outlawed by the International Olympic Committee (IOC), the Olympic governing body, were detected in a sample of the sprinter's urine during a test performed on all Olympic winners.

The drug that Johnson took, called *stanozolol*, belongs to a family of chemicals known as anabolic steroids, which are believed to increase strength and endurance. The IOC prohibits the use of all anabolic steroids for two reasons: They may give athletes who take these drugs an unfair advantage over those who do not, and anabolic steroids have potentially dangerous side effects, including heart disease and liver damage.

Nevertheless, athletes continue to take anabolic steroids in the belief the drugs can increase their muscle mass and enhance their performance. At the Seoul Olympics alone, three other competitors besides Johnson were barred from the games for using stanozolol. At a Canadian government inquiry convened in March 1989 to investigate drug use among athletes, Charlie Francis, Johnson's coach, alleged that anabolic steroids were a routine part of Olympic training programs in the United States, the Soviet Union, and other nations.

But Olympians are not the only athletes to use anabolic steroids. Although the distribution of these steroids without a prescription is illegal in the United States, the drugs are easily available in many gyms and locker rooms, by mail order, and from other sources. Weight lifters and body builders have been using the drugs for nearly three decades to gain weight and increase strength, and to make their bodies look better. Some sports-drug experts estimate that more than half the players in the National Football League (NFL) now use anabolic steroids regularly. Other sports where experts believe steroid use may be widespread include swimming, boxing, wrestling, triathlon, and cycling.

The illicit use of the drugs has even spread to high schools. In December 1988, biologist William Buckley of Pennsylvania State University in University Park, Pa., reported the results of a survey of 3,403 male seniors at 46 high schools across the United States that showed that 6.6 per cent of them had previously used or were still using steroids. Extrapolated across the entire country, Buckley's results indicate that as many as

The author:
Thomas H. Maugh II is a science writer for the *Los Angeles Times*.

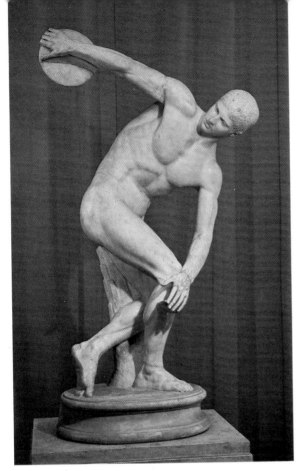

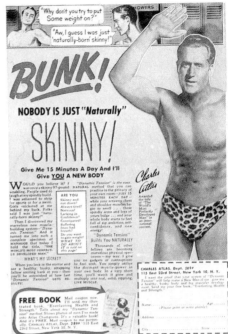

A muscular male physique has been lauded for centuries. In ancient Greece, the well-developed body was the subject of many sculptures; in the 1950's, Charles Atlas touted body-building exercises. In the 1980's, despite health risks, some people who seek more muscular builds are taking anabolic steroids.

500,000 adolescents have used or are now using these drugs.

Most researchers now believe that steroids can increase the strength and endurance of athletes, so one of the questions the widespread use raises is one of fairness—whether individuals taking performance-enhancing drugs should be permitted to compete with individuals relying on their own natural talents. Of even more serious concern, however, are the potentially disastrous health effects of anabolic steroids.

Researchers now maintain that anabolic steroids can increase the risk of heart disease; cause fluid retention and perhaps hypertension, as well as liver problems and perhaps liver cancer; and produce disturbing psychological changes and aggressive tendencies. In men, the drugs can cause the testicles to shrink, the breasts to become enlarged, and the sex drive to diminish. In women, they can produce male-pattern baldness, growth of facial hair, and lowering of the voice. In adolescents, steroids can stunt growth irreversibly by speeding up bone maturation. They also can cause acne.

But despite the hazards of these steroids, demand for them is high. Illicit sales of these drugs in the United States repre-.

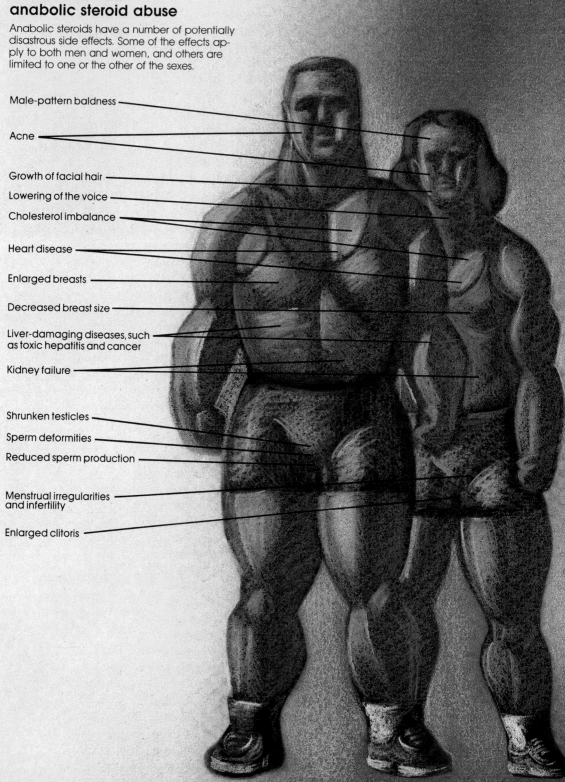

Some health risks associated with anabolic steroid abuse

Anabolic steroids have a number of potentially disastrous side effects. Some of the effects apply to both men and women, and others are limited to one or the other of the sexes.

Male-pattern baldness

Acne

Growth of facial hair

Lowering of the voice

Cholesterol imbalance

Heart disease

Enlarged breasts

Decreased breast size

Liver-damaging diseases, such as toxic hepatitis and cancer

Kidney failure

Shrunken testicles

Sperm deformities

Reduced sperm production

Menstrual irregularities and infertility

Enlarged clitoris

sent a market estimated at more than $100 million annually.

The steroids are two families of hormones that share the same general structure. The *cortical steroids* are produced by the *cortex* (outside) of the adrenal glands, walnut-sized organs that sit on top of the kidneys. Doctors use synthetic forms of cortical steroids to treat arthritis, serious asthma attacks, and other ailments. The cortical steriods are not abused by athletes, because one of their side effects is breakdown of body tissues, causing deterioration of muscles and weight loss—the opposite of the effects sought by users of anabolic steroids.

The second family of steroids, the *anabolic or androgenic steroids*, are derived from the male sex hormone testosterone, which is produced by the testes. These steroids have two kinds of effects—androgenic activities and anabolic activities—associated with them. Androgenic activities cause maleness. For example, they lower the voice and promote the growth of facial and body hair. Anabolic activities stimulate the growth of the body. They encourage the production of red blood cells, promote formation of proteins and tissues, and increase appetite.

Synthetic anabolic steroids are used medically for treating certain forms of *anemia* (a condition in which the number of healthy red blood cells falls below normal), and, in some cases, for promoting weight gain in patients with cancer or other wasting diseases.

Experts recommend the use of synthetic anabolic steroids only if their benefits—as in treating anemia—outweigh their considerable side effects. And of the many side effects of synthetic anabolic steroids, the most serious one, according to medical experts, is liver damage. Because the condition is initially painless, few symptoms may appear until the damage is irreparable. The chief liver-damaging diseases associated with the use of anabolic steroids include *toxic hepatitis* (inflammation of the liver) and liver cancer.

Anabolic steroids also can increase the risk of heart disease because of their effect on the balance of *cholesterol* (a white, fatlike substance) in the bloodstream. Deposits of cholesterol and other substances can narrow the arteries that feed the heart, setting the stage for heart disease. The anabolic steroids produce a rise in the level of substances called *low-density lipoproteins* (LDL's), which help deposit cholesterol in the cells of arteries. At the same time, these drugs reduce the level of substances called *high-density lipoproteins* (HDL's), which help remove cholesterol from cells.

In a normal, healthy individual, the ratio of LDL's to HDL's is between 2.5 to 1 and 3.5 to 1. Physicians consider ratios above 5 or 6 to 1 to represent a significantly higher risk of

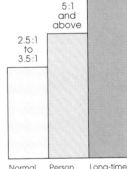

Ratio of LDL to HDL in the bloodstream

Anabolic steroids increase the risk of heart disease by throwing off the balance between two forms of cholesterol in the blood, the "bad" low-density lipoproteins (LDL's) and the "good" high-density lipoproteins (HDL's). A person with an elevated ratio of LDL's to HDL's has a higher risk of heart disease.

heart disease. Long-time users of anabolic steroids frequently have LDL/HDL ratios in the 30's and 40's to 1, according to nutritionist Guy R. Dirkin of the Sandoz Nutrition Corporation, a Minneapolis, Minn.-based firm that makes nutritional products. The drugs also cause retention of sodium and water, which can increase a tendency to high blood pressure.

Steroids also may cause disturbing psychological side effects. Steroid users may become more aggressive and more violent, a phenomenon known as 'roid rage. In an April 1988 report, psychiatrists Harrison G. Pope, Jr., of the McLean Hospital in Belmont, Mass., and David L. Katz of Harvard Medical School found that 15 of 41 steroid-using athletes they studied suffered such symptoms as delusions, hallucinations, manic episodes, and depression. The disorders disappeared when the athletes stopped using the steroids.

A graphic example of the mental effects of steroids was offered in *Sports Illustrated* by Tommy Chaikin, a former lineman on the University of South Carolina football team. Chaikin described pulling a loaded shotgun on a pizza delivery boy because "I thought it was funny," destroying his room, severely battering a marine in a bar, and even attacking his own teammates while under the influence of anabolic steroids. Ultimately, he tried to commit suicide with a handgun before his father persuaded him to enter a hospital for psychiatric care. Psychiatrists attributed his behavior to the anabolic steroids rather than to underlying emotional problems.

Many of the other adverse effects of anabolic steroids result from their effects on hormonal systems. The drugs' androgenic properties cause females to become more masculine in appearance, with growth of facial hair, loss of hair on the scalp, enlargement of the clitoris, and decrease in breast size. These effects are typically not reversible. The drugs can also cause irregularities in the menstrual cycle and even infertility. A loss of sexual desire can also occur.

These steroids generally produce some opposite effects in men, because the body perceives synthetic hormones as natural and therefore reduces or completely shuts down its own production of testosterone. As a result, the testicles begin to shrink, sperm production declines and the sperm themselves become deformed, and the breasts become enlarged. The irony here is that while many males are taking anabolic steroids to increase their external sexual attractiveness, the drugs are actually undermining their physiological sexuality and bringing about a loss of sex drive and a growing impotence. In both men and women, high levels of these drugs produce acne in the same fashion that increased testosterone levels during puberty contribute to acne in males.

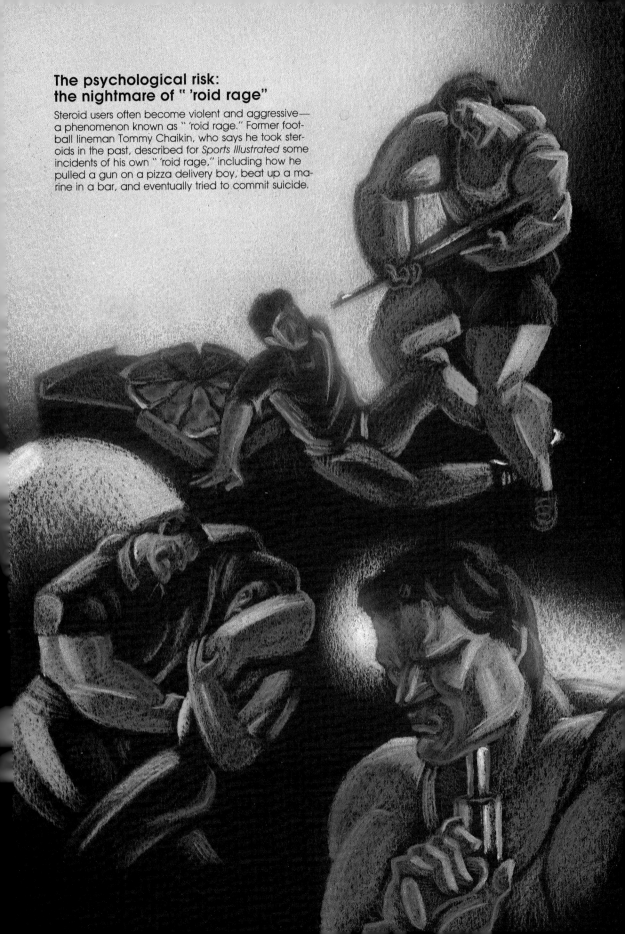

The psychological risk: the nightmare of " 'roid rage"

Steroid users often become violent and aggressive—a phenomenon known as " 'roid rage." Former football lineman Tommy Chaikin, who says he took steroids in the past, described for *Sports Illustrated* some incidents of his own " 'roid rage," including how he pulled a gun on a pizza delivery boy, beat up a marine in a bar, and eventually tried to commit suicide.

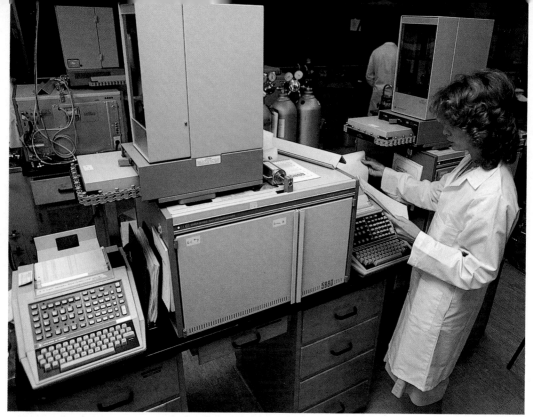

Many sports officials consider frequent and regular drug tests to be the most effective approach against steroid abuse by athletes. But steroid tests require sophisticated equipment, such as that shown above, and the cost—about $200 to test a single specimen—is too high for most high schools and colleges.

Given all the adverse effects of anabolic steroids, why do athletes use them? According to pharmacologist Thomas A. Gossel of Ohio Northern University in Ada, Ohio, their major reasons can generally be put into four categories. First, athletes believe that anabolic steroids increase their muscle mass and strength. They contend that they not only compete better in sports activities but also look better doing so. Second, they believe that the drugs decrease muscle recovery time following exercise. After the athletes have worked out, therefore, less time must elapse before the next workout.

Third, athletes report that anabolic steroids decrease muscle healing time following an injury so that they can begin exercising again more rapidly. Finally, athletes believe that the aggressiveness promoted by the drugs enhances the intensity of their workouts and perhaps their aggressiveness to other people as well—again making them more competitive.

Lurking behind all these rationales, however, is the "winning is everything" mentality, a desire for the riches and prestige that athletic success can bring. The financial rewards for athletic achievement can be tremendous and can blind young competitors to ethical considerations and to any future health risks. Johnson, for example, reportedly had $18 million in various contracts that were lost after he tested positive.

Whether anabolic steroids do improve athletic performance has been a subject of intense debate for at least three decades. Until the last few years, most scientists asserted that the steroids have no effect, and some still do. But the growing consensus among physicians is that the drugs do have some positive effect on performance.

At least 25 separate clinical studies have been conducted to examine the performance-enhancing effects of anabolic steroids, but the results have been mixed, with some studies indicating that the drugs enhance performance and others suggesting that they do not. But critics note that such studies have used steroids only at the concentrations recommended for medical therapy, whereas athletes use them in concentrations 10 to 100 times as high. Most athletes using steroids also "stack" the drugs, combining several different forms to try to obtain the maximum effect.

Another problem with studies of anabolic steroids is the difficulty of isolating steroid use from such other factors as an

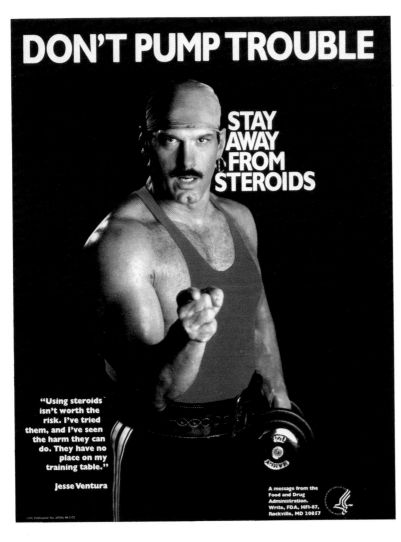

Schools and government agencies have initiated education programs stressing the dangers of steroids. The U.S. Food and Drug Administration, for example, sent copies of this poster, which features wrestler Jesse Ventura, to high school and college coaches across the country.

athlete's diet, intensity of training, and strength of motivation. The American College of Sports Medicine recognized the influence of such factors when in 1984 it reversed its long-held position that steroids have no effect on improving an athlete's performance. The organization concluded that "the gains in muscular strength achieved through high-intensity exercise and proper diet can be increased by the use of anabolic-androgenic steroids in some individuals," but it continued to warn against the health hazards of the drugs.

One telling study performed by researchers at Leeds University in England seems to demonstrate that almost anyone who exercises can gain weight by using anabolic steroids, but only athletes who are already training intensively tend to gain strength as well. The researchers found that men who were not weight lifters gained far more weight when they exercised and took these steroids than when they exercised and took a *placebo* (a pill with an inactive substance). The strength of the men, however, as measured by their ability to raise and lower a barbell while lying on a bench, increased just as much whether the men took steroids or not. But when the researchers studied weight lifters who were already training intensively, they found that those who took anabolic steroids gained both weight and strength at a faster rate than those taking placebos.

Whatever the real performance-enhancing effects of steroids might be, just as important are the perceived effects. If athletes believe that steroids produce at least some benefit and that their competitors are using them, many feel tremendous pressure to use the drugs themselves.

Athletes who want to obtain drugs seem able to get them fairly easily. Some physicians, pharmacists, and veterinarians—who are sympathetic, uninformed, or simply unethical—make anabolic steroids available for athletes who wish to bulk up, providing an estimated one-fifth of the U.S. supply, according to Sandoz Corporation's Dirkin. But the number of such individuals is declining as the adverse health effects of the drugs become more widely known and as state authorities step up enforcement of existing regulations against nonmedical use of the drugs. But even without the aid of physicians, there is a vast underground network of suppliers who make anabolic steroids available.

The black market has been so blatant that major dealers have regularly sent out direct-mail advertising and catalogs listing shipping prices and costs. Most gyms in the country have at least one "connection" who can supply anabolic steroids or who knows of someone who can. Many athletes buy the drugs in quantity and supply them to their friends.

Substances banned in sports

Anabolic steroids may be the most famous of the drugs banned by the International Olympic Committee (IOC), but they are not the only ones. In all, the IOC has forbidden the use of more than 70 drugs in several major categories, including stimulants, narcotic analgesics, tranquilizers, beta-blockers, and diuretics.

Stimulants were the drugs that first led the IOC to establish drug regulations in 1967. Drugs in this category, which include a variety of medications ranging from amphetamines and methamphetamines to caffeine, give the user a feeling of extra energy and could potentially improve performance enough to make a difference in a close competition. Many nonathletes also abuse stimulants in such situations as staying up all night to study for a test.

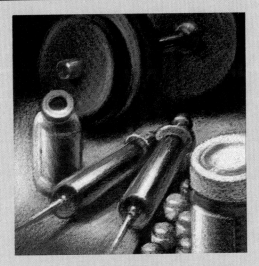

Pharmacologist Don H. Catlin of the University of California at Los Angeles, who is in charge of testing for the United States Olympic Committee, says there used to be "tremendous abuse of stimulants in the 1960's, even deaths among athletes who were given walloping overdoses of stimulants." That abuse has largely abated, a phenomenon that many attribute to the efficacy of testing. Regulations now also prohibit large amounts of caffeine, such as might be obtained by drinking more than a half-dozen cups of coffee.

Narcotic analgesics, such as codeine, deaden pain and thus allow athletes to compete when they are injured. Their prohibition is designed more to protect athletes from serious injury than to prevent performance enhancement. Aspirin and other nonnarcotic analgesics are allowed.

Tranquilizers have a calming effect, and *beta-blockers* slow the heartbeat and reduce tremors. These effects might not seem desirable for competitions in which the athlete should be as alert as possible, but slowing the heartbeat and reducing tremors can be beneficial in archery and riflery, where a steady hand is important.

Diuretics cause the body to excrete more urine than normal. Athletes use them primarily to help flush long-acting drugs, such as steroids, out of the body prior to a sporting competition. The presence of diuretics may also, in some cases, mask the presence of other forbidden drugs.

One technique that is illegal but that cannot yet be detected is *blood doping*. The technique involves removing some blood from an athlete before a competition and storing it, typically by freezing. During the interval before the competition, the athlete's body replaces the lost red blood cells. Shortly before the competition, the stored red blood cells are reinjected into the athlete. Some people believe the additional red blood cells help carry more oxygen to tiring muscles and increase endurance. Because of natural variations in the number of red cells in an individual's blood, blood doping is virtually impossible to detect.

The use of human growth hormone (HGH) by athletes, like blood doping, is illegal but nearly undetectable. A naturally occurring hormone, HGH is produced by the pituitary gland and causes children to grow larger. A synthetic form is made through genetic engineering techniques. When given to adults, particularly those who are on an exercise program, the drug tends to decrease their fat and increase their muscle. In an August 1988 study, researchers found that exercising athletes given HGH for six weeks gained an average of 6 pounds (2.7 kilograms) of muscle.

But physicians warn that large doses of synthetic HGH in adults may produce the same undesirable effects as an excessive production of natural HGH, typically a result of pituitary tumors. High amounts of HGH can lead to *acromegaly*, a deforming condition in which the bones of the hands, feet, and face become enlarged.   [T. H. M.]

According to the U.S. Department of Justice, about one-third of the steroids sold illegally in the United States are imported, principally from Mexico, where they can be bought without a prescription. Another third are produced legally but then diverted to the black market, and the remainder are made in clandestine labs in the United States. (Justice Department officials note that many such "steroids" actually contain no drug at all or are contaminated with toxic chemicals or hazardous microorganisms.)

Since 1985, when the Justice Department stepped up prosecution of individuals involved in the illegal manufacture and distribution of anabolic steroids, more than 100 people have been prosecuted. Also, in October 1988, the U.S. Congress passed the Anti-Drug Abuse Act, which increased penalties for the distribution of steroids without a physician's prescription for the treatment of a disease. The bill, which was signed by President Ronald Reagan in November 1988, upgraded steroid trafficking from a misdemeanor with a penalty of one year in prison to a felony with a three-year prison penalty, which would be doubled if the steroids were sold to minors. The bill also includes a maximum fine of $25,000.

The states are also stepping up their efforts to restrict steroid abuse. As of early 1989, nine states (Alabama, California, Colorado, Florida, Indiana, New Mexico, Ohio, Texas, and Virginia) had passed laws designed to cut down the nonmedical use of anabolic steroids. Several other states were considering similar restrictions. But many authorities believe that such measures—like those prohibiting cocaine and heroin—will have little effect as long as demand remains high.

The first line of defense against steroid abuse, therefore, is education. Potential users need to be alerted to the hazards of anabolic steroids, and coaches need to be convinced of the hazards to the athletes they supervise. But education apparently is not enough, because many athletes are not paying attention to the warnings. According to Gary I. Wadler, clinical professor of medicine at Cornell University Medical College in New York City, this fact is largely attributable to the medical profession's previous attempts to discredit the efficacy of the drugs. Wadler describes the attitude of many users as "First you told me steroids don't work, and now you are trying to scare me, so I don't believe whatever you say."

Most sports officials consequently view frequent and regular testing of athletes as the only effective way to combat steroid abuse. So far, however, testing has been used only on a limited basis, and with very limited results. The National Collegiate Athletic Association (NCAA), which oversees college sports, tests only at bowl games and national championships.

Governing bodies of track and field and other sports affiliated with the U.S. Olympic Committee test only winners, and only at some events.

In the realm of professional sports, testing is even spottier. The National Basketball Association and the National Hockey League do not test their players for steroids, nor does major league baseball. The National Football League (NFL), on the other hand, does test its players—once during training camp and again during the year if there is reasonable cause. The league's tests have yielded questionable results, however. In the 1988 exhibition season, for example, the NFL said 6 per cent of its players tested positive for steroids, but many sports drug experts disputed that figure as being far too low.

The problem with the current testing approach by the NCAA, the NFL, and other sports organizations is that athletes know when testing will be conducted and thus can restrict their steroid use for a few days or weeks before the testing period and allow all traces of the drugs to be flushed out of their bodies. Only those who do not quit soon enough fail to pass such tests.

Many experts think that random tests would be a more effective means of detecting steroid abuse. In December 1988, the International Olympic Committee appointed a commission to develop procedures and logistics that will allow a testing team to travel from country to country administering steroid tests to athletes on short notice during training periods. Prince Alexandre de Merode of Belgium, the chairman of the committee's medical commission, said that about two years would be required before such testing could begin.

Widespread random testing for steroids does have its drawbacks. One is cost. Each individual steroid test runs about $200. That figure translates to at least $20,000 for one round of testing for a college football team, and most schools argue that further testing would be prohibitively expensive.

But until testing becomes more common, athletes seem likely to continue mortgaging their futures for supposed present gains—a tragedy whose full magnitude will begin to become glaringly apparent only when some of the most serious side effects begin to be fully felt, about 20 years from now. And those who are caught, like Ben Johnson, will not be immune to suffering, either. As writer William Oscar Johnson noted in *Sports Illustrated*, the Seoul Olympics transformed Ben Johnson "from a man with one of the brightest, richest futures in all of sport to a man with nothing to look forward to but days of shame."

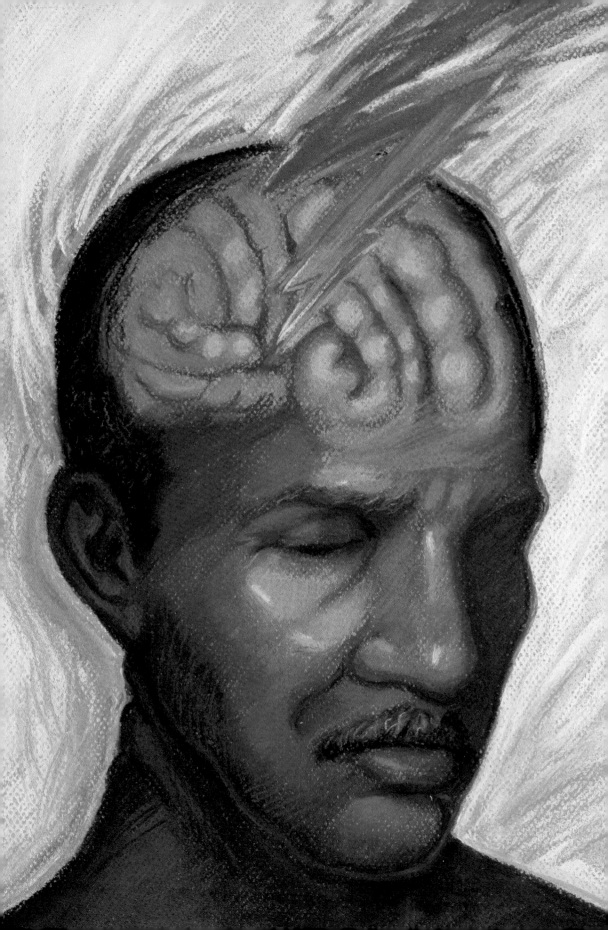

Stroke is the third leading
cause of death in the United
States. Fortunately, much
can be done to prevent it.

What Everyone
Needs to Know
About Stroke

By Beverly Merz

Imagine a cold and rainy November evening. You are nestled
into your favorite chair in front of the fireplace and have just
begun to read the last chapter of a good novel.

Suddenly, the print begins to blur, and you close your eyes.
When you try to open them, you realize that something is
wrong. For a confused moment, you think a shade has been
pulled down over one eye, leaving you half-blind.

You attempt to rub your eyes, but one hand, heavy and
limp, won't cooperate. Now you notice that the leg on which
the limp hand is resting seems to have fallen asleep—but that
may be because your dog has snuggled up against it. You open
your mouth to tell him to get up, but the words won't come.

That is what it might feel like to have a stroke.

A stroke is a frightening medical emergency with a simple
cause: The blood supply to part of the brain is disrupted. Diminished blood flow deprives tissue of the oxygen essential to
life. After as little as 4 to 10 minutes without oxygen, brain
cells begin to die, causing the parts of the body they control to
stop functioning properly. If, for example, the brain cells that
control the left leg die, that limb becomes paralyzed. If the

The author:

Beverly Merz is an associate editor of *The Journal of the American Medical Association.*

brain cells that control a vital bodily function are affected, the stroke may be lethal.

Although dramatic and devastating, stroke is fairly common. Each year, about 500,000 people in the United States—nearly 30 per cent of them under 65 years of age—have a stroke, according to the American Heart Association in Dallas. Luckily, strokes can be prevented, and efforts to do so have caused the death rate from stroke to decline markedly since the 1940's. Today, about one-third of stroke sufferers die, making stroke America's third leading cause of death, after heart disease and cancer. Another one-third are permanently disabled, and the remaining third make a full recovery.

Which category would you fall into if you had actually suffered the stroke described earlier? The answer depends on several factors—including what part of the brain is affected and what type of stroke is suffered.

The types of stroke

There are several types of stroke, which can be grouped into two categories: those caused by *ischemia*, a cutoff in blood flow; and those caused by *hemorrhage*, or bleeding.

Ischemic strokes, which are caused by a blocked artery in the brain, are the more common of the two types. The most common kind of ischemic stroke, *cerebral thrombosis*, occurs when a blood clot forms in—and obstructs—a brain artery already narrowed by *atherosclerosis* (a condition in which fatty substances in the blood build up inside arteries). About 70 to 80 per cent of all strokes are cerebral thromboses. After a period of time that varies from hours to days, natural clot-dissolving substances in the blood may dissolve the blockage so that blood flow is resumed. The affected brain cells may be dead by this time, however.

Cerebral thrombosis can be preceded by *transient ischemic attacks (TIA's)*. These have symptoms similar to strokes, but their effects are temporary. Experts believe that most TIA's are due to clumps of *platelets* (a blood component important in clotting) that form in blood vessels roughened by atherosclerotic build-up; the lumps may then break off and travel downstream, where they may temporarily plug a small vessel.

The symptoms of cerebral thrombosis and TIA are similar. The person may develop visual impairment and weakness, numbness, tingling, or paralysis on one side of the body. *Aphasia*, an inability to speak, read, or associate words with their meanings, is another common symptom. With cerebral thrombosis, the impairment may be permanent. With TIA, normal function returns within 24 hours.

Cerebral embolism is a second, and less common, type of ischemic stroke, accounting for 5 to 14 per cent of all strokes.

It occurs when a blood clot forms in another part of the body (typically in a large blood vessel or in one of the chambers of the heart) and travels through the bloodstream to the brain. When the blood clot reaches a narrower artery in the brain, it creates a plug that instantly cuts off blood flow. The symptoms of such a stroke are virtually identical to those of cerebral thrombosis.

Hemorrhagic strokes are caused by the rupture of one or more of the brain's blood vessels. The most common type of hemorrhagic stroke is *cerebral hemorrhage*, in which the ruptured vessels are located deep within the brain. This type of stroke is often the result of high blood pressure, which can eventually weaken small arteries in the brain so much that they burst. When they burst, the blood supply to certain regions of the brain is diminished and oxygen-deprived cells in those regions die. As blood pools within the brain, it presses on nearby brain cells, disrupting their function. Cerebral hemorrhage accounts for about 10 per cent of all strokes.

Another kind of hemorrhagic stroke is *subarachnoid hemorrhage*, which occurs when blood vessels on the surface of the brain rupture. These vessels bleed into the space between the membranes surrounding the brain (an area called the *subarachnoid space*), putting pressure on brain cells and depriving others of blood. About 7 per cent of strokes are caused by subarachnoid hemorrhages.

This type of hemorrhagic stroke is usually caused by the rupture of an *aneurysm*, an abnormal, balloonlike distention of an artery caused by a weakness in the artery wall. Aneurysms are usually defects present since birth, but they can also be caused by an infection in the wall of an artery.

The symptoms of subarachnoid and cerebral hemorrhages are generally the same as those of ischemic stroke—paralysis, loss of vision, and perhaps loss of consciousness. Because blood may leak slowly in these kinds of strokes, mild symptoms such as headache and vomiting may begin an hour or two before the

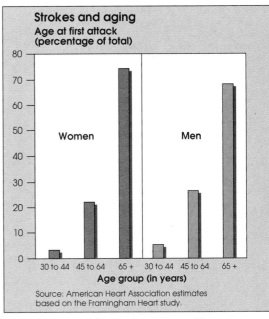

Source: American Heart Association estimates based on the Framingham Heart study.

Most strokes occur in people over age 65—though strokes in younger people are not rare, *above*. The risk of death from stroke differs among racial groups and between the sexes, *below*; the stroke death rate is higher for nonwhites than whites, and men have a higher stroke death rate than women.

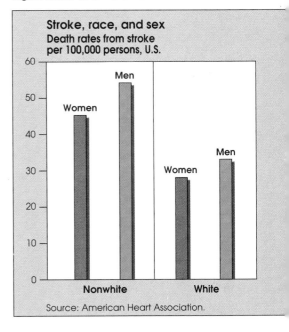

Source: American Heart Association.

Two kinds of stroke

Strokes generally fall into two categories. Ischemic strokes, *below left,* are the result of a blood clot that blocks an artery in or leading to the brain. The blockage deprives brain cells of the bloodborne oxygen and nutrients essential to life. Hemorrhagic strokes, *below right,* occur when one or more blood vessels in the head rupture. The pressure of pooling blood can damage or kill nearby brain cells.

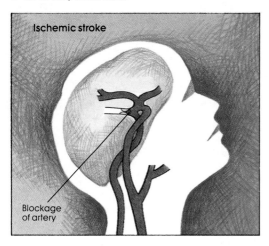

Ischemic stroke

Blockage of artery

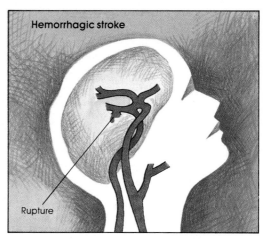

Hemorrhagic stroke

Rupture

Sophisticated imaging techniques reveal the problems that may lead to stroke. An area of blocked blood flow in the neck, *below left* (marked by arrow), may result in an ischemic stroke. An aneurysm, a ballooning of a weakened blood vessel wall, *below right,* may burst, causing a hemorrhagic stroke.

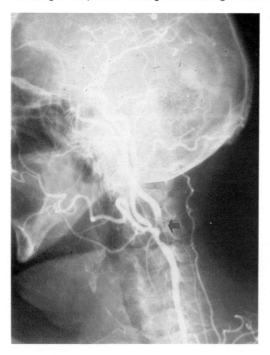

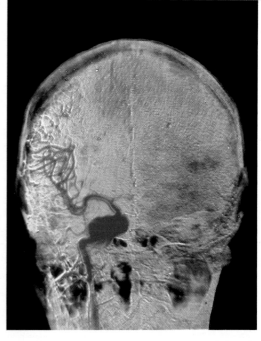

person having the stroke begins to suffer its major effects. If an aneurysm in the brain bursts, the effect is akin to being shot in the head. The person typically feels a sudden, violent flash of pain and loses consciousness.

Both types of hemorrhagic stroke generally occur with little warning, and, because bleeding may continue for a while before stopping naturally, they are the most damaging and most deadly kind of stroke. Approximately 70 per cent of patients with hemorrhagic stroke die within 30 days—most of them succumbing to increased pressure on the brain but some from cell death due to loss of blood supply. Those who survive usually recover more fully than victims of ischemic stroke, however, because the pressure of accumulated blood is less destructive to brain cells than is a complete cutoff in blood flow.

How stroke is diagnosed

It is important to seek medical attention as soon as the symptoms of stroke appear. At most hospitals, a *neurologist* (specialist in the nervous system), other specialists, and an intensive-care nursing staff are available to evaluate and stabilize the patient.

Before deciding on treatment, however, the medical team must know what kind of stroke the patient has suffered. Inappropriate treatment can seriously harm the patient. For example, if a patient suffering from cerebral hemorrhage is given the treatment for cerebral thrombosis—a blood-thinning drug designed to dissolve clots in blocked arteries—the bleeding in the brain will intensify, making the patient worse.

Fortunately, there are several ways to determine the kind of stroke a patient is suffering from. One technique uses *computerized tomography*—called a *CT scan* or *CAT scan*. A CT scan uses a large number of X rays to provide detailed cross-sectional images of the brain. Pools of blood are readily detectable on CT scans, making it possible to diagnose a cerebral hemorrhage soon after it occurs. *Magnetic resonance imaging* (MRI), a diagnostic technique that uses magnetic energy

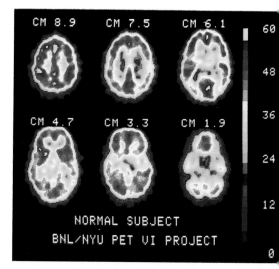

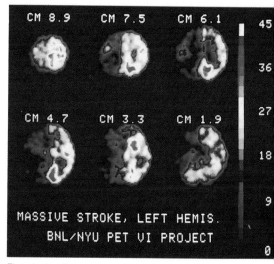

The destructive power of a stroke is clearly revealed by images of the brain made by a technique called positron emission tomography (PET), which detects chemical activity in body tissue. In contrast to the images of a normal brain, *top*, PET scans of the brain of a stroke patient, *above*, reveal extensive areas of damaged tissue (shown in blue).

and radio waves rather than X rays, also helps physicians obtain a visual image of the brain.

If there is no evidence of pooling blood, the medical team may perform a *spinal tap*, a procedure in which a needle is inserted into the spinal column to extract a small amount of the fluid that bathes and cushions the brain and spinal cord. The fluid is then examined for the presence of red blood cells, which may indicate bleeding inside the skull.

CT scans and MRI have made diagnosing hemorrhagic stroke much more accurate than in the past. Unfortunately, it is not so easy to diagnose ischemic stroke. To see a blood clot within a vessel requires injecting a dye into the bloodstream and taking X rays of the head. But this procedure, called *arteriography*, carries a slight risk of causing death, and it is not considered safe for patients undergoing a stroke. Thus, ischemic stroke must often be diagnosed indirectly, by ruling out hemorrhagic stroke.

Limited treatment options

When the medical team is confident that they know what type of stroke the patient is experiencing, they can decide on treatment. In many cases, the team may opt for simply making the patient comfortable while the stroke runs its course.

This is especially true with patients suffering hemorrhagic stroke, because attempts at intervention carry a fairly high risk of triggering more bleeding. Moreover, once the bleeding has stopped naturally, small blood vessels will slowly drain off the accumulated blood, taking pressure off brain cells. If a CT scan reveals large pools of blood exerting life-threatening pressure, however, a surgical operation to drain off the blood may be necessary.

If an ischemic stroke is developing, treatment may involve preventing further clotting through the use of *anticoagulants*, drugs, such as heparin and warfarin, that interfere with the clotting of blood. Because these drugs may cause bleeding at the site of the damage, patients taking them are watched carefully for signs of developing hemorrhagic stroke. Patients who have survived a cerebral thrombosis may be given aspirin, which, if given at the correct dosage, interferes with the clotting function of platelets and may prevent another stroke.

Experimental therapies that may prove more effective than present treatments are being studied by several research groups. Studies are underway to determine if a clot-dissolving substance called *tissue plasminogen activator* (*t-PA*) can dissolve clots responsible for stroke without triggering hemorrhage. In addition, some scientists think that a group of drugs called calcium channel blockers may help people suffering from ischemic stroke because these drugs relax blood vessels, allowing an increase in blood flow. Other researchers are developing treatments to relieve swelling in the brain or provide it with extra oxygen to prevent cell death. These treatments are experimental, however, and their effectiveness has yet to be determined.

The long road back

After the stroke victim's condition has stabilized, the medical team will examine the patient to determine the extent of brain damage. If the patient is alert, he or she will be given a detailed neurological examination to determine the size and location of the damaged area. The patient may be asked to perform a series of exercises designed to test how well different parts of the body function. The medical team can then associate the inability to perform a certain task—grasping with the right hand, for example—with damage to the brain cells that control that action.

If a patient is comatose, physicians can determine how much brain function is left by making an *electroencephalogram* (*EEG*)—a recording of the electrical activity of the brain. The neurologist also may perform an *evoked-response test* to measure how well the brain responds to such stimuli as flashing lights, sounds, and mild electric shocks to the arms and legs.

The team's next step is to design a rehabilitation program based on the knowledge that the brain's function may improve markedly after the stroke. Aphasia, for example, often can be overcome. On the other hand, the rehabilitation program also must take into account the fact that extensive brain damage means that some functions, such as the use of now-paralyzed limbs, may be permanently lost.

With all stroke-related disabilities, the sooner rehabilitation begins, the better the patient's chance for recovery. Some type of rehabilitation usually starts while the patient is still bedridden. Nurses and physical therapists turn the patient frequently to improve circulation and prevent bedsores, and they massage and exercise paralyzed limbs to maintain muscle condition and joint flexibility.

After the patient is well enough to leave the hospital bed, further help can be provided by rehabilitation centers in hospitals or at special rehabilitation facilities. In these centers, nurses, physical therapists, speech therapists, and occupational therapists help patients become as independent as possible by regaining lost functions and by learning skills to compensate for those that cannot be regained. For example, a patient whose hands can no longer grasp may be taught how

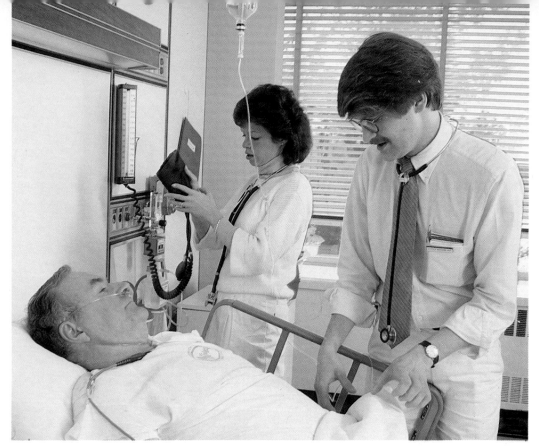

After a stroke patient's condition is stable and the patient is alert, the physician can begin to determine the extent of brain impairment by talking to the patient, *above,* and asking him to perform physical tasks.

to use a mechanical device in order to pick up objects.

To bolster a patient's spirits during this often-difficult process—which can take months or even years—the therapists may enlist the help of the family. Family members are taught to appreciate what the stroke survivor has undergone and to understand how his or her life will be different. They can also be trained to assist with the patient's exercises so that rehabilitation can continue at home.

Family members also need to be aware that the stroke may affect more than the patient's physical abilities; it can alter mental capacity and personality as well. Sometimes stroke patients lose problem-solving skills or have memory lapses. They are likely to have periods of depression—which can be made worse by the difficulty of relearning skills. They may also have mood changes that are beyond their control, and family and friends may need to cope with inappropriate outbursts of laughter or tears.

Prevention—the best answer for today

Despite the efforts of physicians and rehabilitation teams, two-thirds of all strokes cause death or some permanent disability. Thus, many health experts emphasize prevention—by minimizing or eliminating some of the factors that predispose people to stroke—as the best way to combat stroke today.

Since the late 1950's, evidence has accumulated that certain factors increase a person's chances of having a stroke. Much of this evidence has come from long-term research studies in which large numbers of people are followed for many years to see what diseases they develop.

Not surprisingly, these studies show that strokes are more common in people with high blood pressure, atherosclerosis, and certain heart defects. Researchers have also found that the stroke rate for men is 30 per cent higher than for women, and 60 per cent higher for blacks than for whites. These differences may be partially explained by the fact that men are more prone to atherosclerosis and blacks to high blood pressure. Diabetics, who have an increased risk of atherosclerosis, also have an increased risk of stroke.

Other stroke risk factors include a family or personal history of stroke or of the conditions linked to stroke. Another is advanced age, which brings with it an increased risk of atherosclerosis. Although nearly 30 per cent of all stroke victims are younger than 65, the rate of stroke doubles every 10 years after age 55. Smokers also have a higher than average risk of stroke. Finally, women 35 years or older who use oral contraceptives have an increased risk of stroke—which is compounded if they also smoke.

Although you can do nothing about your age, race, sex, or family history, you can eliminate or minimize some underlying causes of stroke. High blood pressure, for example, can be treated successfully. Under a physician's supervision, you may be able to lower your blood pressure by losing weight, quitting smoking, and perhaps maintaining a diet low in sodium. When these measures alone are not successful, a doctor may prescribe medication.

Atherosclerosis doubles the risk of stroke, and one of its principal causes is having elevated levels of cholesterol in the blood. This is one reason all adults should have their cholesterol levels checked—at least once every five years, according to the American Heart Association. Cholesterol is a substance that is produced by the liver and is also found in foods. Although small amounts are necessary for good health, high levels of cholesterol in the blood can be associated with a build-up of substances inside the walls of blood vessels. Most health experts—including the American Heart Association and the National Research Council in Washington, D.C.—agree that the likelihood of developing the condition can be lessened if people maintain a diet that derives no more than 30 per cent

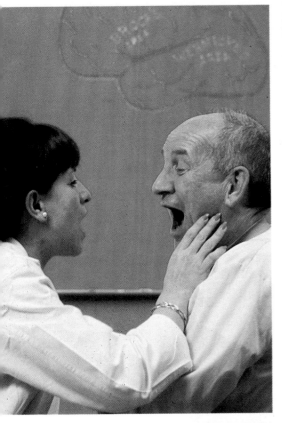

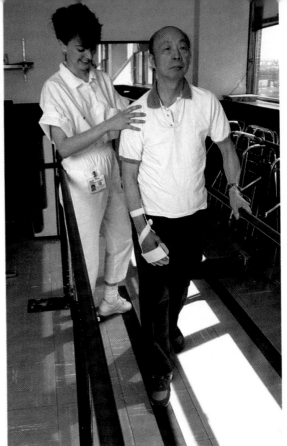

Regaining lost functions

Although some damage may be permanent, physical and speech therapy can help stroke survivors recover as much function as possible. Some stroke patients may be able to regain lost motor skills, *above,* as well as such language skills as speaking, *left,* and reading, *below.*

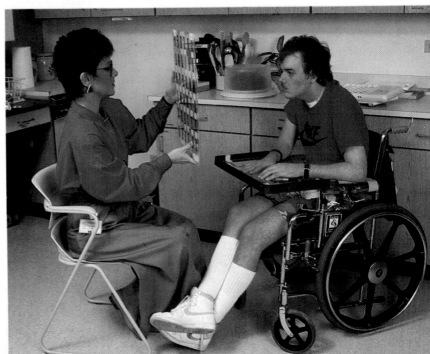

of its calories from fat. Medication may also be needed to lower the cholesterol level if it is abnormally high.

Heart defects increase the risk of stroke caused by embolisms traveling to the brain. Weakened hearts can develop blood clots within them that may break off and travel to the brain with the flow of blood. Another problem is *atrial fibrillation,* a condition in which the upper, or atrial, chamber of the heart twitches rapidly and irregularly rather than contracting rhythmically, slowing steady blood flow in the chamber and allowing the formation of clots, which can then travel to arteries in the brain. In most cases, the condition can be prevented with medication.

Defects in the valves of the heart—as well as the presence of artificial valves that heart surgeons use to replace malfunctioning valves—can also be associated with clot formation and embolisms. Patients with these heart problems can reduce the risk of stroke by taking anticoagulant drugs to reduce the formation of clots.

Stroke risk is also high for people who have a condition called *polycythemia,* in which the blood contains an unusually large number of red blood cells—making clotting more likely. Reducing the risk in these people can be accomplished by removing small amounts of blood periodically to reduce the volume of red blood cells.

Finally, although only about 10 per cent of strokes are preceded by TIA's, these attacks are predictors of a possibly damaging stroke, and anyone who suspects he or she has had a TIA should see a physician immediately. The doctor will use a stethoscope to listen to blood flow in the arteries in the patient's neck and examine the arteries by feeling them. If the physician hears the murmurlike sound of irregular blood flow or if the pulsations are reduced, further examinations may be needed to determine if these arteries are obstructed. Several sophisticated techniques can be used to give the physician an image of the arteries. One is *Doppler ultrasound,*

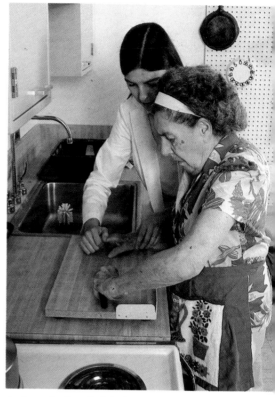

An important part of stroke recovery is learning how to perform everyday tasks despite some impairment. A therapist, *above,* visits a stroke survivor at home to help her regain the ability to handle household chores.

Preventing stroke by reducing risk factors

Some risk factors for stroke—such as being over 65, being male, or having had a prior stroke—cannot be changed. Others can be treated, however, and this may reduce the risk of stroke.

Risk factors	Treatment
Elevated cholesterol level	Maintaining a low-fat diet; cholesterol-level-lowering medication
Heart defects	Anticoagulant medication
High blood pressure	Life style changes such as losing weight and quitting smoking; blood-pressure-lowering medication
History of TIA's (small strokes)	Anticoagulant medication; surgery to remove fatty deposits in arteries
Obesity	Losing weight
Oral contraceptive use	Avoidance of oral contraceptives if the woman is over 35 or a smoker
Smoking	Quitting the habit

Stroke is often preventable. Taking steps to minimize the factors that lead to stroke, *above,* has led to a dramatic drop in the number of people who die from stroke in the United States, *right.*

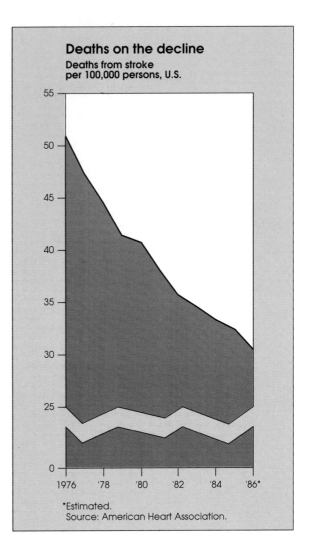

Deaths on the decline

Deaths from stroke per 100,000 persons, U.S.

*Estimated.
Source: American Heart Association.

a procedure that produces pictures by bouncing sound waves off the artery walls.

If the examinations fail to show a substantial narrowing of the arteries in the neck, the physician may assume that the TIA was caused by thromboses or embolisms in other blood vessels, perhaps inside the head. In that case, the physician may prescribe aspirin or some other anticoagulant to reduce the risk of more clotting.

If, on the other hand, the tests show or the physician suspects that there is a substantial narrowing of either artery in the neck, the physician often recommends arteriography to visualize the vessels in the neck. If atherosclerotic build-up is found, the next step may be *carotid endarterectomy*, surgery in which the artery is cut open lengthwise and the fatty deposits are scraped from the artery's inner walls. Thousands of endarterectomies are performed in the United States each year, but the value of the operation seems to vary depending on the expertise of the surgical team and the patient's condition. Many patients have relief from TIA's after surgery, but others do not. Several studies are underway to determine which patients definitely benefit from carotid endarterectomies and which medical centers have the highest success rates with the procedure.

Although the value of endarterectomies is still under study, it's clear that surgery is sometimes vital to correct aneurysms and other malformed vessels in the brain that have ruptured or might in the future. Aneurysm surgery typically involves clamping off the ballooning section of the artery or using lasers to cut it out and then sewing the severed vessel together again. Surgical procedures to correct other malformed vessels vary according to the individual problem. Occasionally, the surgeon may decide to seal off a malformed blood vessel with an injection of a harmless plastic or by directing radiation at the vessel to cause a growth of protective scar tissue.

Looking ahead

Specialists expect to see advances in the treatment and prevention of stroke during the next few decades as more data about stroke are compiled. Even in the absence of breakthroughs, the incidence of fatal stroke in the United States has been declining rapidly. In the 1940's, the death rate from stroke began to fall by 1 per cent each year. In the 1970's, that decline accelerated, reaching a 5 per cent to 6 per cent annual decrease. As a result, although stroke killed 89 of every 100,000 Americans in 1950, it will kill only 34 of 100,000 in 1989.

This remarkable decline may reflect not only the availability of better medical care but also the attention we have begun to pay to the need for treating stroke-causing conditions, particularly high blood pressure. As we await a cure for stroke, we can take courage in the fact that there is much that we can do to prevent it.

For more information, write to:

The American Heart Association
7320 Greenville Avenue
Dallas, TX 75231

The National Stroke Association
300 East Hampden Avenue, Suite 240
Englewood, CO 80110-2622

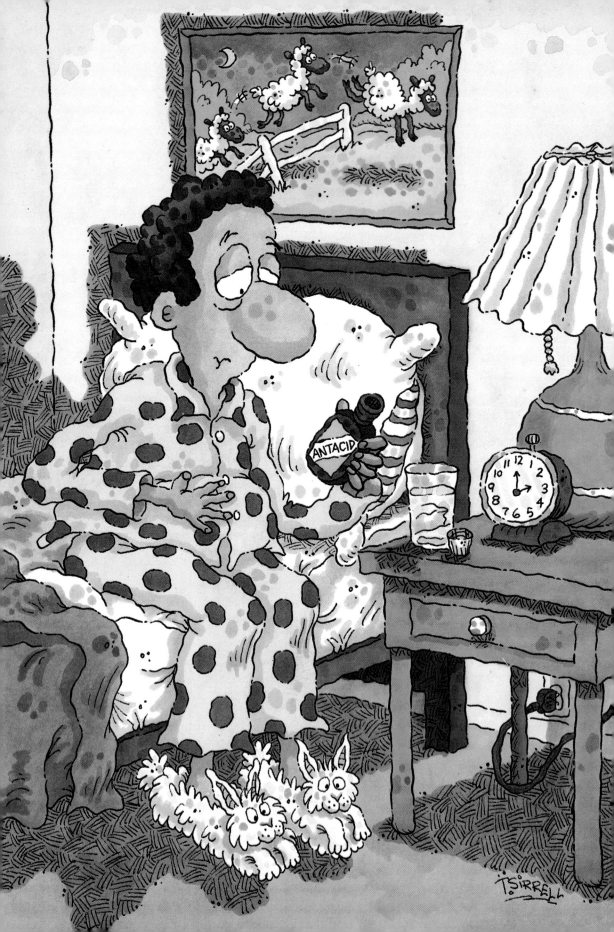

The Inside Story on Ulcers

By John Schaffner

Forget the old ideas about what
causes peptic ulcers. It's not what
you eat—not even what's eating you.

It's after midnight, and you suddenly wake up with a gnawing, burning ache in the middle of your abdomen, just below
the breastbone. You feel hungry. "Indigestion," you say to
yourself and head for the medicine chest to get an antacid.

But after several weeks of this discomfort, you ask yourself,
"Could I have an ulcer?" And you answer, "No, I'm not the
type," because your picture of an ulcer patient is that of a
middle-aged businessman with a stressful job, a hard-driving
workaholic who dines regularly on rich, spicy foods.

But, in fact, a patient with an ulcer might just as likely be a
30-year-old waitress or a 70-year-old retiree who eats bland
food and has little stress. Even children sometimes develop
ulcers. In other words, there really is no such thing as a typical ulcer patient.

As the stereotype of an ulcer patient has fallen by the way-
side, so have many of the old ideas about what causes ulcers
and how to cure them. The old staples of ulcer treatment—a
bland, milky diet and surgery—are seldom used. In their
place, doctors have some remarkably safe and effective new
drugs—and many unanswered questions.

A *peptic ulcer*—as doctors call an ulcer in the stomach or
the first part of the small intestine—is one of the most common diseases and also one of the most mysterious. About 1 of
every 10 Americans will develop an ulcer sometime in life.
But doctors do not know exactly what causes an ulcer and

Glossary

Duodenal ulcer: An open sore in the lining of the small intestine just below the stomach.

Duodenum: The part of the small intestine just below the stomach.

Dyspepsia: Indigestion.

Endoscopy: Examination of the stomach and duodenum with a flexible tube called an *endoscope*, made of optical fibers that transmit light.

Gastric ulcer: An open sore in the lining of the stomach.

Gastroenterology: The branch of medicine dealing with the stomach, intestines, liver, and pancreas.

Pepsin: An enzyme in the stomach's digestive juice that helps to digest meat and other proteins.

Peptic ulcer: An open sore in the lining of the stomach or the duodenum.

Prostaglandins: Hormone-like substances that perform many functions, including preserving the lining of the stomach.

what a person can do to keep from getting one, why many ulcers heal by themselves, or why ulcers flare up again and again. Doctors do not even know whether ulcers are one disease or many.

What is a peptic ulcer?

A peptic ulcer is an open sore in the surface lining of the digestive tract. There are two types of peptic ulcers: *gastric ulcers*, which occur in the stomach, and *duodenal ulcers*, which occur in the duodenum, the part of the small intestine just below the stomach.

Ulcers take an enormous toll in human suffering. Dennis M. Jensen, a *gastroenterologist* (specialist in diseases of the stomach and intestines) at the School of Medicine of the University of California at Los Angeles, has studied the economic impact of peptic ulcer disease. Jensen estimates that 200,000 to 400,000 new cases of duodenal ulcer and almost as many new cases of gastric ulcer develop each year in the United States. In addition, as many as 70 per cent of the patients with duodenal ulcer disease suffer a recurrence within one year after diagnosis.

For unknown reasons, ulcers tend to recur seasonally, appearing most often in spring and fall in temperate climates—that is, in most of the United States and southern Canada. And just as mysteriously as they appear, ulcers also tend to disappear. Without treatment, approximately 40 per cent of all ulcers will heal themselves in six weeks. With treatment, and it doesn't seem to matter which of the standard treatments is used, about 80 per cent heal in six weeks.

The financial costs of this baffling disease are staggering. Jensen estimates the economic burden of ulcer disease at approximately $3.25 billion a year in the United States. This figure includes hospital and physician costs as well as lost productivity. About 1.5 per cent of all days absent from work due to illness can be attributed to peptic ulcer disease.

Despite the misery and expense, peptic ulcer disease is seldom a matter of life and death. In the United States, only about 3 of every 100,000 cases result in death.

Ulcers can cause bleeding, which may be minor or life threatening. They can *perforate* (eat through) the wall of the stomach or duodenum, spilling the contents of the stomach or intestine into the abdominal cavity. Duodenal ulcers will more likely perforate than gastric ulcers.

Ulcers in certain locations also can produce an obstruction that blocks food from moving down the digestive tract. Such blockage may be caused by swelling or by the build-up of scar tissue from recurring ulcers. Obstruction occurs almost exclusively in the duodenum or the narrow section of the stomach.

The author:

John Schaffner is an associate professor of medicine at Rush Medical College in Chicago.

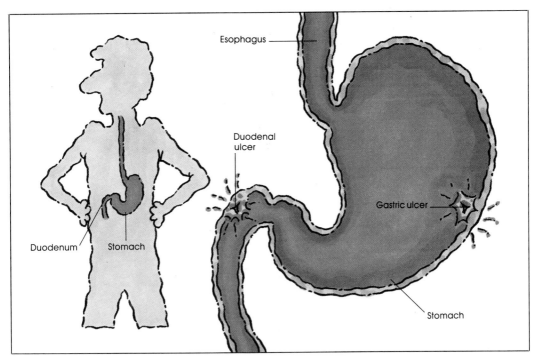

Esophagus

Duodenal ulcer

Gastric ulcer

Duodenum

Stomach

Stomach

Where ulcers occur

There are two main types of peptic ulcers. *Gastric ulcers* form in the stomach. *Duodenal ulcers* develop in the duodenum, the upper part of the small intestine.

What causes an ulcer?

Ulcers in the duodenum and stomach differ in many respects, leading doctors to suspect that ulcers may be many disorders which all produce the same result—a hole in the lining of the digestive tract. Duodenal ulcers tend to occur in patients with too much stomach acid. Gastric ulcers develop in patients with less acid than normal. What the two types of ulcers have in common is that they occur because of an imbalance between the amount of stomach acid and the defenses that protect the digestive system from its own acid.

The stomach produces a powerful digestive juice containing an enzyme called *pepsin* and, in most people, a strong acid called *hydrochloric acid*. The pepsin and acid begin the digestion of meat, eggs, and other protein foods—substances much like the walls of the stomach itself. Acid, however, is not crucial to digestion. Many individuals, particularly elderly people, have no stomach acid but still have normal digestion. In a healthy person, the stomach's own defenses prevent the digestive juices from attacking it.

A breakdown of the stomach's defenses probably accounts for most gastric ulcers. *Bile salts*, substances produced by the

Things that don't cause ulcers

Research has overturned old beliefs about what causes ulcers. There is no evidence, for example, that a diet of hot, spicy food causes ulcers.

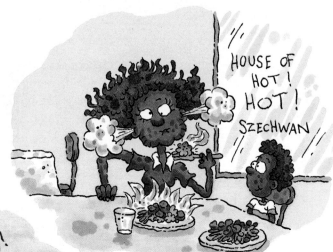

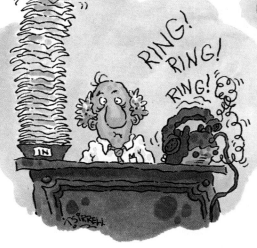

Stress may play a role in peptic ulcer disease, but there is no proof that people with high-pressure jobs or much tension in their lives are more likely to develop ulcers. More important than the amount of stress is how an individual reacts to it.

liver that aid in the digestion of fats, may enter the stomach from the duodenum and damage the stomach lining, allowing acid to penetrate the lining and create an ulcer. Certain drugs, including aspirin and other arthritis drugs, may also damage the lining of the digestive tract. These drugs may irritate the stomach and duodenum by direct contact, causing tiny points of bleeding wherever they touch the organs' lining. They also may promote ulcers by blocking the formation of hormonelike substances called *prostaglandins*. Prostaglandins are found in many tissues, including the stomach, and help perform a variety of jobs, such as promoting production of a thick, protective fluid called *mucus* that covers the stomach lining.

Excess hydrochloric acid is an important factor in duodenal ulcers. Many patients with these ulcers—though not all—produce excess acid when fasting and after eating. All of the factors that cause peptic ulcers are not known.

Things that do cause ulcers

Cigarette smoking not only increases a person's chances of getting an ulcer but also interferes with the healing of ulcers after they develop.

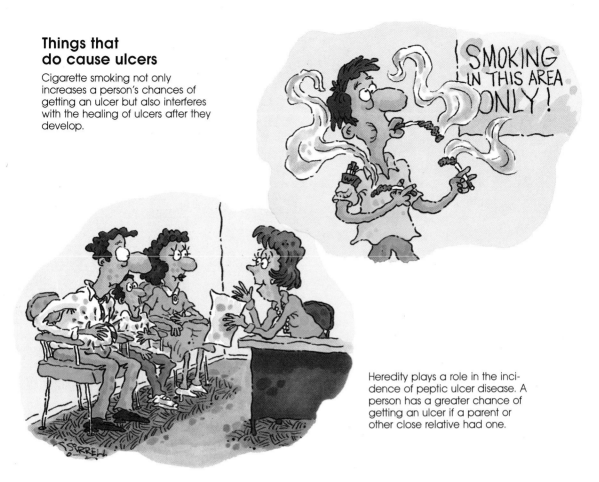

Heredity plays a role in the incidence of peptic ulcer disease. A person has a greater chance of getting an ulcer if a parent or other close relative had one.

In the early 1980's, researchers found links between a bacterium known as *Campylobacter pylori*—abbreviated as *C. pylori*—and certain disorders of the stomach and duodenum. The relationship of *C. pylori* to ulcers remains controversial, though the organism is found in the stomach of 90 per cent of patients with duodenal ulcer. Studies have shown that ulcer recurrence drops dramatically in patients treated with antibiotics to eliminate *C. pylori*.

Who will get an ulcer?

It is difficult to identify patients who are at risk for peptic ulcer disease because the exact cause for most naturally occurring ulcers is unknown. Research has overturned previously held beliefs about diet and life style. The only life-style factor that does seem to contribute to ulcers is smoking, though the mechanism is unknown. Smoking also appears to interfere with ulcer healing.

Stress may play a role in ulcer disease, but its role remains unproven. Probably more important than the amount of stress

75

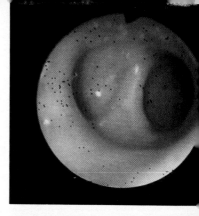

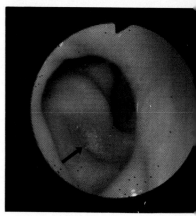

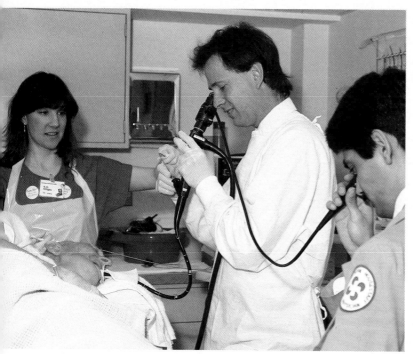

The most advanced technique for diagnosing ulcers is *endoscopy*, performed by passing a thin, flexible tube called an *endoscope* through the patient's mouth into the stomach and duodenum, *above*. The endoscope, made of optical fibers that transmit light, enables the physician to see whether the lining of the upper digestive tract is normal, *top right*, or has an ulcer, *above right* (arrow).

is how an individual reacts to stress, which cannot be measured precisely. Alcohol has not been shown to cause duodenal ulcers, though it can damage the stomach lining and cause inflammation when consumed in high concentrations.

Some patients with ulcer disease may have inherited a tendency to the disorder. But having a family history of ulcers does not mean that everyone in the family will develop one. In addition, for unknown reasons, people with type O blood are at greater risk for ulcers than people with other blood types. Of course, type O blood is the most common blood group, and most people with that blood type never get an ulcer.

What are the symptoms of an ulcer?

The symptoms of ulcer disease are not nearly as specific as was once believed. The majority of patients with ulcer symptoms do not, in fact, have an ulcer but merely indigestion, which doctors call *dyspepsia*.

The typical pain of ulcers is located in the middle of the abdomen below the breastbone. The pain may be sharp, dull, gnawing, or burning. At times, the pain may radiate to the back. The discomfort may be severe enough to awaken the patient at night. The response of pain to eating is variable. Some patients' pain may be aggravated by eating, while others may obtain relief from food. Other symptoms associated with ulcers include nausea, vomiting, lack of appetite, weight loss, heartburn, and bloating. The symptoms alone do not distinguish a duodenal from a gastric ulcer.

Ulcer complications produce additional symptoms. Patients with bleeding ulcers may vomit blood or may pass blood from their rectum. The vomited blood may be bright red, or it may be brown and granular, resembling coffee grounds, due to the action of stomach acid on the blood. Blood passed from the rectum is most frequently black and tarry, though patients with massive hemorrhage may have bright red bleeding from the rectum.

People with perforating ulcers may have more persistent, severe pain. Patients with obstruction from ulcers frequently vomit and fail to hold any food down. If you have any of these symptoms—vomiting of blood or material that looks like coffee grounds, passing stools that have a tarry appearance, severe pain, or repeated vomiting—see a doctor at once.

How is an ulcer diagnosed?

Modern ulcer drugs are so safe and effective that if a patient has symptoms of an ulcer, the doctor may prescribe a drug therapy without trying to confirm the diagnosis. If the patient's symptoms recur or are not relieved by treatment, the physician will seek a definitive diagnosis.

The two chief diagnostic techniques are X rays and a process called *endoscopy*. Both X rays and endoscopy are outpatient procedures, performed without putting a patient in the hospital. Both require the patient to fast for several hours before the test.

The most common procedure for detecting an ulcer is a series of X rays known as an *upper GI* (gastrointestinal) *series*. The patient is asked to swallow a thick, chalky, sometimes fruit-flavored liquid containing barium sulfate, a metallic element that shows up clearly on X rays. Often the patient then swallows an effervescent substance that causes air and barium to better coat the stomach and duodenum. The latter technique is known as an *air-contrast upper GI*. Barium studies of the upper gastrointestinal tract enable doctors to detect as many as 90 per cent of ulcers in the stomach and duodenum. Cancers of the esophagus and stomach can be detected as well by this technique.

If X-ray studies fail to reveal an ulcer and yet symptoms persist, a gastroenterologist or other physician may perform endoscopy. Endoscopy is more expensive but also more accurate. It enables the physician to see the lining of the esophagus, stomach, and duodenum. The examination is performed by passing a thin, flexible tube called an *endoscope*—made of optical fibers that transmit light—through the mouth into the stomach and duodenum. The physician can look directly through the endoscope or have the organ's image projected onto a television screen. Through the tube, the doctor can remove small pieces of tissue for microscopic examination, called a *biopsy*, to determine if tissue is cancerous or not.

Ulcer treatments that don't work

Many old ulcer treatments are no longer used. Researchers have found that a bland diet is no better than a spicy one, and that milk, once a staple for ulcer patients, stimulates secretion of stomach acid. Eating frequent small meals seems to offer little help.

How are ulcers treated?

Despite the mystery that still surrounds the cause of peptic ulcer disease, treatment of the condition has come a long way since the mid-1970's. Many of the old treatments, such as a bland diet and hospitalization, are no longer necessary. Diet plays no role in the management of ulcers unless particular foods bother an individual patient. Researchers have found that a bland diet is no better than a spicy one. Milk, which ulcer patients once drank by the pitcher, is now known to stimulate more stomach acid than does beer or coffee.

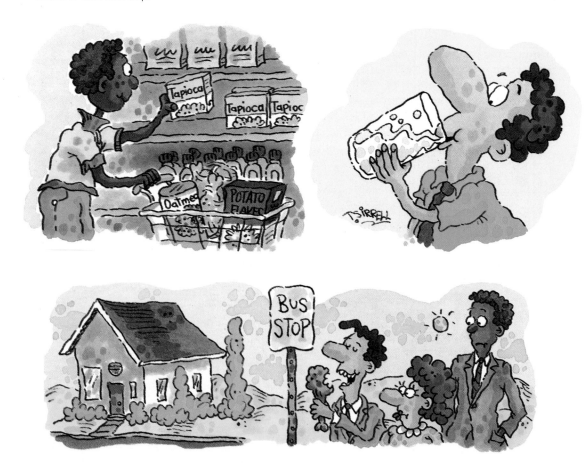

Treatment usually involves several different areas. First, any offending agent that may contribute to the formation of the ulcer should be removed. The patient should avoid ulcer-causing drugs such as aspirin and similar anti-inflammatory drugs and should quit smoking.

Drug treatment may aim at decreasing the stomach's production of acid, neutralizing any acid that is produced, or strengthening the natural defenses of the lining of the digestive tract. Regardless of which approach is employed, ulcers generally heal at the same rate. The side effects of most ulcer drugs are few and rare, making these drugs among the safest available. They are also the most widely prescribed medications in the world. The chart on page 80 lists the most common ulcer drugs, how they act, and their possible side effects. Physicians often recommend antacids, over-the-counter remedies that neutralize acid in the stomach, for use alone or in combination with prescription drugs.

Ulcer treatments that do work

Quitting smoking will aid ulcer healing and help prevent recurrence. Ulcer patients should avoid aspirin and similar anti-inflammatory drugs, which may cause ulcers. Many sufferers get relief from antacids, over-the-counter remedies that neutralize stomach acid. Several prescription drugs safely and effectively help ulcers heal and protect against recurrence.

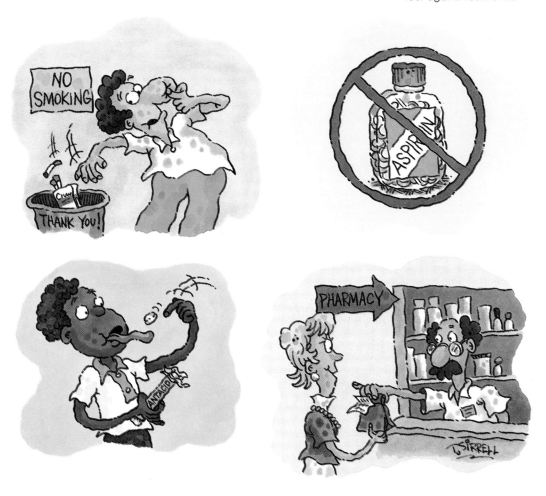

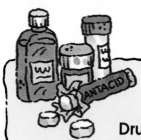

Drugs commonly prescribed for ulcers

Class of drugs	Generic and trade names	Possible side effects
Histamine H$_2$-receptor antagonists These drugs block the stomach's response to a body chemical called *histamine* that triggers secretion of gastric acid.	cimetidine (Tagamet®) ranitidine (Zantac®) famotidine (Pepcid®) nizatidine (Axis®)	Side effects are rare, occurring in about 1 per cent of users. For cimetidine, side effects include mental confusion, especially in elderly patients; breast enlargement; dizziness; diarrhea; skin rashes; and muscle pain. The other drugs may have fewer side effects.
Antacids These medications neutralize acid in the stomach.	magnesium hydroxide (milk of magnesia) aluminum hydroxide (ALternaGEL®, Amphojel®, and others) combinations of magnesium and aluminum hydroxide (Di-Gel®, Maalox®, Mylanta®, and others)	May cause diarrhea (from antacids containing magnesium) or constipation (from antacids containing aluminum). May hinder absorption of certain other drugs in the digestive tract.
Protective coating agent This drug coats the ulcer to shield it from irritation as it heals.	sucralfate (Carafate®)	May cause constipation.
Synthetic prostaglandins This drug makes the lining of the stomach and duodenum more resistant to acid. Used to decrease side effects of aspirin and other anti-inflammatory drugs.	misoprostol (Cytotec®)	May cause diarrhea.

Scientists also are exploring some promising new therapies for peptic ulcers. For example, two new families of drugs are being tested and may become part of the arsenal of ulcer medications. One group of drugs, *proton pump blockers*, may be more effective than currently available medicines in blocking the stomach's production of acid. The second family of drugs, a combination of antibiotics and bismuth compounds designed to eliminate *C. pylori* from the stomach, may help heal ulcers and prevent their recurrence.

One major reason for ulcer surgery, ulcers that will not heal, has almost completely disappeared because of improved drugs. Today, most surgery is performed for ulcer complications such as perforation, bleeding, and obstruction. But despite the advances in drug treatment, a few patients still require surgery for ulcers that fail to respond to medication.

Researchers are testing techniques that may eliminate the need for emergency surgery to treat bleeding peptic ulcers. In March 1989, a panel of experts convened by the National Institutes of Health (NIH) in Bethesda, Md., described two procedures as particularly promising alternatives to surgery. Both techniques use endoscopy to locate the area of bleeding; once the area is pinpointed, the physician inserts an instrument through a special channel in the endoscope. One procedure, *multipolar coagulation*, passes an electric current through the tissue to stop the blood flow. The second method uses a heated aluminum cylinder to achieve the same result.

The diagnosis and treatment of peptic ulcer disease have advanced rapidly in recent years. Doctors now have the means to make accurate diagnoses and to prescribe safe, effective treatment, and we're continuing to make progress in these areas. Perhaps the coming years will provide answers to some of the mysteries that still surround this common but little understood disorder, and we will learn what causes ulcers and how they can be prevented.

For more information, write to:

CURE Foundation
Suite 300
11661 San Vicente Boulevard
Los Angeles, CA 90049

National Digestive Diseases Information Clearinghouse
Box NDDIC
Bethesda, MD 20892
Send a stamped, self-addressed envelope with 45 cents postage.

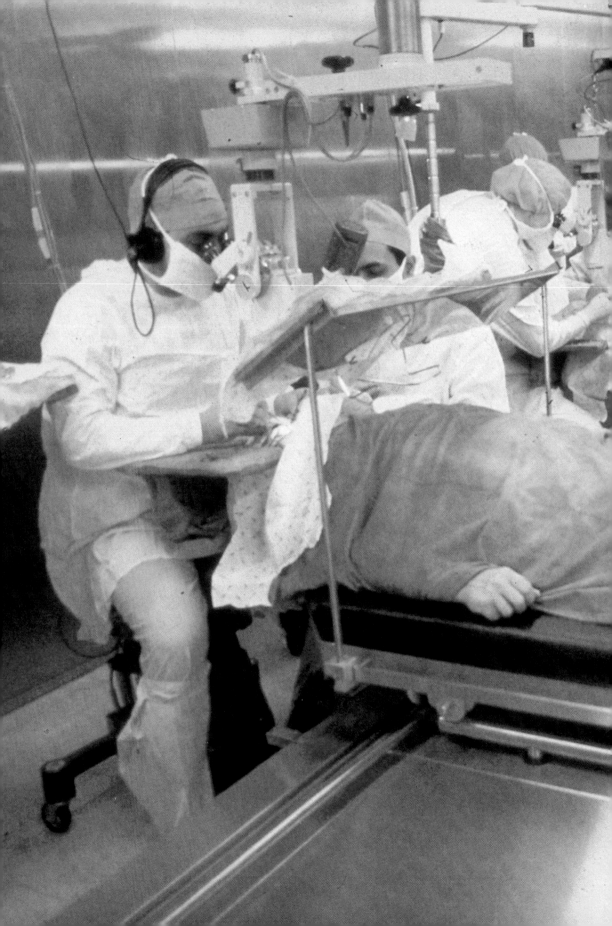

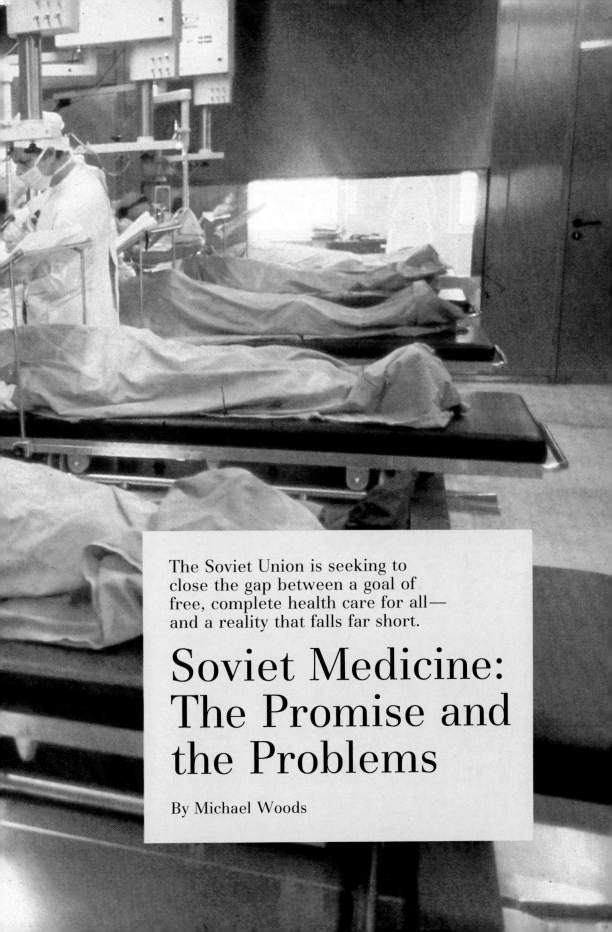

The Soviet Union is seeking to close the gap between a goal of free, complete health care for all— and a reality that falls far short.

Soviet Medicine: The Promise and the Problems

By Michael Woods

Five patients in wrinkled hospital gowns lie on operating tables attached to a metal rail in the floor. The rail runs the length of the modern operating room, through the glass walls at both ends.

A masked surgeon hunches over each patient's eyes, peering into a microscope while manipulating delicate microscalpels. One by one the surgeons finish and raise their heads.

"Who's this?" asks Surgeon No. 3, tilting her head at me.

"American medical journalist," the translator answers.

"You will be surprised," she says, a smile creasing the fabric of her surgical mask. "Nowhere else in the world . . ."

A soft pneumatic hiss intervenes as the glass walls slide open. I stare in utter disbelief as the operating tables and patients move ahead on the rail, like automobiles on a factory conveyor belt. One table exits the room, and the patient gets up and walks away. Another patient rolls in on a table newly coupled to the rail. The glass walls close. The surgeons return to work, each performing one step in an operation to remove cataracts, a clouding of the lens of the eye. Every three to five minutes another patient rolls off the line.

Yes, this *is* assembly-line surgery.

Welcome to the sometimes strange and frequently surprising world of health care in the Soviet Union. This is a world in which medical care is free and easily available, where doctors make house calls and ride in ambulances—but where treatment is so impersonal that patients gladly pay for private care. It is a world in which physicians have a low status in society; most are women who typically are paid less than a farmhand.

Five times since 1985 I've entered this world to interview Nobel Prize winners, top health officials, doctors, nurses, and patients from Moscow to Siberia. Clad in surgical mask and gown, I've watched operations, deliveries, and other procedures in the most prestigious Soviet medical institutes. Wearing muddy rubber boots, I've accompanied physicians on their rounds in remote villages in the Caucasus Mountains, where people supposedly live to extreme old age. I've eaten, drunk, and talked with Soviet doctors long into the night. If these encounters have taught me anything, it is that an enormous gulf exists between the promise and the reality of Soviet medicine.

No other country can claim a deeper commitment to health than the Union of Soviet Socialist Republics (U.S.S.R.). It was the first to make health care a national priority by creating a system of free, universal care financed by the state. The Soviet Constitution guarantees citizens the right to health care. About one-third of all the physicians in the world work in the Soviet Union. The U.S.S.R. leads the world with about 4 million hospital beds, four times more than the United States.

Moreover, as the unusual surgical assembly line at the Moscow Research Institute of Eye Microsurgery suggests, Soviet

The author:

Michael Woods is science editor of the *Toledo Blade*. His articles on scientific and medical topics have appeared in more than 100 newspapers.

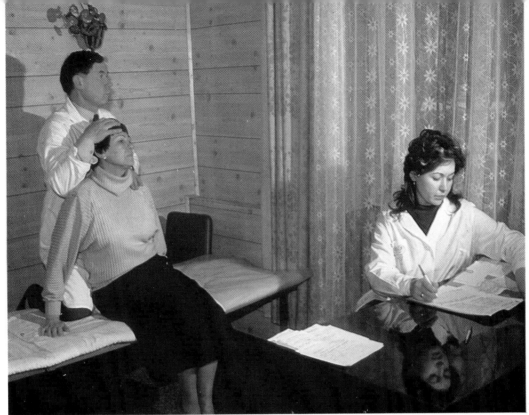

A doctor examines a patient at the Lecheniye i Konsultatsia (Treatment and Consultation) clinic in Moscow, the first medical cooperative established under a 1987 law that made private clinics legal. All Soviet citizens are entitled to free medical care, but many choose to pay for faster, more personal service at the new clinics.

medicine offers numerous examples of innovation and excellence. Soviet physicians have pioneered important procedures—in ophthalmology, surgery, orthopedics, and other fields—that have been widely adopted throughout the world.

Given all this, it's only natural to expect the U.S.S.R. to have one of the best health-care systems and healthiest populations. But just the opposite is true. Decades of inadequate funding have left the Soviet Union ensnared in a health-care crisis perhaps unparalleled in the industrialized world.

Far from trying to conceal the fact, Soviet officials are openly discussing the problems and solutions. "Radical changes are essential," Yevgeni Chazov, minister of health of the U.S.S.R., told me on a cold, snowy Moscow evening in 1989. "I have fired 100,000 doctors for incompetence."

Mikhail Gorbachev, the Soviet leader, appointed Chazov as health minister in 1987 as part of the new government policies of *perestroika*, the restructuring of Soviet society. Chazov— a cardiologist who shared the 1985 Nobel Peace Prize as co-founder of International Physicians for the Prevention of Nuclear War—was given responsibility for restructuring the health-care system. Chazov has said that if he had known in 1987 how bad the system was, he would have refused the job.

The crisis is far-reaching, indeed. There are chronic shortages of basic medicines and medical instruments. Ordinary citizens do not have access to such potentially lifesaving treatments as coronary bypass surgery and organ transplants. Computerized X-ray scans and other diagnostic procedures common in the United States exist in only a few major Soviet hospitals. About one-third of rural hospitals do not even have hot water, and one-fifth have no sewers, according to the Soviet newspaper *Literaturnaya Gazeta*. Figures from other sources differ; some suggest conditions are even worse.

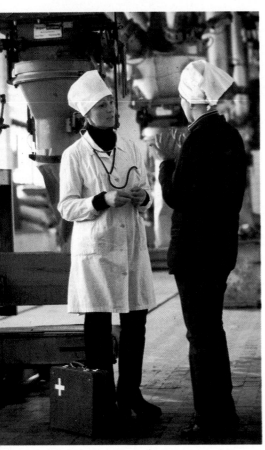

Some large industrial plants operate health clinics for their workers. Here, a doctor speaks to a worker at the Moscow Oil Refinery.

Soviets react with amusement to America's preoccupation with diet, exercise, and avoiding cigarettes. They eat large amounts of saturated fat and cholesterol. Alcohol abuse is rampant, despite an intensive government campaign for sobriety.

Cigarette packages have warning labels, but 70 million of the U.S.S.R.'s 290 million citizens smoke—including 4 out of every 10 children under age 15. Many physicians smoke as well; Soviet cardiologists and cancer specialists have told me that smoking is merely relaxing and harmless. Indeed, Soviet patients seeking more attentive care from a doctor know that few "gifts" are more effective than packs of American cigarettes.

But at the root of the country's health problems is the government's long-term failure to make an adequate financial commitment to health. Indeed, Chazov says that the proportion of the national budget spent on health care declined for 25 straight years until 1986. Even in 1988, the Soviet Union ranked somewhere between 60th and 70th among nations worldwide in terms of the proportion of national income spent on health, Chazov says.

The problems have had a serious impact on the health of Soviet citizens. The infant mortality rate, a measure of the number of children who die in their first year, is perhaps the most telling statistic. Experts see infant mortality as a key index of medical care, nutrition, and other factors that influence health. The United States has long agonized over its infant mortality rate, which was 10.4 deaths per 1,000 live births in 1986 (the most recent year for which data were available). About 20 other industrialized countries have a better record. But Soviet infant mortality rose so sharply in the 1970's that the government banned publication of statistics. When publication resumed with 1985 data, the rate was 26.0 deaths per 1,000 births—identical to the U.S. rate 25 years earlier.

Other statistics tell a similar story. Male life expectancy actually has decreased since the mid-1960's. It is now about 65 years, according to Soviet officials. That is equivalent to the U.S. figure from 1949 and well below the 71.3-year life expectancy for American men today. Soviet officials blame the high male mortality rate largely on accidents and diseases associated with alcohol abuse.

Health conditions have improved dramatically, however, since the 1917 revolution, when the Bolsheviks (Communists) seized power and established Soviet rule. In pre-revolutionary Russia in 1913, the average life span was 32 years, comparable to America in the late 1700's. The infant mortality rate was 269 per 1,000 births, about 2.7 times the U.S. rate at that time. About 43 out of every 100 children died before reaching age 5.

The bad health conditions inherited by the Bolsheviks grew even worse. Fanned by primitive sanitation, poverty, famine, and malnutrition, infectious diseases sickened and killed millions of people. Early Soviet leaders, in fact, viewed the rampaging epidemics of plague, smallpox, typhoid fever, measles, malaria, cholera, and typhus as the most serious threat to their rule. Typhus, spread by fleas and lice, became such a problem that Vladimir I. Lenin, chief founder of the Soviet Union, warned the seventh Communist Party Congress in 1919: "Either the louse defeats socialism or socialism defeats the louse."

The socialist battle for health began in 1918, when Lenin signed a charter to establish a national system of socialized medicine directed and financed by the state. The de-

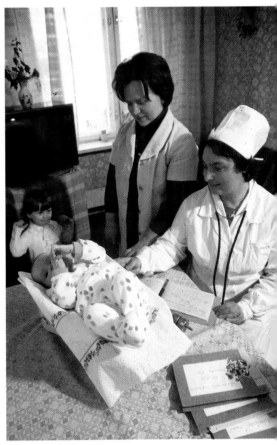

House calls are a routine part of the Soviet system of free medical care. Here, a doctor checks on a child at home.

cree made physicians state employees and created a Commissariat of Health with far-reaching powers.

Today, the Soviet system revolves around three main types of health-care institutions: polyclinics, hospitals (both general and specialized), and sanatoriums.

Polyclinics, where about 80 per cent of all patients receive care, are the cornerstone of the Soviet health-care system. Polyclinics are neighborhood outpatient centers, with medical and dental offices, diagnostic equipment, laboratories, and treatment rooms. A nationwide network of more than 40,000 polyclinics employing 40 per cent of all Soviet medical personnel provides care for more than 10 million patients each day. Some polyclinics serve adults; some, children under age 15.

The Ministry of Health operates most polyclinics. But big industrial plants, scientific research institutes, and other enterprises sometimes have polyclinics for their own workers. There also are a small number of "cooperative" polyclinics that charge a fee but provide more personalized care. The co-ops, which often provide only limited services in accordance with official policy, are operated by individual physicians. The physicians—some of whom are state physicians who moonlight at the co-ops—set fees and divide profits.

Today, I am in City Polyclinic No. 122, a typical state-run polyclinic located in northeastern Moscow. It is 1 of 12 polyclinics—7 for adults, 5 for children—that care for about 350,000 residents of this industrial district. Several industrial enterprises also operate polyclinics here.

The clinic is open from 8 a.m. to 9 p.m. every day except Sunday. Its 250 employees—including 75 doctors and 130 nurses—work two shifts of 6½ hours. The building, like many other Soviet medical facilities, is old, reminiscent of an American hospital built in the 1920's or 1930's and never updated.

A few dozen patients are waiting in the reception area and corridors outside treatment rooms. Jakov I. Vsheptinovskiy, the chief physician, notes that some have appointments, while others simply appeared at the clinic to wait their turn. Care is impersonal. New patients usually cannot select a specific general doctor, and visits tend to be so hurried that strong doctor-patient relationships seldom develop.

Visits are brief partly because the doctors provide little actual care. Vsheptinovskiy says Soviet general practitioners are not trained in procedures routine for American general practitioners—such as reading an electrocardiogram, examining a patient's eyes with an ophthalmoscope, and performing a simple rectal examination for disorders of the prostate gland. Under the Soviet system, such tasks are performed by specialists.

An American with mild high blood pressure, for example,

normally would be treated by a single doctor—perhaps a family physician or general internist. But consider the plight of a comparable Soviet patient. According to Vsheptinovskiy, the polyclinic doctor might refer the patient to a cardiologist for an electrocardiogram; an ophthalmologist to check the retina of the eye; a nerve specialist to determine the role of stress and anxiety; and perhaps several other specialists. Each referral might require a separate visit to the polyclinic, so that weeks may pass before the patient is properly diagnosed and treated.

Vsheptinovskiy cites another persistent problem in Soviet medicine—low pay that gives doctors little incentive to work longer hours, improve their skills, or please patients. As of early 1989, starting pay for a new doctor was 160 rubles per month—about $256, less than the 178-ruble average monthly wage of farmworkers and the 217-ruble average monthly wage of other workers. After seven years in general practice, the same doctor would earn just over 200 rubles per month. Specialists and doctors with advanced degrees earn more. (As of early 1989, one ruble was worth about $1.60.)

Polyclinic physicians spend part of each shift making house calls to patients who are too sick or old to leave their apartments. They also assess patients' ability to work. Clinic doctors issue work excuses—permits for paid sick leave for anywhere from a few days for minor illnesses to several months for more serious conditions. Mothers with sick children can also get a work excuse to stay home and care for the child.

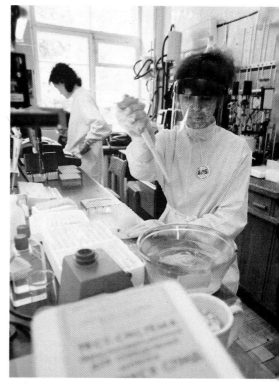

A Soviet researcher prepares serum for an AIDS test. The Soviet Union has adopted some of the world's strictest measures to check the spread of the deadly disease, including testing all members of high-risk groups and imposing prison sentences on people who knowingly spread the virus.

When Soviet patients leave the polyclinic with a prescription, they go to another medical institution most Americans would find peculiar—the Soviet pharmacy. Unlike American drugstores, Soviet pharmacies do not sell cosmetics, candy, or other merchandise. They are spartan, bare-wall stores that carry only drugs and medical supplies and do not permit self-service. Everything—even aspirin, antacids, and thermometers—is kept in a glass display case at the counter or on shelves behind the counter. Customers must elbow through the crowd to determine the price of an item. Then they stand in line at the cashier's station to pay and get a receipt. After waiting in another line, they exchange the receipt for the item.

Although medical care is free, most patients must pay for prescription drugs. With many drugs in short supply, patients sometimes must spend hours going from one pharmacy to another trying to get a prescription filled. Soviet pharmacists ordinarily will not order a drug or telephone another pharmacy to find a particular medication.

Chronic shortages of medicines sometimes deprive patients of the best therapy. At Psychiatric Hospital No. 1 in Moscow, I asked what drugs are used to treat clinical depression.

"Whatever we can get," responded Vladimir N. Kozirev, the hospital's director. "This is a big problem. Effective drugs are available for a few months and then disappear, and we have to resort to less favorable medicines."

Patients with serious illnesses may be referred to a specialized research and treatment center. These big institutions—such as the Moscow-based All-Union Cardiology Research Center, the U.S.S.R. Oncology Research Center, and the U.S.S.R. Surgery Research Center—represent Soviet medicine at its best. They tend to be modern, clean, well equipped, and staffed by extremely competent physicians.

But such centers of excellence exist only in Moscow and a few other big cities. Because their capacity is so limited, the typical patient is more likely to wind up in a general hospital.

Perhaps nowhere else in the Soviet health-care system is the lack of funding more visible, from a Western perspective, than in general hospitals. Those are my first thoughts as I enter Moscow City Hospital No. 6, a 1,000-bed general hospital. The hospital was founded in 1874 and still uses the original buildings, complete with crumbling concrete stairways, sheets of soiled linoleum peeling from the floors, flaking paint and plaster, and unlit corridors.

The Soviets have increased the nation's hospital beds by about 50 per cent during the last 20 years, from 2.7 million in 1970 to almost 4 million today. But as health minister Chazov told me, the emphasis has been on numbers rather than quality. The construction boom has saddled the Soviet Union with an enormous number of hospitals that lack basic equipment taken for granted in the West.

Although Soviet hospitals have some private and semiprivate rooms, most patients stay in wards. There may be four, six, eight, or more small, iron-frame beds crowded into a ward. Patients from several wards may use a single bathroom, which is likely to be small and unimaginably filthy, with no toilet seats or toilet paper.

Chazov himself has acknowledged, and repeatedly condemned, a practice that many patients find essential for obtaining better accommodations and care: bribery. Patients come to the hospital with a supply of cash, knowing that "tips" of a ruble or so to nurses and other attendants can make hospital life much more comfortable. Tips may be necessary to ensure that the bedpan arrives quickly, that dressings and bed linen are changed, or that medication is administered on schedule. Larger payments by the patient or family can bring a better room and food, or care from a renowned doctor.

Hospital No. 6 has a staff of 230 physicians and 500 nurses who treat about 22,000 patients each year. Valentina I. Molotkova, deputy chief physician, tells me that the hospital has several clinical departments so outstanding that doctors in other cities refer patients here. One is the cardiology department.

In the United States, a 1,000-bed hospital with a nationally renowned cardiology department would provide certain basic services essential to diagnosing and treating the underlying cause of most heart attacks, coronary artery disease (the progressive blockage of the blood vessels that serve the heart). These treatments—including procedures for locating and unblocking clogged blood vessels, drugs that can abort a heart attack in progress, and such operations as bypass surgery and heart transplantation—are often performed routinely even at smaller U.S. hospitals. None are available at Hospital No. 6.

The typical Soviet heart attack patient is forbidden to get out of the hospital bed for 12 days. At that point, an American probably would be recuperating at home. In fact, Soviet heart attack patients usually remain in the hospital for four weeks. About 80 per

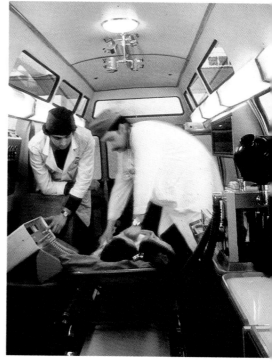

Soviet hospitals do not have emergency rooms; emergency care is provided by specially equipped mobile units, such as the one pictured *above*.

cent of Americans who survive a heart attack return to work within three months, while Soviet survivors do not return for five to six months. The contrast reflects not only a difference in treatment techniques but also a difference in medical philosophy: The Soviets favor long recuperation periods, and U.S. physicians send heart attack patients home sooner than do doctors virtually anywhere else in the world.

The care available for other conditions also is decidedly low-tech. Most general hospitals do not have scanners for computerized tomography (CT) or magnetic resonance imaging (MRI), techniques for "seeing" inside the body that have revolutionized the diagnosis of numerous diseases. Indeed, the hospitals rarely have disposable medical supplies—such as hypodermic needles for injections and plastic tubing for intravenous infusions—that decrease the risk of spreading infections from one patient to another. Soviet hospitals in 1988 needed an estimated 6 billion disposable syringes, according to the Soviet magazine *Ogonyok*, but industry produced only 7 million. Soviet nurses thus must wash and reuse needles and rubber tubing, a practice that contributes to the spread of infections among hospitalized patients. In 1988 and early 1989, 84 infants in two Soviet hospitals contracted the deadly virus for AIDS when nurses reused contaminated syringes.

In the Soviet Union, AIDS remains a relatively minor problem, with officials acknowledging only 8 cases of fully developed AIDS as of early 1989, compared with America's cumulative total of 88,100 at that time. Yet the Soviets have adopted some of the world's most stringent measures to prevent the spread of the AIDS virus, which a person may carry for years before developing the disease.

For example, it is a criminal offense, punishable by a prison term, for an infected person to knowingly spread the AIDS virus. Soviet citizens who live abroad longer than three months must take a blood test for the virus upon their return. Foreigners who plan extended stays in the U.S.S.R. must have a medical certificate verifying that they are not infected. Tests also are mandatory for known homosexuals, prostitutes, and other people at high risk for the disease. In June 1989, Soviet health officials reported that more than 30 million tests had identified 258 infected Soviet citizens, as well as 464 infected resident foreigners (most of whom were deported). By comparison, the U.S. government estimates that about 1 million Americans carry the virus.

Soviet hospitals do not house certain services considered standard in American hospitals. One is the emergency department. People who need immediate care for minor illness or injuries go to their polyclinic. Victims of traffic accidents, poisonings, heart attacks, and other emergencies rely on the *Skoraya Meditsinskaya Pomoshch* (Fast Medical Help).

Emergency care in most countries emphasizes rapid transport of the victim to hospital emergency rooms. But the Skoraya largely replaces Western-style emergency departments with mobile emergency rooms sent to the patient. A Soviet who needs medical assistance dials 03 on the telephone—the counterpart to the 911 emergency number used in many U.S. communities. Calls go to a command center, where a trained dispatcher evaluates the seriousness of the problem. In some cases, a Skoraya physician or nurse may be able to give the patient self-care advice over the phone or refer the patient to the local polyclinic's house-call service. In true emergencies, the dispatcher can send an ambulance, which carries a physician trained in emergency medicine.

Once at the scene, the ambulance physician makes a diagnosis, administers treatment, and decides whether hospitalization is necessary. Patients requiring hospitalization are taken to the nearest hospital equipped for their condition. Others are allowed to remain at home, under care of doctors from their local polyclinic.

General hospitals also have no obstetrical wards; childbirth occurs at separate maternity hospitals. The Soviet approach to pregnancy and childbirth differs from that of America in several other ways as well. For example, while many American hospitals encourage fathers to be present during labor and delivery, Soviet maternity hospitals ban fathers and other visitors entirely. "They're potential sources of infection," says Ekaterina M. Vikhlyaeva, deputy director of the All-Union Research Center for Maternal and Child Health Care. New fathers "visit" their wives and newborn infants from the street in front of the hospital. Mothers hold the baby at the window, while fathers wave and strain for a glimpse.

Prenatal care emphasizes routine visits to the doctor and avoiding excessive weight gain, smoking, alcohol, and other drugs. Proper diet is also stressed, but pregnant women do not routinely receive vitamin and mineral supplements. Soviet obstetricians view the pain of labor and childbirth as a reflex that women can control by assuming the proper mental attitude. But there are no formal classes, like those in the United States, to prepare women and their husbands for natural childbirth. As labor pains increase, Soviet women receive an injection of antispasmodic medication that has a pain-relieving effect. During delivery, they may get a few whiffs of nitrous oxide—"laughing gas"—that provides light anesthesia. The highly effective spinal anesthesia, often administered just prior to delivery in the United States, is not used in routine births.

Soviet women count the distinctly unpleasant experience of childbirth among their reasons for hesitating to have more children. Still, there are relatively few options for couples who want to limit their family size, according to Anatolyi Anatonov, an authority on birth control with the Institute of Sociology of the U.S.S.R. Academy of Sciences in Moscow. Physicians frown on voluntary sterilization and oral contraceptives, the most reliable birth control methods. Anatonov says that Soviet physicians mistakenly equate sterilization with castration and believe that birth control pills are "unwholesome," supposedly causing abnormal brain-wave activity.

Diaphragms and intrauterine devices are produced in a single size, making them unsuitable for many women. There is a nationwide shortage of condoms—and in any case, Soviet-manufactured condoms are so thick and unwieldy that many Soviet men refuse to use them.

Anatonov says the government, concerned about a declining birth rate in the European part of the U.S.S.R., intentionally limits the availability of contraceptives. But he sees such a policy as short-sighted and self-defeating, simply encouraging abortion as the primary method for controlling family size.

"Contraception is an alternative to abortion," Anatonov explains. "But this simple truth evades the bureaucrats. In an effort to increase the birth rate, they increase the abortion rate." He estimates that 10 million to 11 million of the world's 40 million annual abortions are performed in the Soviet Union. "I consider it a horrible, shocking figure."

Psychiatric care is also removed from the general hospital. People with serious emotional disorders obtain care in specialized psychiatric hospitals or clinics. Many Soviets with emotional problems, however, hesitate to seek care because of the pronounced stigma associated with mental illness in the U.S.S.R. The names of people who undergo psychiatric treatment are placed on the *Register*, an official government list of 5 million to 6 million psychiatric patients. People on the list are deprived of certain rights, such as driving a car or working in particular occupations. In most instances in the past, a person's name has remained on the list for life.

Newspaper and magazine articles criticizing psychiatrists have contributed to the public's distrust. "Antipsychiatric tendencies that always existed in society have been inflamed by public discussions of our methods," says Vassily I. Yastrebov, director of the Institute of Preventive Psychiatry at the All-Union Mental Health Research Center in Moscow. "Now patients who genuinely need care hesitate to come forward.

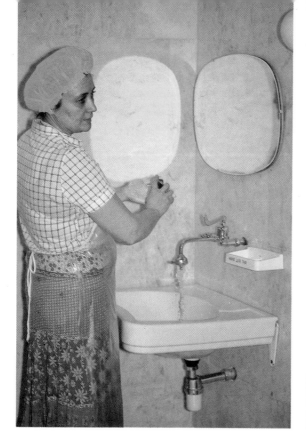

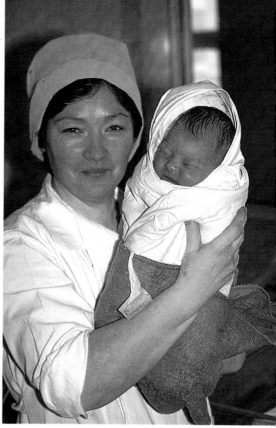

An obstetrician, *above left,* washes up in preparation for a Caesarean delivery at the All-Union Research Center for Maternal and Child Health in Moscow, the Soviet Union's premier institution for maternal and child-health problems, high-risk births, and fertility treatment. *Above right,* a nurse displays a newborn infant.

After the newspaper articles questioning our motives, beds in psychiatric hospitals were empty as never before."

Psychiatrists worry that the lack of care will contribute to already-serious public health problems such as suicide. In 1988, the U.S.S.R. State Committee for Statistics published suicide statistics for the first time in 50 years. The Soviet rate for 1984 was 30 suicides per 100,000 people. That compares with 22 suicides per 100,000 in France, 12 per 100,000 in the United States, and 9 per 100,000 in Great Britain.

The psychiatrists worry for their own safety as well. Psychiatrists solemnly describe incidents in which colleagues were threatened, beaten, stabbed, and shot by patients or patients' relatives. Protesters on the streets of Moscow have distributed leaflets that urged "Death to Psychiatrists!" and named specific psychiatrists they deemed worthy of that fate.

The internal unrest is part of an international controversy about Soviet psychiatry. For more than 20 years, critics in the West have accused the Soviet Union of using psychiatry as a political tool by having people declared mentally ill and forcibly hospitalized and drugged. In 1983, the Soviet Union withdrew from the World Psychiatric Association rather than be expelled from the international society.

Soviet psychiatric officials have always denied the allega-

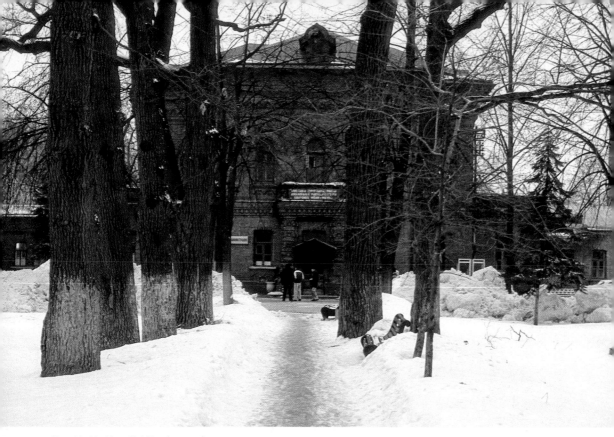

Psychiatric Hospital No. 1, *above*, opened in 1894 in Moscow. With 2,715 beds, it is still one of the largest hospitals in the Soviet Union.

tions. Still, efforts are underway to rehabilitate psychiatry's tarnished image. New laws now provide numerous safeguards against unwarranted hospitalization. Officials are beginning to remove some names from the *Register*. There are plans to provide more psychiatric care on an outpatient basis. And the World Psychiatric Association was scheduled in late 1989 to consider the U.S.S.R.'s application for readmission.

Perhaps no other component of the Soviet health-care system is less familiar in the West than the third major type of health institution—the sanatorium. To most Americans, a sanatorium (or sanitarium) is an old-fashioned institution for tuberculosis patients, invalids, or even the mentally ill. In the Soviet system, a sanatorium stay is the most sought-after of all health-care benefits. People react with absolute delight to a *putevka*, a pass or ticket to one of the 2.5 million sanatorium beds available nationwide. The privilege often goes to people with heart disease, arthritis, emphysema, or other chronic health problems.

Sanatoriums are recuperation centers, usually located in picturesque areas, such as the shore of the Black Sea in the southwest U.S.S.R. Some are the villas, mansions, and castles once used by czars and grand dukes in prerevolutionary Russia. A typical stay lasts 24 days and includes medical tests and therapy, mud and mineral baths, massage, and exercise in the fresh air. At some sanatoriums, patients march down to the beach or onto porches at 11 p.m. to sleep in the open.

"We take the sanatorium system very seriously," says A. F. Gavrilenkoe, director of the Sechenov Clinic in Yalta, a city on the Black Sea. The clinic is a national center for research on sanatorium treatment.

Gavrilenkoe says researchers have found that trees and other vegetation along the Black Sea release "bioactive aerosols." He describes these as airborne chemical compounds that improve the functioning of the body's disease-fighting immune system and have other beneficial effects on health. Gavrilenkoe says there is objective scientific evidence that a sanatorium stay decreases the number of days that workers spend on sick leave.

Soviet officials are convinced that the health-care crisis will ease substantially by the mid-1990's, when the effects of massive spending increases become apparent. Chazov described plans to re-invent much of the health-care system by spending more than 190 billion rubles by 1995. One major construction program will replace 1 million existing hospital beds with new beds in modern, well-equipped buildings. Another will create a nationwide network of 150 new diagnostic centers filled with the most modern instruments for diagnosing diseases. Plans also call for substantial increases in spending to produce adequate quantities of drugs and medical supplies by 1993.

As part of a new emphasis on high-quality care, Chazov required all doctors to take a competency examination. About 100,000 failed and were banned from practice. Changes in medical education will increase emphasis on clinical skills, training doctors to perform the wide range of services available from America's family physicians. The government also plans to raise salaries and provide other incentives for state doctors to deliver care that is more personal.

Major emphasis will be placed on disease prevention, with cigarette smoking a prime target. Officials say that one such offensive—the sobriety campaign—already has yielded great public health benefits. They believe that a decline in alcohol consumption has contributed to recent improvements in life expectancy, infant mortality, and other health indicators cited by the government's State Committee for Statistics.

Chazov and other officials seem to envision a new health-care system that is as efficient and effective as the assembly line at the eye microsurgery institute. But they are also aiming for something else—personal, compassionate care that would finally translate the early Soviet commitment to health into a reality for its citizens.

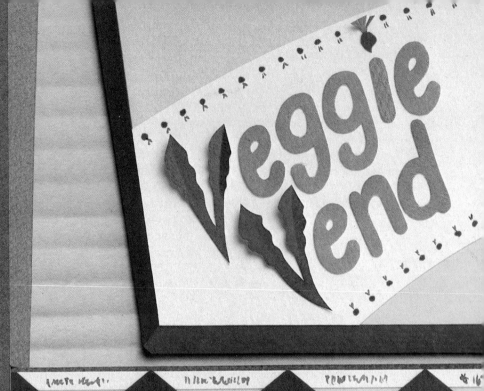
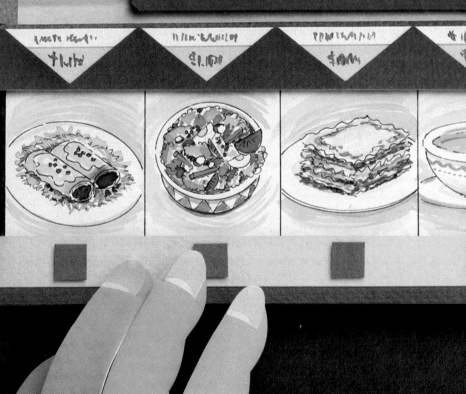

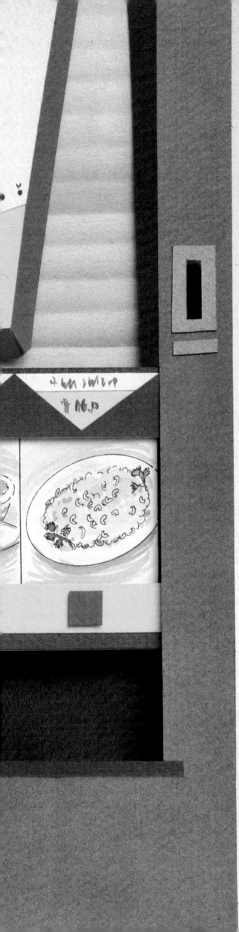

Many people believe
that vegetarian diets can
reduce the risk of some
diseases. But such diets
may not be for everyone.

Make Mine Vegetarian?

By Johanna T. Dwyer

Talk about vegetarianism and most people
probably conjure up images of tofu sandwich-
es sprinkled with sprouts or soybean burgers
topped with sunflower seeds—exotic fare
eaten by people who decline to eat meat and
other animal products for moral or religious
reasons. By and large, many of us who have
been raised to assume that meat, eggs, or
dairy products are an integral part of every
meal find the idea of eating a diet restricted
to vegetables, grains, and fruits a bit odd.

But since the early 1980's, the public's perception of vegetarianism has begun to change.
Scientific evidence linking a diet high in animal fats to heart disease, cancer, and other
illnesses, coupled with reports that vegetarians appear to be at lower risk than nonvege-

tarians for these diseases, have convinced many people that they should modify their eating habits. Thus, many believe that a carefully planned meatless—or semimeatless—diet, aimed at reducing or eliminating animal fats from the menu, may help them maintain good health.

Such a shift in eating habits in the United States has had an impact on the marketplace. Comparisons of two U.S. Department of Agriculture surveys—one taken in 1977 and the other in 1985—show a marked decline in the average per person consumption of red meat, eggs, and whole-fat dairy products (such as whole milk) and a significant jump in the consumption of vegetables, fruits, grains, fish, and low-fat milk.

The medical community endorses dietary changes of this nature. For example, in July 1988, U.S. Surgeon General C. Everett Koop in his *Report on Nutrition and Health* stated that many of the major causes of death in the United States—including cancer, heart disease, stroke, and diabetes—have been linked to diet. He urged Americans to reduce their intake of animal fats and increase their consumption of vegetables, fruits, and whole grains. Similar eating habits have been recommended by the American Cancer Society and the American Heart Association.

But vegetarianism should not be attempted without careful planning. People who abstain from meat and dairy products can develop serious—and possibly life threatening—nutritional deficiencies unless they plan a diet that supplies all the vital nutrients.

A centuries-old practice

Although the word *vegetarian* was first coined in the mid-1800's, the idea of a diet composed only of vegetables, fruits, and grains dates back to ancient times. Vegetarians were once referred to as "flesh abstainers" or "Pythagoreans," after Pythagoras, an ancient Greek philosopher and mathematician who is often called the father of vegetarianism.

Throughout history, many well-known people have embraced vegetarianism. Italian painter and scientist Leonardo da Vinci, English scientist and mathematician Sir Isaac Newton, American statesman and inventor Benjamin Franklin, and Irish-born playwright George Bernard Shaw were confirmed vegetarians. So were Mohandas K. Gandhi, the spiritual and political leader of India, and German philosopher and missionary Albert Schweitzer.

For centuries, many of the world's religions—including Hinduism, Buddhism, and Jainism—have advocated vegetarian diets. Eating animal foods goes against the belief these religions have in *reincarnation* (the survival of the soul after death and its rebirth in the body of another person or living

The author:

Johanna T. Dwyer is professor of medicine at Tufts University Medical School in Boston.

thing) and in the sanctity of animal life. The Seventh-day Adventist Church, a Christian group, advises its followers to abstain from meat and certain other kinds of food and drink because they might be harmful to the body, which Seventh-day Adventists believe to be the temple of the Holy Spirit.

Vegetarian options: Where's the beef?

There are several different kinds—or degrees—of vegetarian diets that people can follow. The most restrictive diet is the *strict vegetarian* or *vegan* diet, which excludes all animal foods—meat, poultry, fish, eggs, and dairy products. Less restrictive are the *lactovegetarian* and the *lacto-ovovegetarian* diets, which exclude meat, poultry, and fish, but allow dairy products. The lacto-ovovegetarian diet also includes eggs.

Many health-conscious Americans, however, follow what some call a *semivegetarian* or *part-time vegetarian* diet. Semivegetarians eat little or no red meat, but occasionally consume poultry, fish, eggs, and dairy products.

Vegetarian diets—if they are carefully planned with an eye toward nutrition—can be healthful. But some vegetarian diets—such as one form of *macrobiotics* (a dietary system derived from principles of Zen Buddhism)—are so limited in the kinds of foods they allow that they can be very unhealthy. One type of macrobiotic diet consists only of brown rice. Because brown rice does not contain all the nutrients the body needs, people on this diet develop serious, potentially fatal nutritional deficiencies.

Cutting out fats

Why do some nutritionists consider a well-planned vegetarian diet healthier than a diet that overemphasizes meat, eggs, and dairy products? One reason is that many animal foods are high in fat and cholesterol. Both fat and cholesterol are vital to good health, but a diet too rich in either of them can play a role in certain illnesses.

Cholesterol, a fatlike substance found in blood and body tissues, is necessary for digestion and the production of hormones. It is also a part of the membranes of all the cells in the body. The body acquires cholesterol in two ways: It is made by the liver, and it is obtained from animal foods. If the liver produces too much of this substance or if a person eats cholesterol-rich foods, high levels of blood cholesterol may occur. Such high blood levels may play a role in *atherosclerosis*, a build-up of deposits of cholesterol, calcium, cells, and other substances along the inner walls of the arteries. If the

The benefits and risks of vegetarian diets

There are four kinds of vegetarian diets: strict vegetarian or vegan, lacto-vegetarian, lacto-ovo-vegetarian, and semivegetarian. Each diet includes different types of food. Many people believe that vegetarian diets reduce the risk of some diseases, but the more restrictive vegetarian diets may actually pose health risks. If carefully planned, however, with an eye toward nutrition, vegetarian diets can be healthful.

Are vegetarian diets good for you?

Many people believe that a well-planned vegetarian or semivegetarian diet can help decrease an individual's risk of a variety of diseases. These diets usually contain less animal foods than a nonvegetarian diet. Many animal foods are high in cholesterol and certain fats, substances that scientists have linked to some diseases. At the same time, vegetarian diets are rich in grains, vegetables, and fruits—foods that contain dietary fiber, which is believed to protect against constipation and certain diseases. Scientific evidence supports some of the health claims made about vegetarian diets; other claims, however, still lack solid support.

Heart disease: There is evidence that vegetarians—especially those who eat no animal foods—have a lower risk of heart disease. This lower risk, however, may also be due to other healthy practices followed by some vegetarians, such as regular exercise and abstaining from smoking and drinking.

Cancer: There is no strong evidence linking a vegetarian diet to a lower incidence of cancer. Some scientists believe vegetarians may have a lower risk of breast cancer and cancer of the colon (the main part of the large intestine).

Diverticulosis: There is strong scientific evidence that fiber-rich vegetarian diets may prevent complications of diverticulosis, a colon disorder.

Obesity: There is strong evidence that vegetarians—especially those who eat no animal foods—are less likely to be obese than nonvegetarians. Some scientists believe this is because vegetarian diets are full of fibrous foods, which add bulk to the stomach and prevent overeating. Scientific research has linked obesity to a variety of serious health problems, including high blood pressure, diabetes, and heart disease.

Osteoporosis: There is little scientific evidence to support the theory that a vegetarian diet can help prevent osteoporosis, a disorder that causes bones to become brittle and break easily.

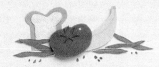

Strict vegetarian diet

A strict vegetarian or vegan diet includes only plant foods—vegetables, grains, fruits, seeds, and nuts. It excludes meat, fish, poultry, milk products, eggs, and all foods containing ingredients of animal origin. An improperly planned vegan diet can cause deficiencies in protein, iron, zinc, calcium, and vitamins D, B_2 (riboflavin), and B_{12}. Strict vegetarians may also find it difficult to consume enough calories to maintain their proper weight.

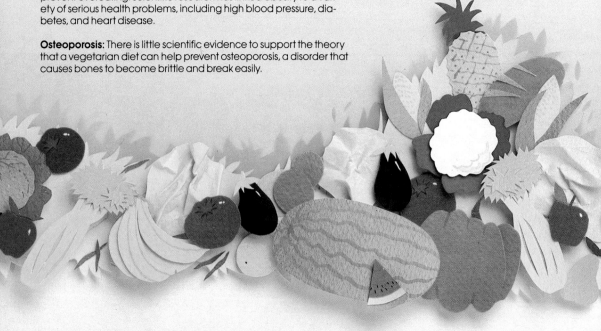

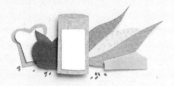

Lacto-vegetarian diet

A lacto-vegetarian diet includes plant foods and milk and dairy products. It excludes all meat, fish, poultry, and eggs. An improperly planned lacto-vegetarian diet can cause deficiencies in iron, zinc, and vitamins D, B_2, and B_{12}.

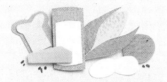

Lacto-ovo-vegetarian diet

A lacto-ovo-vegetarian diet includes plant foods, milk and dairy products, and eggs. It excludes all meat, fish, and poultry. People following this type of diet rarely experience nutritional deficiencies. An improperly planned diet, however, may not provide enough iron.

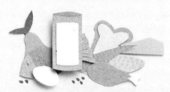

Semivegetarian diet

A semivegetarian diet includes plant foods, milk and dairy products, eggs, and some fish and poultry. Red meat is avoided or eaten only occasionally. Semivegetarian diets pose little or no nutritional risk.

arteries that feed blood to the heart muscle become narrowed and clogged with such deposits, a condition called coronary artery disease develops—and the eventual result can be a heart attack.

Fat, which is found in both plant and animal food, is an important source of energy. It is also necessary for the growth and maintenance of the body. Most scientists, however, believe that one type of fat—called *saturated fat*—plays a key role in coronary artery disease. Saturated fat is found in red meats, eggs, such whole-fat dairy products as whole milk and butter, lard, and such oils as coconut oil and palm oil. Studies suggest it may increase the amount of cholesterol in the blood and may also increase the risk of obesity.

Because of the strong relationship between a diet high in cholesterol and saturated fat with coronary artery disease and other disorders, the American Heart Association, the American Cancer Society, and other health groups urge adults to reduce their consumption of foods containing these substances. They recommend that only 30 per cent of an adult's daily caloric intake come from fat and that no more than one-third of this intake—or 10 per cent of daily calories—should be saturated fat.

Another reason well-planned vegetarian diets may be healthier than some nonvegetarian diets is that they contain greater amounts of vegetables, *legumes* (plants in the pea family, such as soybeans and peanuts), fruits, nuts, and grains—foods that are low in fat. Such foods are also rich in *carbohydrates* (sugar and starches) that provide energy and help build and repair body tissues. And some plant foods, such as rice, wheat, corn, and potatoes, not only are rich sources of carbohydrates but also provide dietary fiber, the parts of plant foods that are not broken down by the digestive system. Although fiber is not essential to health, many health experts believe that it may help relieve constipation and may prevent complications of *diverticulosis*, a disorder in which pouches form along weakened areas of the colon wall. Some forms of fiber also appear to help control diabetes and may help lower blood sugar and cholesterol levels.

Vegetarian diets—especially strict vegetarian diets—may provide a way for people to maintain their proper weight. Vegetables and fruits are lower in calories than other types of food. Vegetarians often claim that bulky plant foods satisfy their hunger and cause them to stop eating sooner than nonvegetarians. As a result, they do not consume excess calories, which can cause obesity. This benefit, however, can also pose health problems. Vegetarians who stop eating before they consume enough calories to meet their energy needs could develop malnutrition. To make sure they receive enough calories, strict vegetarians—especially children—should eat many small meals a day rather than a few large meals.

Avoiding nutritional pitfalls

People who choose to follow a vegetarian diet must carefully plan their meals to provide all the nutrients they need to remain healthy. In the early 1970's, the Food and Nutrition Board of the National Academy of Sciences (NAS) in Washington, D.C., stated that all vegetarians—even those following strict vegetarian diets—can be well nourished if they select their foods carefully. Health experts recommend that vegetarians follow a few basic principles when planning meals. They should eat a variety of foods, making sure not to eat too much of one food at the expense of another. Experts also warn against adopting severely restrictive vegetarian diets or any extreme diet that relies on just one type of food. Most important, vegetarians should eat plant foods that provide the same essential nutrients as animal foods.

People who may have special vitamin, mineral, and energy needs run the greatest risk of developing nutritional deficiencies if their vegetarian diet is not properly planned. Such people include infants and children, whose bodies are growing rapidly; pregnant women; people who are recovering from illness; and the elderly. These people should consult with their physician before starting any vegetarian diet. Some health experts also question whether children, especially children under the age of 2, should ever be put on diets that are low in fat and cholesterol—typical attributes of vegetarian diets. Again, parents should always consult a physician before placing a child on a diet that is restricted in any way.

In the mid-1970's, my colleagues and I at Tufts University School of Medicine and at New England Medical Center Hospital, both in Boston, conducted a study to determine the impact of poorly planned vegetarian diets on children. We compared the health of children ranging in age from a few weeks to 6 years. Some of the children were from macrobiotic vegetarian families. The others were from lactovegetarian and lacto-ovovegetarian families. The children on lactovegetarian or lacto-ovovegetarian diets were healthy and were the normal size and weight for their age. The children who were fed a macrobiotic diet with little or no animal foods and no vitamin or mineral supplements, however, were smaller than average in height and weight.

In addition, we found that the children on the macrobiotic diet had vitamin and mineral intakes that were significantly lower than the Recommended Dietary Allowances (RDA's) for essential nutrients. The RDA's, which are set by the Food and Nutrition Board of the NAS, are the amounts of each essential nutrient recommended daily for the majority of healthy adults and children in the United States.

Getting enough protein

People who adopt a vegetarian diet must plan their meals carefully to make sure they receive all the essential vitamins, minerals, and other nutrients they need. One nutrient that vegetarians must be sure to get enough of in their diet is protein. The body breaks down protein from foods into smaller molecules called *amino acids*, which are then used as building blocks to make the thousands of proteins needed to build and maintain all the body's cells.

A diet that is deficient in protein can cause *kwashiorkor* (protein-calorie malnutrition), a condition characterized by anemia, fatigue, skin lesions, and changes in skin and hair color. Thus, it is important that the body have a sufficient supply of amino acids to assemble the protein it needs. This supply must include *essential amino acids* and *nonessential amino acids*. Because our bodies cannot make essential amino acids, they must be obtained from the food we eat. Nonessential amino acids can be manufactured by the body from the essential amino acids or they can be obtained from food.

Proteins found in animal foods, such as meat, poultry, fish, cheese, milk, and eggs, are *complete proteins*—that is, they contain all the essential and nonessential amino acids the body needs for making protein. Proteins found in plant foods, however, contain some but not all of the essential amino acids needed to make proteins. For this reason, they are called *incomplete proteins*. But strict vegetarians or those who eat only small amounts of animal foods can combine plants containing different combinations of incomplete proteins to create a mixture that satisfies all the body's protein needs. In other words, plant foods that are low in or lack certain amino acids must be eaten in combination with plant foods low in or lacking different amino acids to create a complete—or complementary—protein mixture.

Simply eating different types of legumes, such as soybeans and peanuts, will not provide a complete protein mixture because all legumes lack the same amino acids. But combining legumes with grains, nuts, or seeds will create complete proteins because grains, nuts, and seeds contain the amino acids that are lacking in legumes—and vice versa. Food combinations, such as a peanut butter and raisin sandwich on whole-wheat bread or meatless chili with beans and corn bread, provide complete protein mixtures. Because the body does not

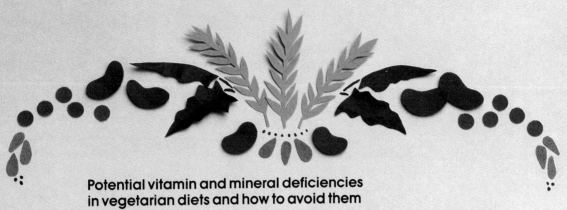

Potential vitamin and mineral deficiencies in vegetarian diets and how to avoid them

People who follow a strict vegetarian diet or a lacto-vegetarian diet run the risk of developing vitamin and mineral deficiencies. To prevent this, they should take care to plan meals that include plant sources of these important nutrients. Below are descriptions of the vitamins and minerals that are most often missing from vegetarian diets, as well as some plant foods that provide these nutrients.

Nutrient	Functions	Symptoms of deficiency	Plant sources
Vitamin D	Promotes mineralization of bones and teeth. Essential for the absorption and regulation of calcium and phosphorus.	*Rickets* or *osteomalacia* (softening and bending of bones).	Vitamin D-fortified soy milk *; cod liver oil.
Vitamin B_2 (riboflavin)	Promotes healthy skin and tissue repair.	*Cheilosis* (cracks at the corners of the mouth); poor growth.	Vitamin B_2 enriched cereals; green leafy vegetables.
Vitamin B_{12}	Maintains normal blood formation and nerve tissue.	Pernicious anemia; neurological disorders.	Vitamin B_{12} fortified cereals and soy milk.
Calcium	Building material for bones and teeth; helps regulate nerve impulses, muscle contractions, and blood clotting.	Rickets; osteoporosis.	Calcium-fortified soy milk; dark green leafy vegetables; legumes.
Iron	A component of hemoglobin, the oxygen-carrying molecule in red blood cells.	Iron deficiency anemia.	Iron-fortified cereals and grains; legumes.
Zinc	Involved in wound healing, building proteins, and other cell processes.	Poor wound healing; loss of appetite; failure to mature sexually.	Whole-grain products; legumes; seeds.

*Soy milk is a by-product of soybeans. Soy milk may—or may not—be fortified with vitamins D, B_{12}, and calcium, so check soy milk labels carefully.

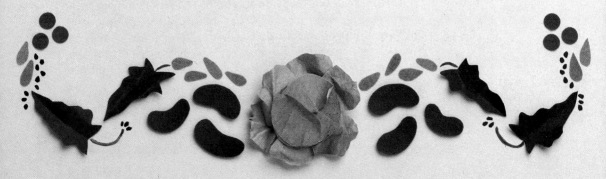

store protein, nutritionists recommend people eat complete protein mixtures at the same meal.

Vegetarians who eat eggs, dairy products, and some animal foods do not have to be as vigilant as strict vegetarians in making sure they obtain enough complete proteins. Just small amounts of these foods provide enough essential amino acids to satisfy the body's needs.

Maximizing minerals

Vegetarians who eat very few or no animal products must also take care that their diet supplies them with enough iron, zinc, and calcium, three minerals essential for good health. These minerals are found in meats, milk, and dairy products. Unfortunately, plant foods that contain iron, zinc, and calcium also have substances that bind up these minerals into large compounds that are not easily absorbed by the body.

Iron is a component of *hemoglobin*, the oxygen-carrying molecule in red blood cells. People with too little iron in their diet may develop *iron deficiency anemia*, a condition in which the number of red blood cells decreases. This can cause fatigue, rapid heartbeat, and other symptoms.

To get enough iron, vegetarians—especially strict vegetarians—should eat foods made with whole grains and cereals and breads that are *fortified* with iron. (In fortified foods, manufacturers have added nutrients that do not occur naturally in the foods or have increased the amounts of nutrients that occur naturally.) Vegetarians should also plan meals that include plenty of oranges, tomatoes, cabbages, and other plant foods rich in vitamin C. This vitamin increases the amount of iron the body absorbs from plant foods. Milk and other dairy products contain very little iron, but the animal protein in these foods helps the body to absorb what little iron is there.

Zinc, another mineral that may be lacking in a vegetarian diet, is important for wound healing, for the building of proteins, and for many other cell functions. Good sources of zinc are seafood, fish, poultry, whole grains, peanuts, dairy products, and eggs.

Unfortunately, whole-grain foods lose most of their zinc during processing, and manufacturers do not put this mineral back into the product. So strict vegetarians should choose minimally processed whole-grain products that retain more zinc. Soybean products, dried peas and beans, and sunflower and sesame seeds are also good sources of zinc.

Vegetarians must also make sure they get enough calcium in their diet. Calcium is vital for building strong bones and teeth. Because the best sources of calcium are milk, cheese, and other dairy products, lactovegetarians, lacto-ovovegetarians, and semivegetarians usually have no problem getting enough

Putting together complementary proteins

People who adopt a vegetarian diet must be sure they receive enough protein. Proteins are made up of molecules called *amino acids*. Some amino acids are made by the body, but others, called *essential amino acids,* are obtained only from food. Meat, dairy products, and eggs provide complete proteins because they contain all the necessary essential amino acids. But plant foods, lacking in certain essential amino acids,

provide only incomplete proteins. Fortunately, the essential amino acids lacking in some plant foods can be provided by other plant foods. Thus, proper combinations of plant foods or plant foods and dairy products can create complete—or complementary—protein. Below are the four groups of foods that vegetarians can combine to create complementary protein along with some possible dishes and snacks.

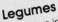

Legumes
This group includes soybeans, peanuts, lentils, kidney beans, black-eyed peas, lima beans, and chickpeas (garbanzo beans).

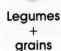

Legumes + grains
Corn tortillas with kidney bean filling; pea soup with rye bread; rice and lentil casserole.

Legumes + seeds
Kidney bean soup topped with sesame seeds; peanut and sunflower seed snack mix.

Grains
This group includes wheat, rice, oats, barley, rye, and corn.

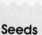

Seeds
This group includes sunflower and sesame seeds.

Grains + dairy products
Cheese pizza with wheat crust; macaroni and cheese; poached egg on toast; quiche.

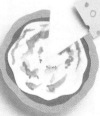

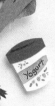

Dairy products + other vegetables
Vegetable salad with yogurt dressing; cauliflower with cheese sauce; vegetable omelet.

Dairy products
This group includes milk, cheese, yogurt, and other dairy products, as well as eggs.

of this mineral. It is a different story for strict vegetarians, however. Most plant foods are low in calcium, and what calcium is available is not easily absorbed by the body. Strict vegetarians should eat plenty of plant foods and products that do contain calcium, such as dark green leafy vegetables, calcium-fortified soy milk, and calcium supplements.

Vitamin concerns

Because their vegetarian diet may be deficient in vitamins D, B_{12}, and B_2 (riboflavin), vegetarians must plan their menus carefully to include foods that contain these vitamins. This is especially true for vegetarians who do not take daily vitamin supplements.

Vitamin D is present only in animal foods and is also made by the skin in the presence of sunlight. This vitamin is necessary for strong bones and teeth and is essential for the absorption and regulation of calcium and phosphorus in other body processes. Vegetarians develop a vitamin D deficiency if they consume little or no milk or dairy products, do not use vitamin supplements, and have limited exposure to the sun. Children may suffer from *rickets* and adults from *osteomalacia*, disorders in which the bones soften and bend.

To make sure they get enough vitamin D, vegetarians can add vitamin D-fortified soybean milk and cod-liver oil to their diet and also take vitamin D supplements. Some people may choose to boost their vitamin D intake by increasing their exposure to the sun, but they should exercise caution since overexposure to the sun may increase the risk of skin cancer.

A strict vegetarian diet also can be low in vitamin B_{12} and riboflavin because these vitamins are found only in animal foods. Vitamin B_{12} is important in blood production and in the function of nerve tissue, while riboflavin is essential for skin health and tissue repair. Since eggs, milk, and other dairy products provide adequate amounts of both vitamins, lactovegetarians, lacto-ovovegetarians, and semivegetarians rarely experience vitamin B_{12} or riboflavin deficiencies.

Because there is no good plant source of vitamin B_{12}, strict vegetarians must take a daily vitamin supplement or add vitamin B_{12}-fortified soy milk to their diet. Some vegetarians choose to eat seaweed or take a vitamin B_{12} nasal gel to obtain this nutrient, but neither source is recommended because these substances do not supply consistent doses of vitamin B_{12}. Oral vitamin supplements are less expensive and more reliable.

The richest sources of riboflavin include liver, kidneys, and other red meats. But cheese and eggs are also good sources, so vegetarians who eat these foods get an adequate supply of this vitamin. Strict vegetarians, however, may consume barely enough of the RDA for riboflavin unless their diet includes such foods as riboflavin-enriched cereals and green leafy vegetables. *Brewers' yeast,* a by-product of beer and ale brewing that is available in pill or powder form, can also provide sufficient riboflavin.

Should you be a vegetarian?

The adoption of a vegetarian diet requires time and thought. The more restrictive the diet, the more time it takes to plan and follow. You must develop meals and menus that provide all the essential nutrients your body needs. To do this, you have to be willing to learn about the nutrient contents of different foods. Vegetarian diets are also time consuming because most meals have to be prepared from scratch, since convenience foods often contain animal products. In addition, such foods as tofu, soy milk, and certain varieties of seeds and nuts might be difficult to find in supermarkets and may require trips to health-food stores or other specialty shops. Eating out may also be more difficult because some restaurants may not offer vegetarian meals.

Unless you are motivated by religious or moral beliefs, it is really not necessary to avoid all animal foods to ensure a healthy diet. A diet that includes animal foods can be beneficial—if these foods are eaten in moderation and contain only modest amounts of saturated fat and cholesterol. This can be accomplished by drinking skim or low-fat milk instead of whole-fat milk and choosing meats that are lower in fat, such as fish or chicken and turkey (with the fatty skin removed), rather than high-fat meats, such as prime rib. People who eat fatty red meats should avoid the white, fatty part and eat only small portions of the flesh. Meats and other foods should be cooked by methods that do not require oil or fats, such as broiling or braising instead of frying.

With a little planning, eating the vegetarian way can be nutritious and delicious, as anyone who has eaten at a first-rate vegetarian restaurant could confirm. And even those of us who are not prepared to forsake our hamburgers and T-bone steaks for all time are learning that a semimeatless diet may help us maintain our good health.

For further reading:
Katzen, Mollie. *The Moosewood Cookbook.* Ten Speed Press, 1977.
Lappe, Frances M. *Diet for a Small Planet.* Ballantine Books, 1975.
Robertson, Laurel. *New Laurel's Kitchen.* Ten Speed Press, 1986.

Medical Ethics and the AIDS Epidemic

By Carol Levine

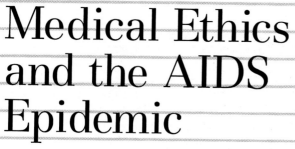

- Should AIDS testing be mandatory?

- Should people with AIDS be isolated from the rest of society?

- Should intravenous drug addicts be given free needles?

- Should health-care workers be required to treat AIDS patients?

AIDS took the modern world by surprise. Unknown and unforeseen when it made its appearance less than 10 years ago, this fatal infectious disease has raised a wide range of questions—medical questions about the disease itself and ethical questions concerning how society should respond to those infected with the agent that causes AIDS.

Although many medical questions remain, such as how AIDS can be treated effectively and prevented, some have been answered. For example, we now know that AIDS is caused by a virus, called the human immunodeficiency virus (HIV). We also know the virus is spread through blood, most commonly through needles used by drug abusers; through sexual intercourse; and from infected mothers to newborns.

As knowledge of the unique nature of AIDS grew—particularly that it is spread through intimate private acts—so did the number of ethical issues the disease presented. These issues have required and continue to require the analysis of *bioethicists*. These specialists in *biomedical ethics* or *bioethics* (the study of ethical problems in biology and health care) have managed to reach a consensus in resolving some of the ethical issues surrounding AIDS. But the AIDS epidemic continues to raise many questions, and bioethicists, such as myself, face the challenge of trying to find answers.

AIDS prompts these troubling bioethical questions mainly because it is an infectious disease that has not yet been conquered. LeRoy Walters, director of the Center for Bioethics at Georgetown University in Washington, D.C., puts the central ethical problem created by AIDS this way: "How can we control the epidemic and the harm it causes without unjustly discriminating against particular social groups and without unnecessarily infringing on the freedom of individuals?"

This central issue gives rise to numerous bioethical questions: Should expensive technology be used to improve the quality of a patient's life even though it cannot offer a cure? Who should pay for such technology? Should the standards of research to develop new drugs and treatments be changed because dying people are willing to be experimental subjects? The list could go on, because no other disease has presented such a range of issues—dilemmas for individuals and for society as well as for bioethicists.

The scope of bioethics

Bioethics originated in the 1950's, when a small group of physicians and religious leaders began to examine the questions raised by new medical technologies that were emerging after World War II. Today, bioethics is a distinct, though interdisciplinary, field. Bioethicists serve on hospital ethics committees, as expert witnesses in court cases, and as consultants to legislatures. Writings by bioethicists help guide debates on public policy and help form public opinion.

Bioethicists use their skills in analyzing problems to help clarify the issues, sort out fact from emotional reaction, and present options. They then apply the basic ethical principles that guide decision making in other areas to determine which principles are relevant to the issue under discussion. Finally, they offer solutions that uphold these principles in ways that also meet the test of practicality.

Bioethicists ask some of the most basic questions about human life: What is right? What is good? What are individuals' responsibilities to one another? How should government and other institutions act toward individuals? When two rights or interests are in conflict, which should be given priority? And what are the reasons to justify a proposed action?

But bioethical analysis of a problem is not limited to just these sweeping and often unanswerable questions. It also is based on the best available factual evidence, whether it comes from law, sociology, public policy, or medicine. Bioethicists must keep up to date on all the issues they discuss. Facts, as

The author:

Carol Levine is a bioethicist and executive director of the Citizens Commission on AIDS in New York City.

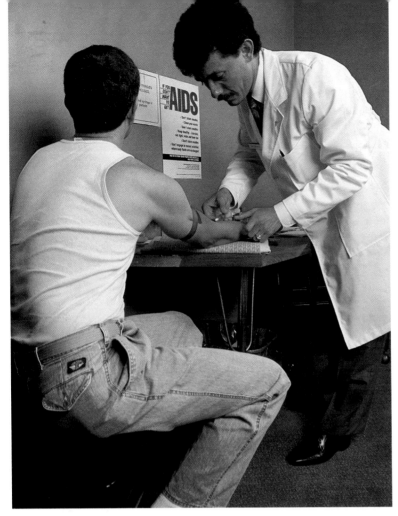

Who should be tested?

One controversial issue surrounding AIDS is the question of testing people for infection with the virus that causes the disease. Bioethicists agree that voluntary testing, *left,* is good for both the infected person—who can then obtain life-prolonging treatment—and for society—because infected people may then avoid spreading the virus to others. Confidential testing of all blood donors, *below,* also helps society while preserving the rights of the individual. Compulsory testing poses a more difficult question, however, because it deprives individuals of privacy and personal freedom.

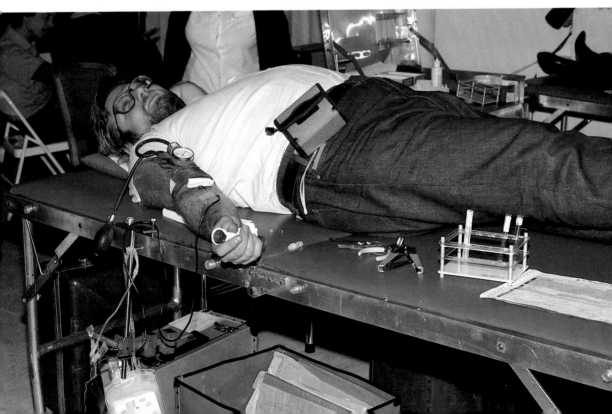

well as ethical principles, influence their conclusions.

Furthermore, the conclusions of bioethicists are not always translated into law. Ethical standards represent society's conclusions about what *should* be appropriate behavior. They are not necessarily enforced by legal means.

AIDS, ethics, and public health

Bioethicists generally use some common philosophical principles, some of which conflict. For instance, *autonomy*—the freedom to act in one's own best interests—is a primary value, but so is a prohibition against harming others. A third value considered by bioethicists is *beneficence*—acting to promote the welfare of others. Still another important value is justice or fairness.

Bioethicists have been called upon to analyze proposals to control the spread of AIDS, ranging from screening blood donations to prevent blood contaminated with HIV from being used for transfusion, to isolating all people infected with the virus. Bioethicists analyze such proposals from several points of view: First, they ask, does the proposal address one of the known ways the virus is spread? Second, would the particular proposal in fact control transmission? Third, what are the important ethical values that might be either promoted or jeopardized by the proposal? Finally, after weighing the pros and cons, should the proposal be adopted?

Should AIDS patients be isolated?

Isolating people with infectious diseases often has been used to prevent the spread of illness. But is such action warranted in the case of AIDS, which is not communicable through casual contact? Is it ethical, as some people advocate, to bar AIDS patients from public schools, *below*? Is it right to quarantine AIDS patients for life, as is the case in Cuba, *below right*?

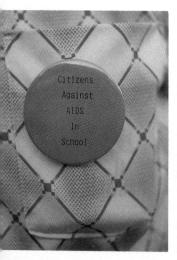

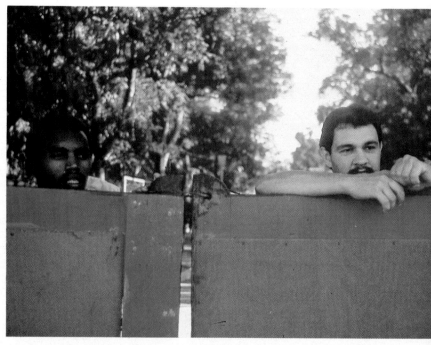

Consider the example of blood screening first. There is considerable evidence that HIV can be transmitted through transfused blood. Therefore, proposals to screen donated blood, using an accurate (though imperfect) test address a known way the virus is spread. Screening blood and discarding contaminated units thus greatly reduces the likelihood of contracting AIDS through a blood transfusion.

Screening follows the ethical principle of beneficence, because it promotes the welfare of blood recipients. But what of the need to protect the interests of blood donors? Only if donors are informed of the test and the results are treated with confidentiality do we avoid violating the needs of blood donors. Under these circumstances, screening blood is considered ethically acceptable.

On the other hand, consider isolation, a technique used in the past—often without any evidence that it works—to keep people with infectious diseases away from the rest of the population. And it has been tried with AIDS. Officials at the Western Middle School in Kokomo, Ind., for example, barred 13-year-old Ryan White from attending classes for several months in 1985, because the boy had AIDS and the board feared that he would transmit it to other students. He was eventually allowed to return to school after a hearing officer ruled he did not pose a health threat to his classmates.

Ryan White's case points up an important consideration in analyzing whether isolation would be effective in controlling HIV: the method of transmission. HIV is not spread through the air, water, or food, or through any casual contact. Therefore, people infected with HIV do not pose a threat to others in the same way that, for example, a person with measles or chicken pox does.

Compounding the problem, currently available blood screening tests are not perfect. In some cases, they fail to identify HIV-infected people; in others, they give "false-positive" results—that is, they falsely label some uninfected people as being carriers of the virus. (False-positive results do not undermine the tests' usefulness in screening blood donations; at worst, some uncontaminated blood is discarded.) The massive screening that would be required to identify all the infected people in the United States—1½ million, according to estimates by federal health experts—undoubtedly would result in significant errors of identification.

Finally, unlike most infectious diseases, in which the period of contagion is a matter of days or weeks, infection with the AIDS virus is considered to be lifelong. Isolation would also have to be lifelong. This and other practical problems, as well as the costs associated with establishing isolation centers, would seem to rule out isolation as a realistic means of controlling the spread of AIDS. The overriding reason most bioethicists oppose isolation, however, is that it would deprive large numbers of people of their liberty without sufficient compensating public health value.

Among the nations of the world today, only Cuba has established a system of screening the entire population—about 10½ million people—for HIV and isolating those found to be infected. Cuba alone has decided that the costs of isolation, both in economic terms and in terms of disrupting lives, are worth paying if such a measure increases the possibility of preventing transmission of the disease.

Blood screening and the forced isolation of HIV-infected individuals present the most extreme ends of the spectrum of possible public health interventions. In-between are many other possible measures, including voluntary HIV testing and counseling; mandatory screening of certain groups, such as military recruits; and tracing of sexual or needle-sharing contacts of an infected person to inform them of their possible exposure to the AIDS virus. Each of these measures can be weighed according to its potential benefits and risks, using the same criteria as those applied to blood screening, mandatory testing, and isolation. But this does not mean that bioethicists are in complete agreement on all these measures. Like the Supreme Court of the United States, bioethicists often reach a consensus rather than unanimity.

Principles in conflict:
The case of needle-exchange programs

Some measures aimed at stopping the spread of the AIDS virus require a choice between conflicting principles. For example, HIV transmission among homosexual men has been markedly reduced in the United States as a result of intensive education. But the virus is now spreading rapidly among intravenous (IV) drug users and their sexual partners. If drug users share needles, they have a high risk of injecting contaminated blood into their veins. Therefore, some public health officials have suggested that if it is not possible to stop needle use—and in most major cities, IV drug users who want to stop are put on long waiting lists for treatment—giving out clean needles is preferable to doing nothing.

Such programs have been established in Europe and Australia, with some success and little controversy. There is no consensus among bioethicists on these programs, but many of those who oppose them do so because they believe, on princi-

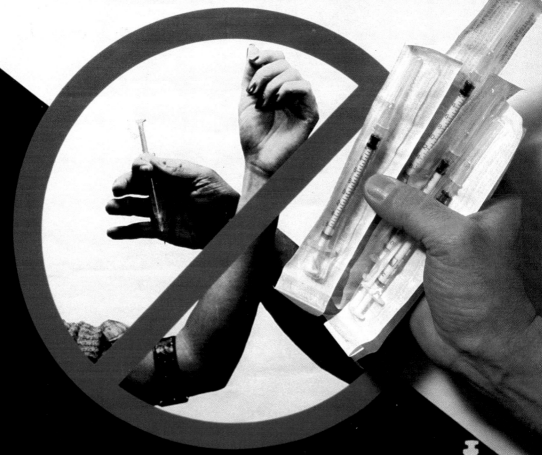

AIDS
IS DEADLY

Don't Pass the Spike!

FOR YOUR DRUG PROBLEM
522-5353

STATE OF NEW YORK
stance Abuse Services
ez, Director

Should health-care workers be required to treat AIDS patients?

Most people agree that everyone, including people with AIDS, has the right to receive medical care—but what of the right of health-care workers to avoid infection with AIDS? The problem is thorniest in the case of bloody procedures, *right,* which put workers at the greatest risk, but masks, gloves, and other precautions can minimize the danger, *below.* Another difficult question is: Should physicians with AIDS be barred from their profession even though they present little or no danger to their patients?

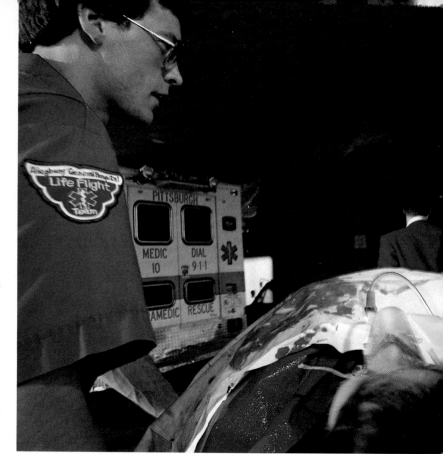

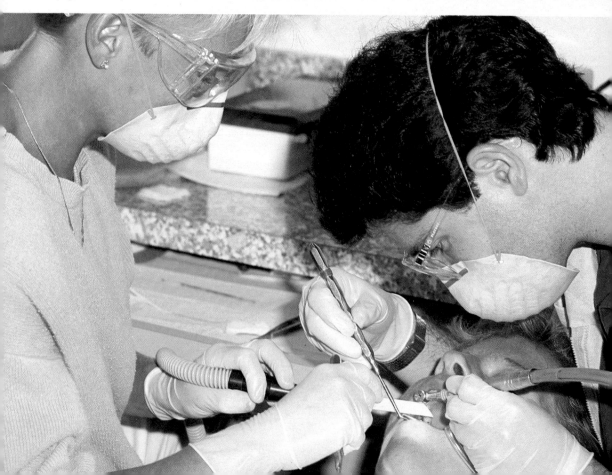

ple, that drug use is harmful and cannot be condoned under any circumstances. Only a few cities in the United States have established needle-exchange programs, and these are only small, pilot ones. Their success or failure in reducing the spread of AIDS among IV drug users surely will have an impact on whether other cities put such programs in place.

AIDS and the health-care worker

AIDS presents particular challenges to health-care workers. Because AIDS can be transmitted through accidental needle sticks and exposure to contaminated blood, some health-care workers now face a small occupational risk of becoming infected. Health-care workers whose jobs regularly involve exposure to large amounts of blood, such as heart surgeons and emergency room nurses, are at increased risk. But the risk of occupational exposure can be reduced considerably if workers wear gloves and other protective materials and follow strict infection-control procedures at all times.

Given the existence of this risk, are health-care workers justified in refusing to treat AIDS patients? Most bioethicists, as well as the American Medical Association (AMA) and all other major medical associations, say that professional obligations to provide care outweigh considerations of personal risk. This broad generalization does not address all the issues, however.

There is still considerable controversy, and no consensus, over many questions. Should all hospital patients, particularly surgery patients, be tested for HIV infection? Should health-care workers who have accidentally been exposed to a patient's blood be allowed to request that the patient be tested for HIV infection without his or her consent? Do patients have the right to know if a doctor has AIDS, and, if so, to refuse treatment from that physician? A bioethical analysis of these questions would involve weighing the benefits to be gained against the risks of invasion of privacy or breach of confidentiality. As in many such questions, policies should be developed that respect both patients' and health-care workers' interests.

In bioethics, a compromise that balances basic values can often be reached. For instance, the AMA's policy on warning the spouse or other known sexual partners of an AIDS carrier of the danger of exposure is a bioethical compromise. The policy recommends that doctors should first encourage AIDS carriers to inform their sexual partners and only then alert public health officials. If those two options fail, then doctors themselves should notify the carrier's sexual contacts.

The AMA's policy represents a reasonable bioethical compromise, because it attempts to protect the welfare of people who have been exposed to the AIDS carrier. At the same

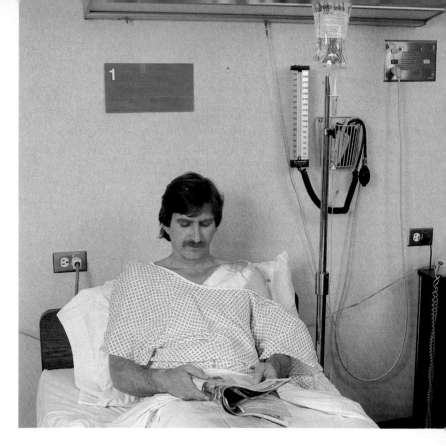

time, although it calls for a breach of patient confidentiality, the policy makes it clear that such a breach should occur only as a last resort.

Ethical dilemmas in patient care

Difficult questions often arise in the course of treating a person with AIDS. For example, when a patient is not responding to treatment, should it be stopped, even if that will result in the patient's death? Should beneficial but very expensive therapies be used indefinitely? When a patient is unable to make decisions for himself or herself because of illness, who should make those decisions?

A group of bioethicists called *clinical bioethicists* has special expertise in dealing with these "bedside" decisions. Most work side by side with doctors and nurses and participate in consultations with other hospital workers. And many hospitals are setting up ethics committees—commonly including bioethicists, doctors, nurses, lawyers, and social workers—to discuss troubling cases. Bioethicists play an important role on these committees by analyzing the facts of each case and presenting various options.

In approaching individual cases, bioethicists ask doctors for a clear presentation of the medical facts, as best as they are known. Then they try to determine the patient's own wishes.

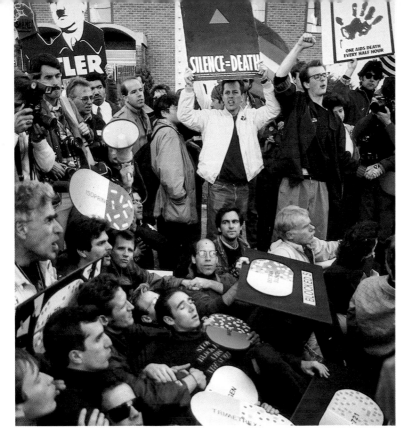

Who should receive experimental treatments?

The process for approving the use of new drugs is typically slow in the United States. Months or years of scientific research are required to prove the safety and effectiveness of a drug. Some people, *left*, charge that this process deprives AIDS patients of access to potentially life-prolonging or lifesaving treatments. A difficult question is: How can AIDS patients be given access to such treatments without compromising the research process that keeps unsafe and ineffective drugs off the market?

Often, however, the patient has not told anyone what his or her wishes are, and others must make the decisions. Here again, bioethicists must balance benefits and risks to arrive at a decision that keeps harm at a minimum and the welfare of the patient at a maximum.

Decisions about withholding treatment in AIDS cases are particularly difficult for several reasons. Many patients in the terminal stages of AIDS suffer from severe neurological complications that impair their memories and judgment skills, including their ability to make decisions. In such cases, physicians normally seek guidance from the patients' families. Some homosexual men with AIDS want their partner or close friend to make decisions about withholding treatment, but these individuals cannot legally make these decisions unless specifically authorized to do so. Sometimes bitter disputes arise between a patient's chosen representative and the patient's family.

When the first cases of AIDS were diagnosed, decisions about offering or withholding treatment were less consequential because there were no treatments that offered any real benefit. Now that situation has changed, as several drugs and treatments have been shown to prolong life, even if nothing yet approaches a cure for the disease.

The availability of these beneficial treatments raises a number of difficult questions. Here is just one example. Severe weight loss often accompanies AIDS. Patients who are given *total parenteral nutrition* (TPN)—a form of feeding through a tube that is permanently implanted in a vein—often gain weight and feel much better. This therapy cannot save a patient's life, however, and its temporary benefits are also very expensive, costing up to $500 a day. Many private insurance companies will pay for the treatment and will likely pass the cost to other policyholders in the form of higher premiums. But Medicaid, the federal-state governmental program that pays for health care for low-income patients, generally does not pay for TPN.

Should TPN be provided to patients? From society's point of view, providing the therapy could be seen as a poor allocation of scarce resources that could be better spent elsewhere. But from the patient's point of view, the benefits of an improved quality of life may outweigh the costs. And from the bioethicist's point of view, the decision to start or stop TPN is one that should be made by the patient after full discussion of what the procedure will mean.

But a bioethicist's consideration of this question does not end there, because this example raises another bioethical principle—that of justice. Is it fair to offer TPN to patients who can afford it but deny it to poor people? As in many bioethical questions, there is no easy answer. In general, however, bioethicists would oppose, on grounds of fairness, withholding beneficial treatment from people on the basis of their economic or social status.

Dilemmas of clinical research

The hope for better AIDS treatments and eventually a cure and vaccine lies in biomedical research. Promising drugs must be tested in human beings; worthless or extremely toxic drugs must be discarded. This complicated and lengthy process presents ethical dilemmas at every stage. Some measures aimed at protecting subjects of research studies in the United States include a process of research review that involves federal regulations, as well as institutional review boards (IRB's) to consider subjects' welfare.

One of these dilemmas concerns how drugs are tested. In most large-scale drug trials, some patients receive the drug while others, called *controls*, receive an inactive substance called a *placebo*. Many scientists assert that a comparison of the two groups is necessary to show whether a drug really has any effect. But many bioethicists argue that in the case of a life-threatening illness such as AIDS, it is unethical to withhold a promising drug from a subject.

The placebo issue is one bioethical controversy that is unlikely to be resolved on grounds of principle. Instead, each trial will have to be considered on its own merits. In some cases, such as trials in early stages of the disease where subjects could be switched to the drug if it turned out to be effective, a placebo group may be appropriate.

But in other situations, many people feel that requiring a placebo group would be unethical. For example, when the Community Research Initiative, a group of AIDS patients and their physicians in New York City, conducted trials in 1988 of a drug called *aerosolized pentamidine*, it did so without a placebo. The group's IRB considered it unethical to withhold the drug from patients who were at risk of death, because considerable preliminary evidence had shown the drug to be effective in preventing the recurrence of a form of pneumonia that is the most frequent cause of death in AIDS. Instead of a placebo, two dosages of the drug were compared. Other IRB's, however, allowed placebo trials of the same drug.

The continuing debate

Bioethicists have been able to reach a consensus on many issues. For example, the right of patients to make personal medical decisions is well accepted in bioethics and law. On other matters, though, such as abortion, there is no consensus now, and there is not likely to be one for some time.

What will the outcome be with AIDS? The evidence so far suggests that consensus has already been reached on some questions, such as isolation of those infected with HIV, but not on others, such as testing hospital patients without their consent. One thing is certain, however: AIDS will keep on posing new ethical questions even while others remain unanswered.

For further reading:
Three reports, "AIDS: The Emerging Ethical Dilemmas," "AIDS: Public Health and Civil Liberties," and "AIDS: The Responsibilities of Health Professionals," have been published by the Hastings Center, a research and educational organization devoted to ethical problems. For information about ordering the reports, write to the Hastings Center, 255 Elm Road, Briarcliff Manor, NY 10510.

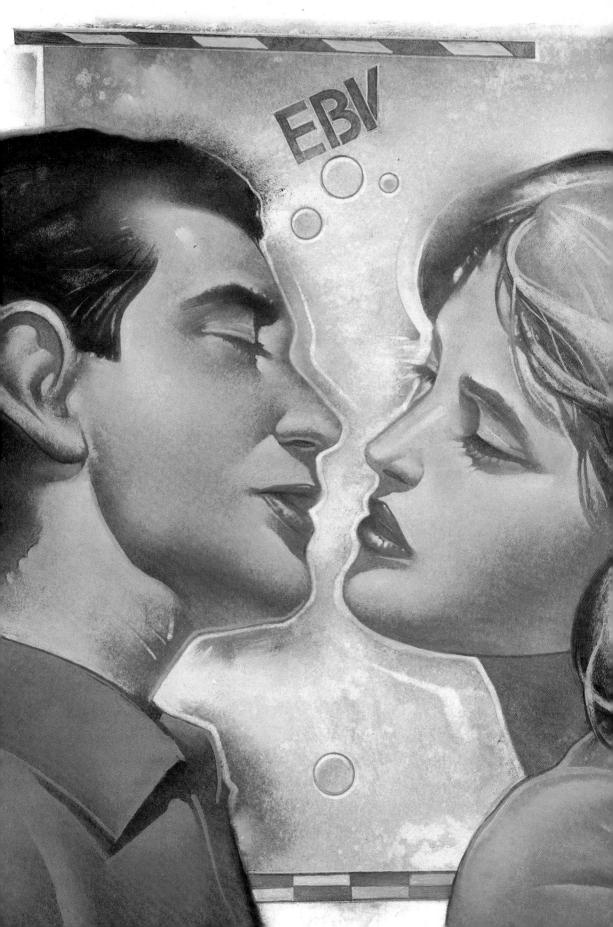

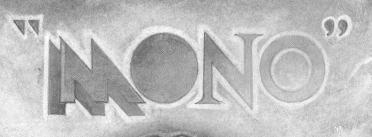

"MONO"

The mononucleosis
virus touches nearly
everyone—and for
some, it brings weeks
or months of illness.

When a Kiss Can
Make You Sick

By Patricia Thomas

$\mathbf{M}$atthew knew something was wrong the moment he woke up. As he glanced toward his bedside clock, sharp pains jarred his eyeballs, as though they were being squeezed by cruel metallic tongs. But all he saw in the bathroom mirror was a little puffiness around his eyes.

Two days later, the 17-year-old high-school junior came home from school at midday, feeling feverish and light-headed. He was sweating profusely despite the crisp fall weather, and he could feel swollen lumps in his neck—a sign that his body was fighting an infection. Matthew's doctor ordered blood tests and told the teen-ager to go home and get some rest. But Matthew, a strapping athlete who'd just finished soccer season and was gearing up for basketball, still tried to do his usual 100 sit-ups. He stopped after 10.

When the lab report on the blood tests came back, Matthew learned why he felt so tired. The tests showed he had infectious mononucleosis, or mono—a strength-sapping flulike illness known best for striking teen-agers and young adults. For the next 10 days, Matthew's most strenuous activity was switching TV channels with the remote control. After that, though, he felt much better, and assumed he was ready for school and sports.

Matthew's doctor was more cautious, however. By carefully feeling Matthew's stomach, the doctor determined that Matthew's spleen (an organ that works to fight infection) was swollen. If Matthew were elbowed during a basketball game, the tender spleen might rupture—a potentially fatal complication.

It was another month before Matthew was allowed off the bench. But the day he returned to action, he scored 25 points, pulled in 15 rebounds, and blocked 6 shots in the best game of his career.

A few blocks away, in the same Boston suburb, 23-year-old Evelyn had a very different experience with mono. Her illness began slowly, like an ordinary cold or flu. The doctor she saw at the university health clinic ordered a mono test "just in case." It came back negative, and the doctor reassured Evelyn that she probably just had a cold.

For the next week Evelyn dragged herself to her job as a receptionist. "I had trouble walking up stairs," she remembers. Her neck swelled and her appetite disappeared. She felt feverish on and off—and tired all the time.

When she developed an acutely painful sore throat, Evelyn went back to the clinic. This time the mono test was positive. She abandoned her apartment for her parents' home, where she spent three weeks in bed before returning to work. Three months later, Evelyn still didn't feel well. She worked only half-time and seemed to catch every bug that came along.

Few people die from infectious mononucleosis. But every year the disease causes some miserable weeks or months for

The author:

Patricia Thomas is Boston correspondent for *Medical World News.*

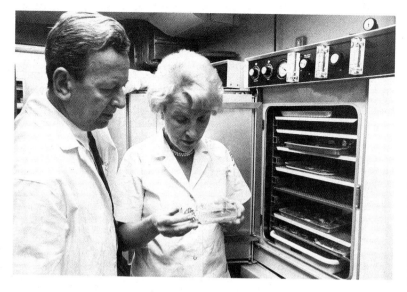

Physicians Werner and Gertrude Henle began research on the newly discovered Epstein-Barr virus in 1967, thinking it might be a cause of cancer. By accident, the husband-and-wife team found that the virus was the long-sought agent of mononucleosis.

about 1 per cent of all Americans aged 15 to 25 and for some older people as well. Since 1968, doctors have known that all these people are infected with a single, common bug, the Epstein-Barr virus (EBV). But they don't know why some bounce back quickly, like Matthew, while others have a lingering illness like Evelyn's.

In the early stages of the illness, mono sufferers often feel tired and out-of-sorts—vague symptoms that could signal a cold or a mild viral infection. In the late 1880's, German doctors described such patients as having *Drüsenfieber* (glandular fever). The designation referred to one of the most common mono symptoms, "swollen glands." Actually, the swollen lumps in the neck, armpits, and groin are not glands at all, but *lymph nodes*—small organs that produce white blood cells and other substances that help the body fight infections.

Although these physicians wrote the first description of the disease we now call infectious mononucleosis, they couldn't accurately predict its course; the doctors couldn't distinguish Drüsenfieber patients from others who would eventually die of leukemia, a cancer of the blood. The diseases had similar early symptoms, and in both cases, samples of patients' blood showed an excess of certain white blood cells. When the Drüsenfieber patients got better on their own, doctors mistakenly thought they had witnessed recoveries from cancer.

It wasn't until 1920 that two physicians at Johns Hopkins University in Baltimore found a sure way to tell the difference between leukemia patients and those with a temporary syndrome of fever, swollen lymph nodes, and fatigue. Thomas P.

Sprunt and Frank A. Evans drew blood samples from six students with those symptoms and examined the samples under a microscope. Not only did they see an excessive number of a type of white blood cells called *mononuclear lymphocytes*, but the cells themselves looked strange—they were larger than normal and had an unusually prominent *nucleus* (the structure that directs the activities of the cell). These special mononuclear cells give infectious mononucleosis its name.

Sprunt and Evans' discovery enabled doctors to reassure many patients that they did not have leukemia, but rather a much less serious illness that would get better on its own. But although accuracy of diagnosis improved, the cause of mononucleosis remained a question for nearly 50 years.

The answer was found by accident. In 1967, Gertrude and Werner Henle, physicians at Children's Hospital in Philadelphia, were studying EBV—a newly discovered virus whose effects were unknown. The Henles thought that EBV might be an infectious agent that caused cancer. They developed a test that allowed them to pinpoint the presence of this virus in blood by identifying particular *antibodies*—disease-fighting proteins produced by the body in response to a bacterium or virus. The scientists then began looking for EBV antibodies in blood from cancer patients.

As it happened, a technician in the Henles' lab became ill. She was diagnosed as having German measles, stayed home for about a week, and returned to the lab. Soon after, she suffered a relapse. Before she went home again, the Henles drew a sample of her blood. They compared it with a routine blood sample she'd given earlier, before her illness.

What they found told nothing about cancer—but it solved the 80-year-old mystery of Drüsenfieber. The earlier specimen of the technician's blood contained no antibodies to EBV, meaning she had not yet been exposed to the virus. But the specimen taken during her illness was rich in such antibodies. In addition, the technician's blood also showed the mononuclear cells that Sprunt and Evans had described 48 years earlier. The technician had mono, not German measles—and her case linked infectious mononucleosis with EBV infection.

Since that time, both EBV antibody tests and microscopic examination of blood cells have been used to diagnose mono. And those tests also have helped researchers figure out how EBV spreads and who it affects.

Although we think of mono as a disease of young adults, studies show that many people are infected with EBV during childhood. Still, EBV infection doesn't automatically mean a

How mono spreads

By age 40, about 90 per cent of Americans have caught the virus that causes mononucleosis, though many never develop any symptoms. But once you're infected, you carry the virus for life and may pass it to others.

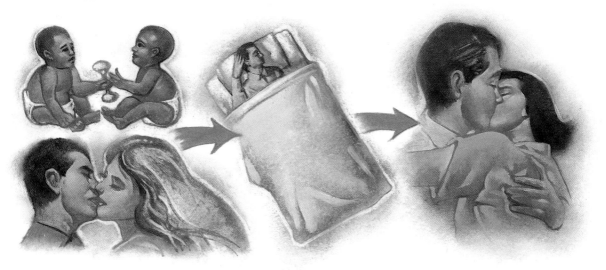

The mono virus typically spreads in saliva. Many people catch it in childhood, often when one baby or toddler chews on a toy and passes it, still wet, to another child. Among teen-agers and adults, the most common method of spreading the virus is through kissing.

Children rarely show symptoms of mononucleosis. But people who catch the virus when they are older may fall ill with mono. In some, the illness will pass in a week or two. Among others, it may linger for months. Once recovered, the person is immune to further attacks of illness.

The mono virus stays in your body for life. Occasionally it becomes active in your blood and the lining of your throat. At those times, you may spread the virus to others when you kiss. But since most people are already immune, few will catch the virus or develop mono.

case of infectious mononucleosis. Most infected children simply make antibodies against the virus without developing any symptoms. The antibodies stay in their blood for life, and this protects them from coming down with mono later.

Because childhood infections have protected so many people, a relatively small percentage of young adults are candidates for EBV infection—and the case of mono that might come with it. Mono usually strikes in the teens and early 20's, with a peak in the 15-to-19 age group. Girls who catch mono are most likely to do so between ages 14 and 16, while the peak years for boys are 16 to 18.

Most of what we know about how mono and EBV affect young adults has been gained by studies of college students. In 1974, epidemiologist James Neiderman of Yale University in New Haven, Conn., reported the results of a four-year study of cadets who entered the U.S. Military Academy at West Point, N.Y., in 1969. Neiderman found that 63.5 per cent of the cadets already had antibodies to EBV when they arrived on campus. Of the 400 or so who had not been infected before they entered the academy, almost half showed evidence of infection by the time they graduated in 1973.

Neiderman's later studies of freshmen at Yale showed that by the late 1980's, the proportion of previously exposed freshmen was between 70 per cent and 80 per cent—somewhat higher than at West Point 20 years earlier. Other studies have revealed that by age 40, as many as 90 per cent of Americans have EBV antibodies—and are thus immune to mono.

Reports of mono cases in the late 1980's have suggested that mono might be rising among people over age 60, but most public health experts say this represents better diagnosis by doctors instead of an actual increase in the number of cases. Mono is more difficult to diagnose in older people because for unknown reasons they're less likely to have the classic symptoms of sore throat, swollen lymph nodes, and enlarged spleens. Instead, they tend to show a vague fatigue and fever, sometimes with such symptoms as abdominal pain. Physicians are also less likely to suspect mono in older people simply because they know most adults are immune.

T he mono virus typically spreads from person to person in saliva. Among preschool children, transmission usually occurs when a baby or toddler chews on a toy and passes it along, still wet, to another child. In teen-agers and young adults, the typical route is kissing. (The fact that girls tend to begin dating—and kissing—slightly younger than boys do may explain why the peak years of mono are earlier for girls than for boys.) It's also possible to be infected by sharing a drinking vessel or from a blood transfusion, but few cases actually spread in those ways. Volumes of research confirm that mono deserves its nickname: "the kissing disease."

It's obvious, however, that the number of people who get mono is far smaller than the number who kiss. New infections happen only when a person who has the virus passes it to a previously unexposed person. But "having the virus" doesn't mean being sick at the moment of contact. This virus belongs to the *herpesvirus* family, which includes the viruses that cause chicken pox and cold sores as well as genital herpes, a sexually transmitted disease. People who have been infected with a herpesvirus carry the virus, usually in a dormant form, for a lifetime. (For more detail on herpesviruses, see EPSTEIN-BARR: A VIRUS OF MANY FACES on page 136.)

In the case of EBV, the virus periodically becomes active, reproducing itself in the blood and the lining of the throat. During those times it's especially easy to share with a friend. Studies show that on any given day, EBV can be found in the throats of 15 per cent to 25 per cent of healthy, symptomless people who have developed antibodies to the virus from a past infection. That means that every time we sit in a classroom, say, or a theater, as many as 1 in every 4 of the people around us are actively "shedding" EBV from the surfaces of their throats.

Yet we never see headlines about outbreaks of mononucleosis, nor do subway posters warn us against the ravages of the kissing disease. There are no mono epidemics for several reasons. Perhaps the most important is that the number of susceptible people falls steadily at the same time as sexual activity—and thus kissing—increases. Only about 20 per cent of college freshmen are susceptible. By the time people are in their 30's or 40's, only about 10 per cent could still get sick.

Another consideration is that not everyone who comes into contact with the virus develops symptoms of mono. In Neiderman's study of West Point cadets, only 26.4 per cent of those whose blood tests showed they were infected during their four years at the academy were ever diagnosed as having infectious mono. The majority never sought medical attention—either because they showed no signs of illness or assumed they had a minor cold or other infection.

The West Point study also supported the idea that intimate contact is required for virus transmission. Susceptible roommates of infected cadets were no more likely to catch the virus than cadets who lived in uninfected pairs. If EBV was an airborne virus, like the ones that cause common colds, roommates of mono victims would be more likely to develop illness. Nor have researchers ever found that the likelihood of infection is higher among family members of patients.

When a susceptible person does develop mono, symptoms generally appear between 30 and 60 days from the time of exposure to the virus. But the exact combination of symptoms can vary, and mono can easily be misdiagnosed at first—not only as a common viral infection but also as other illnesses such as strep throat, German measles, or hepatitis.

Like Evelyn, many people recall that their mono started with vague symptoms and progressed to a sore throat that motivated them to see a doctor. When physicians examine patients in the acute phase of mono, they find that the vast majority have not only a severe sore throat but also fever and swollen lymph nodes in the neck and sometimes the armpits and groin. They feel overwhelmingly tired, lose their appetite, and in some cases can't bear bright light. They may also complain of headache, chills, or sweating.

Half to three-quarters of all patients show swelling of the spleen. A slightly smaller proportion have an enlarged and sometimes tender liver. About half have raised bumps on their tongues, and, like Matthew, about one-third have puffy and painful eyes. Some patients—fewer than one-tenth—show a rash like that of German measles.

Fortunately, most of these symptoms don't last long. The painful sore throat usually gets better after about one week. Fevers usually last for less than two weeks, and lymph nodes rarely stay swollen for more than three weeks.

The spleen's swelling reaches its peak during the second or third week of illness. Liver abnormalities, if any, usually occur during the first three to five weeks of illness, but also resolve of their own accord. About 5 per cent of mono patients develop signs of *jaundice*, a yellowish tinge of the skin and tissues associated with liver disorders; this also resolves on its own as the illness passes.

The single most persistent symptom of mono is *malaise*— the pervasive feeling of being tired. Malaise lingers for months for some people, as Evelyn's experience illustrates. But most, like Matthew, feel well enough to go back to work or school after three to four weeks—or even sooner.

Over the years, doctors have reported a long list of complications associated with infectious mononucleosis. The illness can affect many parts of the body, but fortunately such problems are rare. Deaths from complications of mono are even rarer—so uncommon, in fact, that no formal statistics exist.

The most serious complication, which accounts for many of the infrequent deaths associated with mono, is rupture of the spleen. When the spleen swells during acute mononucleosis, it can rupture on its own or from a sudden blow. That's why doctors tell athletes like Matthew to avoid contact sports while the spleen is enlarged. If the spleen ruptures, the patient needs large blood transfusions and the organ must be surgically removed immediately. Ruptures do not occur often, and few prove fatal. Rarer complications include inflammation of the brain or nervous system, heart problems, pneumonia, and blockage of the breathing passages from swelling of the lymph nodes and other tissue.

At least one drug—the antibiotic *ampicillin*—causes a rash in some mononucleosis patients. This typically happens when a doctor mistakes a case of mono for strep throat—a bacterial infection for which ampicillin is a treatment.

When today's doctors diagnose infectious mononucleosis, they use techniques with deep historic roots. They evaluate physical signs much as German doctors did in the Drüsenfieber era, look for the abnormal blood cells discovered in

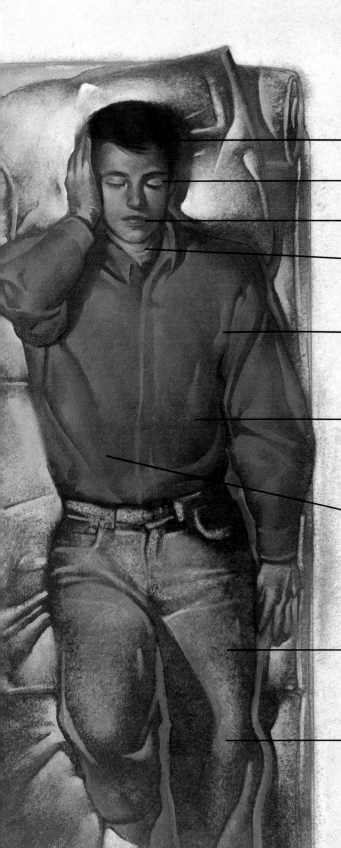

Where mono strikes

Mononucleosis has been called "the great masquerader" because its symptoms resemble those of many other diseases—some of which, like leukemia or hepatitis, are much more serious. Mono's hallmarks are fever and *malaise*—overwhelming fatigue and a general ill feeling. These may be combined with any or all of the following:

Headache and light-headedness often mark the onset of mono.

Painful or puffy eyes, and sometimes a dislike of bright light, may occur.

Bumps on the tongue appear in about half of all mono cases.

A severe sore throat occurs in most patients and may be the first clue that the problem is mono.

Swollen lymph nodes in the neck, armpits, or groin are one of the most common symptoms of mono. The lymph nodes produce white blood cells and other substances that help the body fight infections.

The spleen, an organ that helps fight infection, becomes swollen and tender in half to three-fourths of all patients. A ruptured spleen is the most serious complication of mono. Ruptures require emergency surgery to remove the spleen, and in rare cases they are fatal.

The liver swells in about half of all patients, and a few show *jaundice*, a yellowish skin coloring that comes from liver disorders.

A rash like that of German measles appears in a small proportion of cases. Some mono patients develop a rash when the antibiotic drug ampicillin is administered.

Aches and pains, chills, sweating, and other vague symptoms that affect the whole body may contribute to the difficulty in pinpointing mono early in the course of the illness.

Epstein-Barr:
A virus of many faces

The virus responsible for infectious mononucleosis belongs to the family of herpesviruses, and its relatives cause problems ranging from cold sores and chicken pox to birth defects. These viruses take their name from the Greek word *herpeto*, which means "a creeping thing." The same root word gave rise to *herpetology*, the name for the branch of zoology that deals with reptiles and amphibians.

Inside our bodies, herpesviruses behave much as snakes and salamanders do in the outside world. Like those animals, the virus is able to lie hidden and inactive for long periods of time. Then, when conditions are right, the virus—like the animals—surfaces in a frenzy of activity.

The Epstein-Barr virus, which causes mononucleosis, has also been linked with other diseases since its discovery in 1964 by two British cancer researchers. Pathologist M. Anthony Epstein and his assistant, Yvonne M. Barr, were using a powerful microscope to look at cells grown from a tumor of *Burkitt's lymphoma*, a cancer that is common among children in central Africa but rare elsewhere. Lymphomas are cancers of the lymphatic system, the network of vessels that lubricates body tissues. Quite unexpectedly, they spotted an unfamiliar virus shaped much like the known herpesviruses. They sent a sample to virus researchers in Philadelphia, who soon confirmed that this was indeed a herpesvirus, and a new one at that.

The American scientists first thought the Epstein-Barr virus was an infectious agent that caused cancer. But that possibility dimmed as it gradually became clear that most of the earth's adult inhabitants have been infected with EBV, and only a tiny percentage—most of whom live in certain areas—have cancers associated with the virus. Before long, the researchers were able to connect the same virus with the more common—and noncancerous—infectious mononucleosis.

Scientists have found high levels of antibodies to EBV in patients with Burkitt's lymphoma in certain hot and humid regions of central Africa. In some parts of southern China, and among Chinese who have immigrated to Malaysia and Singapore, there is a strong link between EBV infection and *nasopharyngeal carcinoma*, a cancer of the nasal passages. In neither case do scientists claim that the virus causes cancer all by itself, but they're certain it plays an important role.

These EBV-linked cancers are almost unheard of in the United States and other industrialized nations. Why does Epstein-Barr virus, which is the same the world over, cause cancer in some populations and infectious mononucleosis in others?

Scientists don't know the answer, but they hope to find it by studying the basic processes of viral infection. A virus infects its host by finding a type of cell it can attach to, penetrating the cell, and transforming the cell's own machinery into a virus factory. Virologists have known for some years that EBV thrives in certain white blood cells called *B lymphocytes;* in the 1980's they found evidence that it also reproduces in the lining of the throat and the salivary glands.

Just as a snake may be more successful

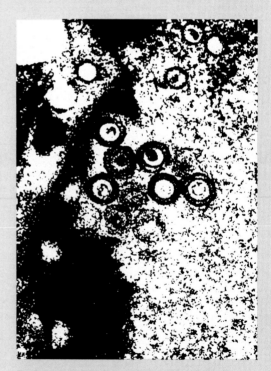

The Epstein-Barr virus (the "bull's-eye" shapes, *above*) hides in white blood cells for an infected person's life, periodically emerging and reproducing in the throat.

raising its young in a burrow than in an old tire, some people's cells may be better homes for a virus than others. Scientists believe that such differences, which they call *host factors*, may someday explain why EBV causes cancer in certain African and Asian peoples and mononucleosis in American teen-agers.

One important host factor is the status of the person's immune system—his or her innate ability to resist disease. For example, people whose immune systems have been damaged by AIDS often develop oral lesions called *hairy leukoplakia* after being infected with EBV. In transplant patients who have received immune-suppressing drugs to keep their bodies from rejecting the new organs, EBV infections can lead to lymphomas.

Another major host factor is a person's genetic makeup. For example, EBV infections seem to prompt cancer in children with a rare genetic disorder called *X-linked*

Burkitt's lymphoma, a form of cancer that most often strikes children in central Africa, is one of several rare diseases linked to Epstein-Barr virus.

lymphoproliferative syndrome. These children—all of them boys—are defenseless against infection, and they almost always develop fatal complications when exposed to EBV.

After more than two decades, scientists are still trying to pin down EBV's role in cancer development. But for a few years in the mid-1980's, they also thought the virus might cause a very different type of disease.

In 1985, two doctors in Incline Village, Nev., made headlines by reporting that 80 to 90 patients in their practices suffered from mysterious fatigue that lasted for months. Many patients had swollen lymph nodes, sore throats, and swollen spleens or livers. They also showed evidence of infection with EBV. The presence of the virus, plus the similarity of the symptoms to those of mono, led the doctors to label the condition "chronic Epstein-Barr infection" or "chronic mononucleosis."

As news of the Nevada observations spread in newspapers and on television, similar clusters were reported elsewhere. Because many victims were middle-class professionals in their 30's, reporters dubbed the mysterious ailment "Yuppie flu." Scientists from the federal Centers for Disease Control (CDC) in Atlanta, Ga., were dispatched to investigate the clusters, and they confirmed that the patients' symptoms were real. But they could not prove that EBV—which normally occurs in as many as 90 per cent of adults in this age group—was anything more than an innocent bystander to the disease.

In May of 1987, in the *Journal of the American Medical Association*, CDC scientists concluded that "the currently popular descriptive terms *chronic EBV disease* and *chronic mononucleosis* are inappropriately specific." The mysterious illness is now called *chronic fatigue syndrome*, and criteria that doctors use to identify patients make no mention of EBV.

Experts are split over whether it is even useful to test these patients for EBV antibodies. Many say the proposed connection between EBV and this syndrome was illogical from the start, simply because almost everyone has been infected with the virus at some time. If EBV caused long-lasting and debilitating fatigue, civilization would long ago have ground to a halt.   [P. T.]

Within 10 minutes, a simple blood test called a *monospot, right,* can reveal the presence of an active mono infection. Signs of mono can also be seen by examining blood through a microscope. A normal white blood cell, *below,* can easily be distinguished from a mono-infected blood cell, *bottom,* with its oversize nucleus.

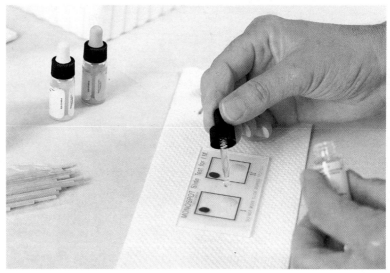

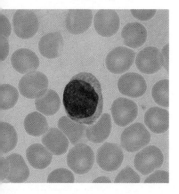

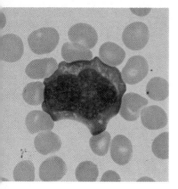

1920 by Sprunt and Evans, and use EBV antibody tests descended from those the Henles developed in 1968.

A doctor who suspects you have mono will ask you about your symptoms, take your temperature, inspect your throat, and feel your lymph nodes and spleen. He or she will draw a blood sample that will be used for at least two tests. The most widely used test for EBV infection is the *monospot,* a test for a particular antibody that occurs with cases of mono. In most cases, these antibodies are present within a week after symptoms first appear. But up to 15 per cent of mono cases—like Evelyn's—won't show up on tests during the first week.

The monospot test is very simple and takes only about 10 minutes to perform. A drop of blood is put onto a card coated with dry materials derived from animal blood cells, mixed in, and watched. If the material forms clumps, the antibodies are present and mononucleosis is the most likely diagnosis.

Another clue to the diagnosis can be obtained by the second test, which is done by smearing blood on a glass slide and examining it through a microscope. If you have mono, the slide will usually show excessive numbers of white blood cells and the large mononuclear cells typical of the disease.

If your doctor has a laboratory in the office or in the same building, your test results may be available during your visit. If your blood has to be sent to an off-site laboratory, the doctor will usually have an answer for you in one or two days.

If the monospot test is negative but your symptoms strongly suggest mono, the doctor may want to retest you after a week to see if antibodies have formed. Or you may be asked to have a more sophisticated blood test to detect a different type of EBV antibody that does not show up on the monospot. These results should also be available within one or two days.

There is no specific medical treatment for mono. Although military personnel or college students who are away from home are sometimes hospitalized, most other people are not. There's not much to do for the illness except rest and wait to feel better. Doctors often advise taking aspirin or other analgesics to relieve headache, fever, and sore throat, and recommend gargling with salt water to ease throat pain.

Many doctors recommend that people with mono not rush back to work or school until their symptoms have disappeared and their energy is back to normal. Some believe that what people do during the first two weeks of illness may be crucial and that stress during this period can substantially lengthen recovery. People who insist on taking a test or meeting a deadline at this time may run the risk of having a relapse that will send them back to bed. (No evidence exists, however, that mono can develop into a long-term tiring illness lasting many months or years. Such a condition, called "chronic mononucleosis" or "chronic EBV infection" in 1985, was later shown to have no real connection to EBV or mono.)

Mono patients with enlarged spleens often get their energy back before their spleens return to normal. It's important to stay away from strenuous activity until a doctor confirms that all signs of swelling have disappeared.

Even at a time when much health practice is focused on stopping disease before it starts, researchers have turned up no breakthroughs in preventing mono. Doctors see no evidence that strategies for boosting the immune system, such as having injections of *gamma globulin* (a component of blood serum that contains antibodies), have any value against mono.

Common sense tells us it's a bad idea to kiss someone who has an active case of mono or is just recovering from the disease. But because all the people who've ever been exposed to EBV are intermittently infectious for the rest of their lives, the only sure way for a susceptible person to avoid mono would be to avoid kissing altogether. That tactic has little appeal. But there's comfort in knowing that the majority of us are immune to the disease by the time we finish high school and that most of those who aren't soon will be—either with or without the illness itself.

For more information:

The book *Herpes Diseases and Your Health*, by Henry H. Balfour (1984, University of Minnesota), includes a good discussion of infectious mononucleosis. Most college and university health services offer students brochures or other information about mono.

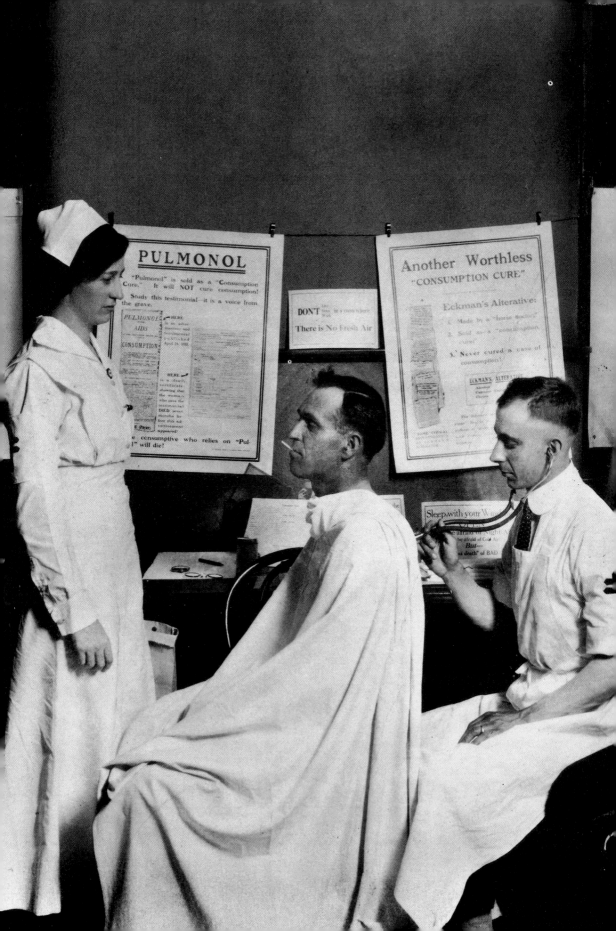

The insidious disease that struck
Chopin, Keats, Poe—and millions of
people living today—has long been
the subject of myth and misconception.

The Great
White Plague:
A History of TB

By William H. Allen

The history of tuberculosis is a record of mistaken notions.
Although the disease seems as antiquated as the various
names given to it over the centuries—*consumption, scrofula,
white plague*—tuberculosis is very much a modern illness,
with millions of new cases diagnosed each year in the developing countries alone. About 23,000 people develop tuberculosis (TB) in the United States annually, and, despite the fact
that we have both a cure and a vaccine, the incidence of TB in
the United States has begun to increase.

Most of us nonetheless think of TB as a disease of the
1800's, depicted in romantic images: pale maidens coughing
delicately into lace handkerchiefs and tubercular poets pen-
ning melancholy verses about death. In fact, because the skeletal remains of prehistoric human beings show signs of TB, we
know that this often-fatal disease—caused by a bacterium and
usually spread by coughing or sneezing—has afflicted people
for thousands of years. On their stone tablets, the Babylonians
in the 100's B.C. described its unromantic symptoms—fatigue,
weight loss, fever, and coughing fits that produce blood and
quantities of pus-filled phlegm. In the 300's B.C., the Greeks

Opposite page: A tuber-
culosis (TB) patient is examined at Sunny Acres
sanitarium in Cleveland
in 1918.

141

(who gave TB the name *phthisis*, which means *to shrink up and wither away*) recorded that it was the most prevalent disease of that time.

History has been punctuated with attempts, some of them bizarre, to find a cure for TB. Because the disease typically affects the lungs and produces great weariness, physicians have since the earliest times recommended fresh air and rest as a treatment. During the first 200 years of the Christian Era, physicians of the Roman Empire encouraged sufferers to take long sea voyages. Those who could not afford such an extravagance turned to folk remedies. Some traveled to Mount Vesuvius, near Naples, Italy, to breathe the volcano's fumes. Others drank elephant's blood, ate mice boiled in salt and oil, or inhaled the smoke of burning dried cow dung.

Unfortunately, none of these remedies worked, and the disease became the most feared of illnesses. In London in the mid-1600's, TB caused 20 per cent of all deaths. In the 1700's and 1800's, consumption (the disease's common name at the time, because of its characteristic symptom of weight loss) killed 25 per cent of all Europeans, according to some estimates. In the United States, as in Europe, TB was the primary cause of death. Because most physicians felt TB was a hopeless disease, quacks filled the void with "miracle cures" developed in "barber shops, taverns, and stables," as one medical-school teacher of the day wrote.

In 1859, a German botanist who had found relief from his TB on a plant-collecting trip in the Himalaya opened a facility called a *sanitarium* for other TB patients. At the facility, which was located in a pine forest in the mountains of Silesia in eastern Europe, consumptives were given "nature's cure" — good food, prolonged rest, and fresh air—conditions erroneously believed to "dry out" the lungs. In 1885, Edward L. Trudeau opened the first TB sanitarium in the United States at Saranac Lake in the Adirondack Mountains of New York. In less than three decades, more than 400 sanitariums were operating throughout the nation. Sites in Florida, the Carolinas, and the Caribbean islands were other favorite spots for American "lungers," as TB victims of the period were often called.

Whether sanitarium treatment was an effective cure is difficult to say. At least sanitariums took infectious patients away from the crowded urban environment that encouraged the spread of the disease. Exposure to sunlight also might have helped some TB patients, because sunlight is necessary for the human body to synthesize vitamin D. Researchers at the University of Colorado Health Sciences Center in Denver reported in 1988 that vitamin D appeared to help patients combat TB.

But the regimens at some sanitariums were radical, includ-

The author:

William H. Allen is a science reporter for the *St. Louis* (Mo.) *Post-Dispatch*.

ing strenuous exercise, horseback riding, exposure to extreme cold, and forced overeating. Few studies of the success of sanitarium treatment have been undertaken, but it is likely that the treatment made little difference in patients' survival rates.

As TB raged out of control throughout Europe and America, it numbered among its victims scores of famous writers and artists. Like today's epidemic of AIDS, TB had a profound impact on the world of arts and letters. Included in the list of famous TB sufferers were such writers and poets as Charlotte and Emily Brontë, Lord Byron, Anton Chekhov, John Keats, D. H. Lawrence, Eugene O'Neill, Edgar Allan Poe, Percy Bysshe Shelley, and Robert Louis Stevenson; composers and musicians such as Frédéric Chopin and Niccolò Paganini; artists Amedeo Modigliani, Paul Gauguin, and Aubrey Beardsley; and philosophers Baruch Spinoza and Voltaire.

Today it is clear that TB killed so many artists and thinkers simply because it was the major killer of all people. But during the 1800's, the lack of understanding about what caused the disease led some people to the erroneous conclusion that there was a link between TB and creativity. Early historians thought TB might be an inherited trait that appeared in geniuses. Others theorized that whatever caused TB secreted substances that stimulated mental activity. Writing in 1925, a historian described the belief that mild cases of TB stimulated parts of the body that accounted for "the enjoyment of life." In the minds of many, the disease thus "enabled poets to sing more sweetly, musicians to give finer music to the world, artists to portray life on their canvasses more clearly."

These theories led to one of the oddest periods in social history, when many people embraced the notion of having a fatal disease, and some artists came to feel that having TB was virtually a requirement. In the 1800's, the French author Théophile Gautier wrote, "When I was young, I could not have accepted as a lyrical poet anyone weighing more than ninety-nine pounds," referring to the underweight condition associated with consumption. Shelley once reassured the stricken Keats that "this consumption is a disease particularly fond of people who write such good verses as you have done." Alexandre Dumas, a French author whose works include *The Three Musketeers* (1844), wrote that in the 1820's "it was good form to spit blood after each emotion that was at all sensational and to die before reaching the age of 30." In 1828, Byron said that he wished he would die of consumption "because the ladies would all say, 'Look at that poor Byron, how interesting he looks in dying.'"

The "fashionable" disease

In the 1800's, when the cause of TB was a mystery, the disease was glamorized in arts and literature. The pale and delicate appearance of the TB sufferer was considered an outward sign of the person's inner refinement of spirit and sensibility.

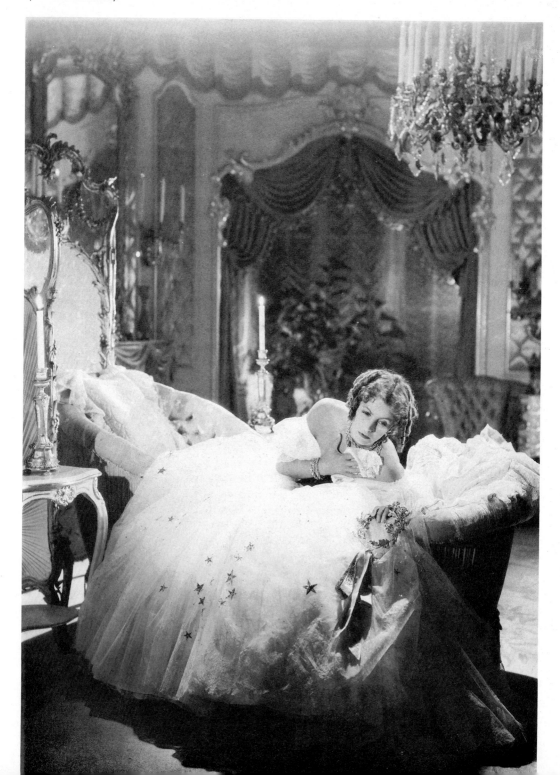

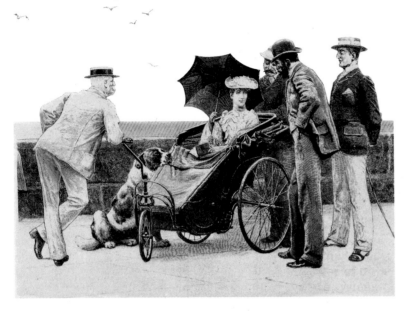

A star-bedecked Greta Garbo, *opposite page*, portrays an ethereal beauty dying of TB in the 1936 movie version of *Camille,* Alexandre Dumas's 1852 play. Fashionable and aristocratic-looking convalescents are depicted in engravings made in 1892, *left,* and 1901, *below.*

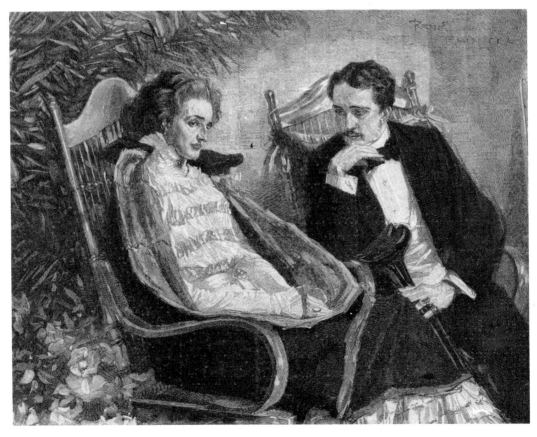

Although society embraced some aspects of the illness, victims were still subject to discrimination and even physical violence. Paganini was thrown out into the street when his landlord guessed the musician had TB. Chopin, who fought TB for most of his life, caused a wave of panic on the Mediterranean island of Majorca when he moved there in the 1830's.

Such reactions were of course rooted in the suspicion that TB, like plague, was contagious. Although the Greek philosopher Aristotle had suggested in the 300's B.C. that TB could be spread from a sick person to a well one, the idea went in and out of fashion as the centuries passed. In the 1500's, physicians again began to insist that TB was contagious, and regulations were enacted in some places to prevent its spread by infection. By the 1600's, however, European medical authorities, noting that TB often affected several members of the same family, concluded that the disease was inherited.

The heredity theory did not fall until 1865 when Jean Antoine Villemin, a French military surgeon, demonstrated that TB could pass from a man to a rabbit—an indication that a disease-causing microbe was transferred. The next major breakthrough in understanding TB came in 1882, when the German scientist Robert Koch identified the microbe as a rod-shaped bacterium, the tubercle bacillus.

Koch's work for the first time provided humanity with a realistic understanding of TB. Today we know that in human beings TB is caused by two strains of the bacteria species *Mycobacterium tuberculosis*. These bacteria are usually transmitted from person to person by airborne droplets. Typically, a patient whose lungs are infected will by coughing spread the infection to others who breathe the contaminated air. The disease is only mildly contagious, so those at greatest risk of contracting TB are people who live in very crowded conditions—generally the poor. Because livestock are also susceptible to TB, contaminated foods, such as unpasteurized milk, can also provide a vehicle for infection. In developed countries, however, where animals are tested for infection and milk is pasteurized, infection from contaminated foods rarely occurs.

The course of a TB infection has two phases. In the initial phase, the bacteria are thwarted by the body's disease-fighting immune system, which does not kill the bacteria but surrounds them with tough capsules of scar tissue known as *tubercles*. The great majority of people infected with the bacte-

"Nature's cure"

Resortlike facilities called sanitariums became the most popular mode of treatment for TB patients in the late 1800's and early 1900's. Sanitariums promoted fresh air—no matter how harsh the climate—as a means of "drying out" congested lungs. Whether such treatment actually helped people is unclear.

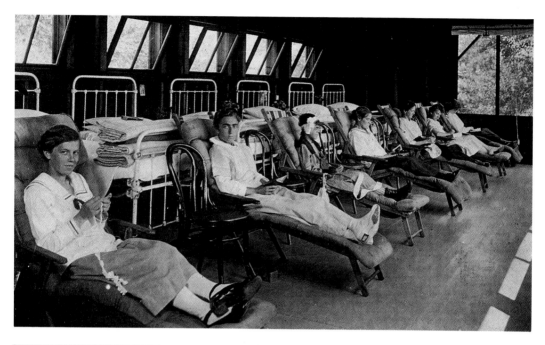

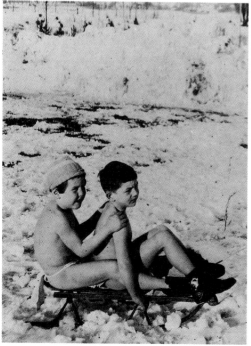

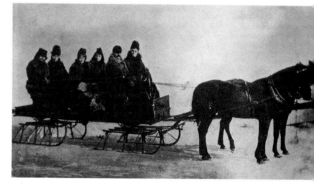

Turn-of-the-century TB sufferers, *top,* rest in open-air barracks at a sanitarium, while young patients play virtually unclothed in the snow, *left.* In an 1886 photograph taken at the first American sanitarium, at Saranac Lake in upstate New York, patients begin an outing in the dead of winter, *above.*

Desperate measures

Until a drug to combat the bacterium that causes TB was discovered in 1943, physicians had little to offer patients other than fresh air or some means of manipulating or stimulating the lungs. Some of these treatments may have provided relief; others were outright frauds.

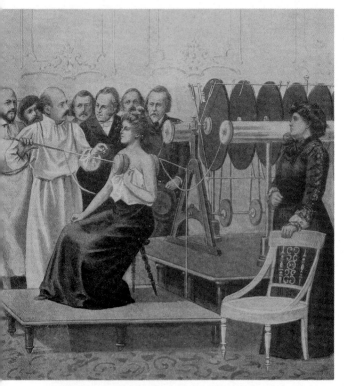

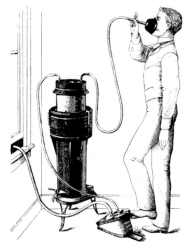

A turn-of-the-century illustration depicts a bizarre treatment for tuberculosis: the application of an electrical contraption to the patient's chest, *left*. An 1891 engraving shows a TB sufferer using a compressed-air apparatus, *above*. Pneumothorax, *below*, a surgical procedure developed in the 1890's and widely used in the 1930's and early 1940's, pumped air into the chest cavity to collapse one lung, resting it temporarily and perhaps slowing the growth of TB bacteria.

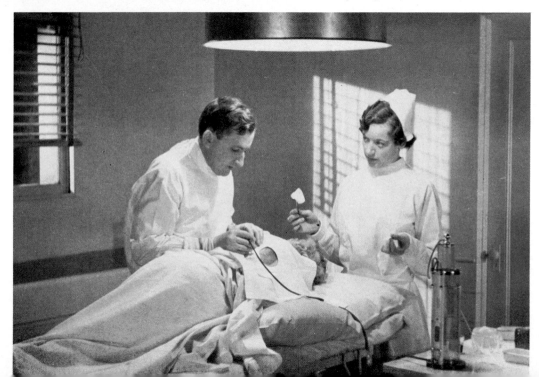

ria never progress beyond this stage and remain healthy and symptom-free. In some of those infected, the bacteria break out of the tubercles months or even years after the primary infection, an action that begins the second phase of the disease. The bacteria may then enter the bloodstream and spread to other organs throughout the body. In advanced stages of untreated TB, the bacteria may destroy the function of infected organs to the point of death.

Koch also attempted to concoct a cure from preparations of the bacteria, but these efforts failed. He did succeed, however, in developing a skin test to detect a person exposed to the bacillus, and for this and his other work on TB he won a Nobel Prize in 1905. As other researchers refined it over the decades, this skin test became a widely used method for screening the general population for infection. A small amount of *tuberculin* (a liquid made from the bacillus) is injected under the skin. Developing a swelling or other reaction at the site of the injection indicates that the person has been exposed to the bacillus, even though he or she may not have the active disease.

A second important method of TB detection was the X ray, developed in 1895 by the German physicist Wilhelm Konrad Roentgen. Beginning in 1936, after a way of producing X-ray film at low cost was discovered, chest X rays were given to large groups of people to detect tubercles on the lungs at an early stage. Today, because we know that the radiation from having many X rays can slightly increase a person's risk of developing cancer, X rays are used only to look for lung damage in people who have a positive TB skin test, rather than as a means of screening the general population. A laboratory examination of the person's *sputum* (saliva mixed with mucus coughed up from the respiratory tract, commonly called *phlegm*) can often verify that the patient has the disease.

Finding effective treatments for patients with active TB proved more difficult than developing ways of detecting those who had been infected. In the 1890's, an Italian physician named Carlo Forlanini pioneered surgical *pneumothorax*, a procedure in which air is pumped into the chest cavity, forcing a lung to collapse. Pneumothorax became a widely practiced, and somewhat effective, method of treatment because collapsing a diseased lung allowed it to rest and for a time deprived the bacillus of the oxygen it needed to thrive. By the early 1940's, collapse therapy was given to about 70 per cent of TB patients.

A real breakthrough in treatment did not come until 1943, when biologist Selman A. Waksman of Rutgers University in New Brunswick, N.J., discovered streptomycin, the first antibi-

Dawn of understanding

"I have undertaken my investigations in the interests of public health," wrote the German scientist Robert Koch when he began studying tuberculosis in 1881. Koch's work eliminated many of the misconceptions about TB and earned him a Nobel Prize in 1905.

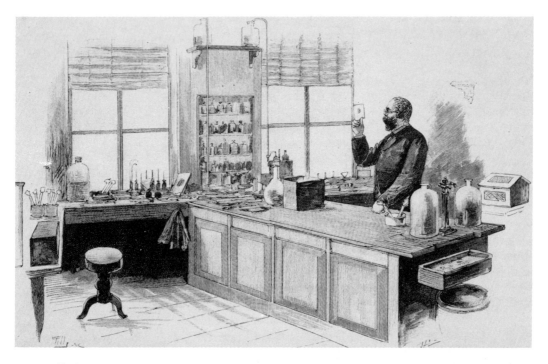

Koch, *above,* discovered that TB was caused by a bacterium and could be spread from person to person. He developed and tested an experimental TB vaccine, *right.* The attempt failed, but the work led to the development of the TB skin test, *opposite page,* which is still used for diagnosis of the disease.

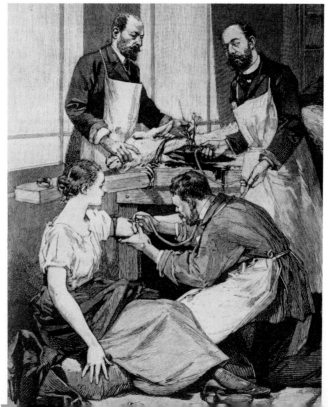

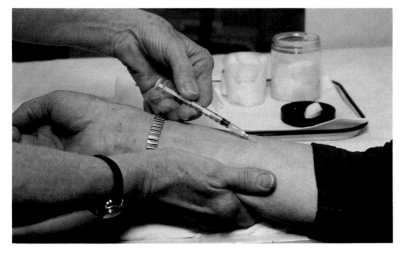

The TB skin test involves injecting *tuberculin,* a preparation made from killed tuberculosis bacteria, under the skin. A swelling at the site of the injection indicates that the person has been infected in the past, but it does not necessarily mean that the person has an active case of TB.

otic effective against the disease. The TB death rate immediately dropped, and Waksman won a Nobel Prize for his discovery in 1952.

That same year, isoniazid, another effective drug for TB patients, was introduced, and the death rate declined even more sharply. During the 1950's, the overall death rate from TB for children under age 15 dropped 88 per cent in the United States and more than 90 per cent in Canada, England, France, and Wales. The death rate for people age 15 and older dropped 68 per cent in the United States during the same period. Similar drops were reported in other developed countries. The need for hospital treatment was reduced, and sanitariums began to close or were converted to other purposes. Newer antibiotics such as rifampin proved to be even more effective in treating TB. The disease seemed to be conquered.

But one of the tragic ironies about TB is that hundreds of thousands of people still die of it every year. The problem is most severe in the developing world, where drugs are difficult to obtain.

A vaccine for TB is available, but it has met with only limited success. Called BCG, the vaccine was developed by researchers Albert Calmette and Camille Guérin at the Pasteur Institute in Lille, France, and was first administered in humans in 1921. Different preparations of the vaccine vary in their effectiveness, however, and in rare instances they can cause complications. In the United States, where there is a low risk of catching the disease, the vaccine is rarely used. Sadly, in the developing world, where the risk of TB is high

TB today

Despite the existence of treatments, TB remains a major health threat—especially in developing countries, where poor sanitation and overcrowding are problems. Even in industrialized nations such as the United States, however, TB still strikes thousands.

Reported annual number of cases of TB, worldwide*	
Africa	115,495
Americas	224,903
Europe	283,308
Middle East	209,541
Southeast Asia	1,100,339
Western Pacific	582,758

*Statistics are for 1984, with 84 per cent of nations reporting. The actual number of cases may be three to four times higher.

Source: World Health Organization.

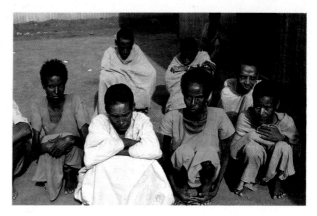

Tuberculosis is especially severe in developing nations, *above*. Ethiopians with advanced cases of TB, some too feeble to stand, await treatment, *above right*.

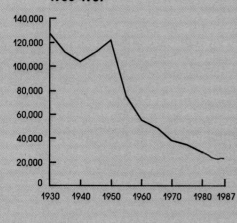

Annual number of cases of TB in the United States 1930-1987

Source: Centers for Disease Control.

1980-1987

In the United States, improvements in sanitation brought a gradual reduction in the incidence of TB, *above*. But the number of cases began to rise in the late 1980's, *above right*, fueled by increases among recent immigrants, prison inmates, AIDS patients, the homeless, and the urban poor. A TB sufferer is examined in an inner-city clinic, *right*.

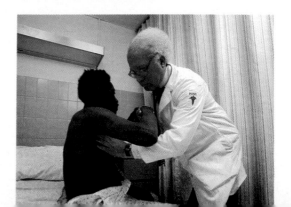

enough to justify its widespread use, the vaccine, like the cure, is difficult to obtain.

A postscript to the story of TB is its recent reemergence as a public health problem in the United States. In 1986, cases of the disease increased for the first time in the three decades since complete national records have been kept. Epidemiologists at the federal Centers for Disease Control in Atlanta, Ga., say that TB has "tremendous potential" for becoming an even larger problem. Many experts think that cases of TB will continue to increase, fed largely by the AIDS epidemic. People with AIDS are especially susceptible to the bacillus because their immune systems are impaired. Immigration from developing countries where TB is not controlled contributes to the problem, as does poverty, with its attendant overcrowding and malnutrition.

It is not unheard of for U.S. TB patients, like those in the developing world, to die of the disease. Nearly 1,800 people died of tuberculosis in the United States in 1986, the latest year for which complete death-rate statistics have been compiled. Many TB sufferers die because they are impoverished and out of the reach of medical care. Another problem is the difficulty of getting patients who do seek treatment to complete it—which may require taking daily doses of antibiotics for as long as two years. New York City's health commissioner reported in 1988 that 60 per cent of the TB patients admitted to that city's public hospitals never complete their treatment. Newly developed regimens that attempt to shorten the course of treatment may eventually solve this problem.

It's clear that the battle against this old-fashioned-sounding disease is ongoing. More than a century after its cause was discovered, researchers are still trying to answer some basic questions about the disease. Why does the infection progress rapidly in some people, but does not develop into the second phase in most patients? Why do the majority of TB cases involve people in whom the bacteria remained dormant for years before causing illness? And what other factors influence the behavior of the bacteria?

The battle against misconceptions about TB also continues. Few people idealize TB victims today, but many are unnecessarily frightened of them. And members of the general population are not the only ones who harbor false notions about TB. One of the greatest worries of public health officials is that some physicians, assuming TB was conquered long ago, are not taking the disease as seriously as they should. Like the bacillus itself, which can lie dormant in the body for years before suddenly bursting forth, TB has proved to be a stubborn and long-lived scourge.

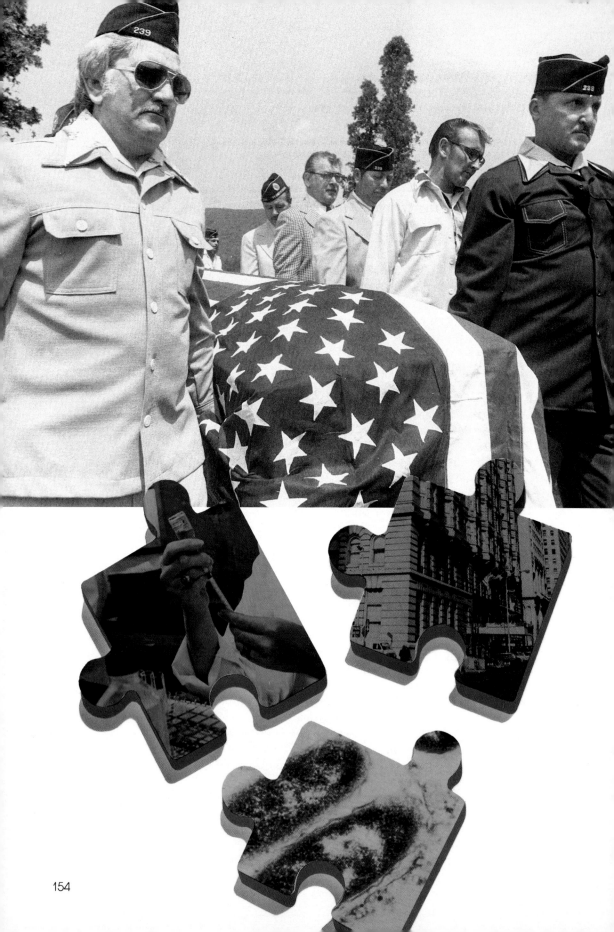

The Puzzle of Legionnaires' Disease

By John Camper

What caused the deadly disease that surfaced at a 1976 American Legion convention? It took the largest epidemiological investigation in U.S. history to find out.

On Sunday, Aug. 1, 1976, Edward T. Hoak, an official of the American Legion in Pennsylvania, received unsettling news. Several Pennsylvania members of the American Legion had suddenly become ill, and two had died.

Alarmed, he called Legion posts around the state and received more bad news: At least five Legionnaires in Pennsylvania cities had been killed by a strange illness. They had been stricken with fever as high as 107°F. (42°C), a dry cough, headache, chills, muscle aches, and chest pain. These symptoms appeared to be those of pneumonia—an inflammation of the lungs usually caused by viruses, bacteria, or other infectious agents. The Legionnaires' physicians hospitalized them, placed them under oxygen tents, and prescribed antibiotics such as penicillin. But nothing had seemed to help.

As Hoak tallied the names of the ill and the dead, he realized that all the victims had one thing in common: They had attended the Legion's state convention, which had been held in downtown Philadelphia two weeks earlier.

Early Monday morning, Hoak conferred with the Pennsylvania Department of Health, which immediately issued a state-

Opposite page: Members of the American Legion bear the coffin of fellow Legionnaire J. B. Ralph at his Aug. 5, 1976, funeral in Williamstown, Pa. Ralph was one of 34 people killed by a mysterious illness.

wide health alert. One of those notified was Leonard Bachman, Pennsylvania's secretary of health. Bachman promptly contacted the Centers for Disease Control (CDC) in Atlanta, Ga., the federal agency that investigates epidemics and unexplained illnesses.

Officials at the CDC gave immediate attention to the report because they feared it might be the beginning of an epidemic of swine flu, a particularly deadly type of *influenza* (a highly contagious viral infection that affects the respiratory system) thought to originate in pigs. Some health experts had been predicting such an outbreak for six months, ever since a young Army recruit in New Jersey died of swine flu. This was a serious matter: A similar type of flu killed 10 million people worldwide in 1918 and 1919.

The CDC put together the largest epidemic investigation team it had ever assembled—comprising 23 experts, who began traveling to Harrisburg, the capital of Pennsylvania, the same day. "I came in with the belief that the most important thing to determine was whether or not this was swine flu," said David W. Fraser, an epidemiologist who led the CDC team. "If it was swine flu, it might have been the beginning of a worldwide epidemic."

Upon arrival in Pennsylvania, Fraser and the other investigators were confronted with an ominous set of statistics. Bachman's office had confirmed 18 cases of the disease, 6 of them fatal. American Legion officials knew of 49 cases, 14 of them fatal—and new cases were being reported by the hour. By Tuesday, authorities had confirmed 20 deaths and 135 cases.

The investigation quickly moved into high gear, beginning the biggest epidemiological inquiry in U.S. history. The investigation had two parts. A group of state and federal scientists performed laboratory tests on blood, throat cultures, feces, and urine from living victims and on tissue samples removed during autopsies of the dead. Their aim was to find and identify a microbe—a bacterium, virus, or other organism too small to be seen with the naked eye—or poison in the victims' bodies. Some of the specimens were tested in Philadelphia labs and others were shipped to the CDC labs in Atlanta.

Because looking for microscopic evidence of the thousands of possible causes of the disease was difficult and time-consuming, a second group of epidemiologists tried a different approach. They looked for overall patterns in the spread of the disease in order to discover what the victims had in common. If these "disease detectives" found that all the victims had eaten a certain food, for example, the lab workers could narrow their search to microbes typical in food poisoning.

The epidemiologists' first order of business was finding out

The author:

John Camper is a reporter for the *Chicago Tribune.*

156

who had developed the disease, and where and when they had taken ill. Authorities set up a telephone hot line and asked people to report any instance of a pneumonialike illness. Some 300 state and local public health workers also fanned out across Pennsylvania to search for cases. The epidemiologists' second step was finding the people in similar circumstances who did not get ill.

"You need to know what the sick people did that was different from those who did not get sick," said Fraser. "Finding the 'non-cases' turned out to be a very tricky issue, because the American Legion didn't have a list of who was at the convention and who wasn't." So the investigators sent packets of questionnaires to all 1,002 state Legion posts. The Legionnaires were asked whether they had gone to the convention, what they had done there, and whether they had become ill.

One of the first discoveries the disease detectives made was that the epidemic appeared to be slowing down. The number of new cases fell off sharply after July 25 through 27, when 79 people came down with the disease. Furthermore, the epidemiologists discovered that the only family members of Legionnaires who became ill had been at the convention, indicating that the disease did not spread from one person to another. People who worked in the hotels and businesses in downtown Philadelphia that had been frequented by the Legionnaires were not getting sick either.

The information was of critical importance, according to Fraser. "That led us to have some confidence that the epidemic was a local phenomenon that was not going to become national," he said. When the number of new cases began dropping, health officials realized they weren't going to have to shut down businesses in downtown Philadelphia.

The absence of person-to-person spread of the disease seemed to reduce the likelihood that they were dealing with the swine flu, but investigators still waited anxiously to see if laboratory tests uncovered a virus—if not the virus that causes swine flu, then perhaps one that causes pneumonia. Using a test commonly used to isolate influenza viruses so that they can be examined and identified, lab technicians injected ground-up tissue from the disease victims into fertilized chicken eggs. If viruses—which grow only in living cells— were present in the specimen, they would multiply within the eggs. This procedure, known as *culturing*, allows a tiny amount of viruses in a specimen to increase in number until they are more easily detectable. The scientists then withdrew fluid from the eggs and mixed it with red blood cells because if flu viruses are present, the blood cells will visibly clump to-gether. But in test after test, the cells failed to clump. The mystery disease was not the swine flu.

The lab workers then performed tests to detect the pres-ence of other types of viruses. Again, the results were nega-tive. The disease did not appear to be caused by a virus. The investigators were relieved to be able to rule out swine flu, but they were discouraged that the disease did not lend itself to an easy identification.

Now the laboratory scientists considered the possibility that the disease was caused by a bacterium. In contrast to viruses, most bacteria are rather easily isolated and identified. A sam-ple of diseased tissue is mounted on a microscope slide and treated with one of several colored stains that adhere only to bacteria. Usually, when such a slide is examined under a mi-croscope, the bacteria are easily detected because the stained bacterial cells are a different color from the tissue cells. But when tissue specimens from the Legionnaires were treated with the commonly used stains, no bacteria were visible.

The scientists also attempted to culture any bacteria that were in the specimens. Most bacteria can be cultured in non-living substances, such as nutrient broth, blood serum, and *agar*, a gel made from seaweed. But when specimens were added to these substances, nothing grew.

After virtually ruling out viruses and common types of bac-teria, the laboratory investigators considered the possibility that the culprit was a *rickettsia*. These microorganisms are parasites similar in some ways to bacteria, but they are smaller and must be cultured in living media. One candidate, a rickettsial disease called *Q fever*, which is caused by inhal-ing infected dust or drinking tainted milk, has symptoms simi-lar to the Legionnaires' and seemed a reasonable possibility. Laboratory workers thus performed the standard tests for iso-lating rickettsia, which involved culturing the specimens in guinea pigs as well as staining the specimens and then exam-ining them under a microscope. But these procedures failed to turn up any rickettsia.

The researchers also performed tests to detect *fungi*, tiny plantlike organisms. Again, the tests were negative.

Within two weeks, then—with the number of cases now totaling 169—the CDC investigators had ruled out all known microbes and were forced to consider that the Legionnaires might have been poisoned by some toxic substance. But searching for a toxin was a daunting task. There are literally thousands of poisonous substances, and detecting them re-quires thousands of different tests.

Despite the difficulties, investigators quickly ruled out 17

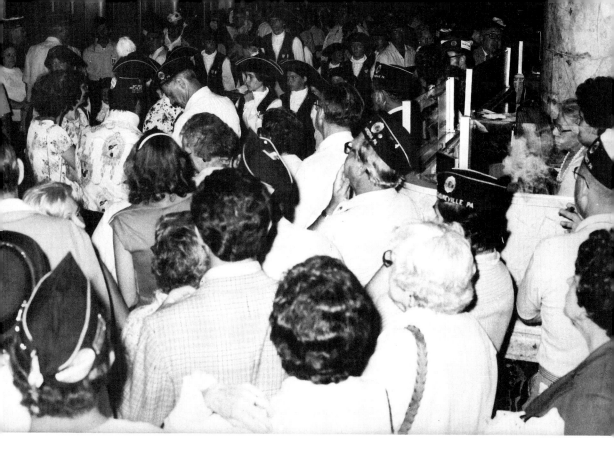

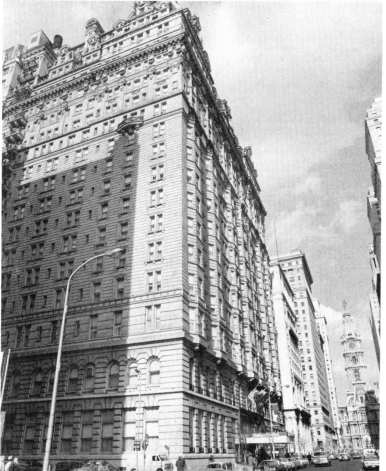

The first clue
Health authorities quickly realize that those who were stricken with the mysterious illness had recently attended an American Legion convention in Philadelphia, *above*. Most of the Legionnaires had stayed at the Bellevue Stratford hotel in downtown Philadelphia, *left*.

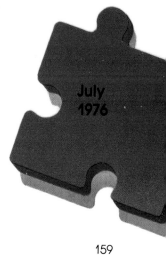

July 1976

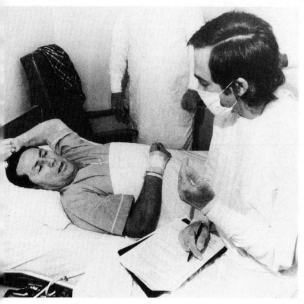
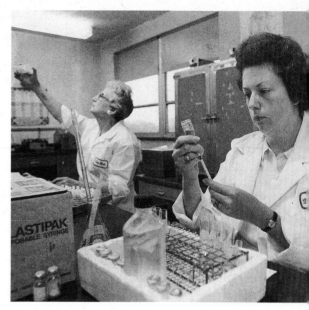

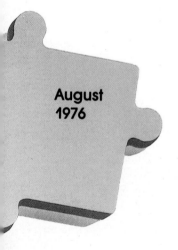

**August
1976**

metals, including arsenic and mercury and even silver and
gold. As they continued to test for the presence of toxins in
the tissue taken from the victims, one chemical became a
prime suspect. F. William Sunderman, director of the Institute
for Clinical Sciences in Philadelphia, and his son, F. William
Sunderman, Jr., a professor of laboratory medicine at the University of Connecticut Medical School in Farmington, noted
that the symptoms of the Legionnaires closely resembled those
of people who have been poisoned by nickel carbonyl, a chemical used to make certain plastics and paints.

Most of the investigators were skeptical about this possibility, however, because nickel carbonyl was seldom used even
in manufacturing, and they could not imagine why it would
have appeared in downtown Philadelphia in large enough
amounts to cause illness and death. But when the younger
Sunderman tested tissue samples of the victims, he found high
levels of nickel carbonyl. Unfortunately, he also found high
levels in samples of tissues from people who had died of other
causes. He concluded that the tissue samples had all been
contaminated, possibly by surgical knives containing nickel.
Looking for uncontaminated samples and testing them for
nickel carbonyl dragged on for weeks, and eventually the
chemical was ruled out.

By this time—the middle of September, six weeks after the
investigation had begun and one month after the last new case
had been reported—it appeared that the search was going to
be much more difficult than almost anyone had expected. The
course and symptoms of the disease had begun to resemble

previous epidemics that had proved impossible to explain. One was an outbreak of pneumonia at St. Elizabeth's Hospital in Washington, D.C., that killed 14 people and infected 67 others in 1965. Another occurred in 1968, when an outbreak of high fever, headache, and muscle aches at a county health department building in Pontiac, Mich., sickened 95 people, all of whom recovered.

During the Legionnaires' disease investigation, doctors also learned of a similar unexplained illness that struck at least 18 people and killed 2 during a convention of the Independent Association of Odd Fellows in Philadelphia in 1974. Interestingly, the Odd Fellows had stayed at the same hotel that was headquarters for the American Legion convention, the Bellevue Stratford.

While laboratory workers did the frustrating work of performing test after test, always with negative results, the epidemiologists had continued to gather information from the victims and their families, looking for patterns that would provide a clue to the nature of the illness. They asked question after question: At what hotel did you stay during the convention? Where and what did you eat? Did you watch the parade—and if you did, where did you stand? Did you drink the water in your hotel? Were you bitten by an insect?

The investigators then fed the answers into computers linked with the Pennsylvania Department of Health in Harrisburg and the CDC in Atlanta. Computers are useful tools in such investigations because they help uncover patterns in seemingly random information. And the computer analysis turned up an important finding: All the victims had either stayed at the Bellevue Stratford or spent a considerable

Deserted hotel
After the investigation fingers the Bellevue Stratford as the likely source of the illness, the hotel's business fails, as a nearly deserted dining room testifies. The hotel closed on Nov. 18, 1976.

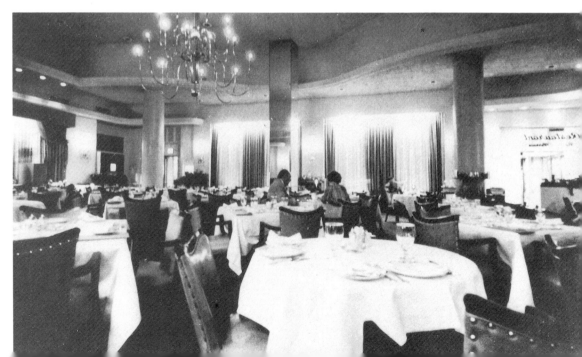

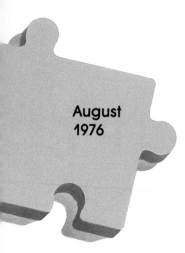

August 1976

A case of poisoning?
After laboratory tests rule out all known microbes, laboratory pathologist F. William Sunderman, Jr., finds a poison called nickel carbonyl in tissue samples from victims of the mystery disease. But he also detects traces of the compound in tissue samples from people who had not developed Legionnaires' disease. The likely explanation: Nickel-containing surgical knives had contaminated all the samples.

amount of time in the hotel or on Broad Street outside it.

The epidemiologists also discovered that those who became ill were more likely than nonvictims to have visited a hospitality room on the 14th floor of the Bellevue Stratford, to have drunk water at the hotel, and to have spent some time in the hotel lobby. Among those who watched a Legion parade on July 23, those who contracted the disease were more likely to have watched from directly in front of the hotel. But, surprisingly, the data showed that only one hotel employee, an air-conditioner repairman, had contracted the disease.

The evidence implicating the Bellevue Stratford was so overwhelming that the epidemiologists decided to make the hotel part of their definition of the disease. The 182 people who contracted the illness and had attended the Legion convention or entered the Bellevue Stratford were described as victims of *Legionnaires' disease*. The 39 victims who had been within one block of the Bellevue Stratford but had not entered the hotel or been a part of the convention were considered victims of *Broad Street pneumonia*.

Searching for more clues, the investigators swarmed over the hotel. They checked the cleaning agents used by the maids and the pesticides used by exterminators. They scraped dust out of the ventilating system and paint off the walls. They asked survivors to return to the hotel to retrace their steps throughout the entire four-day convention. The medical sleuths inspected the hotel's kitchen, the water supply, the ice machines, and the heating and air-conditioning systems.

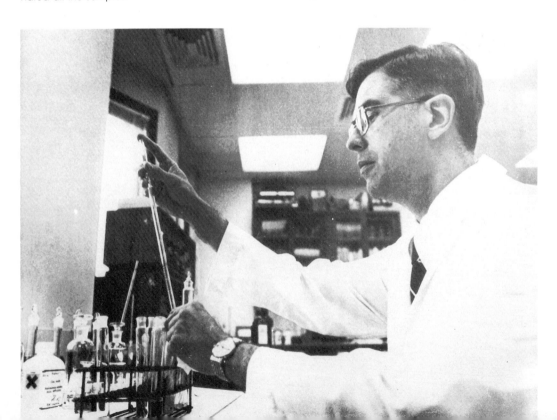

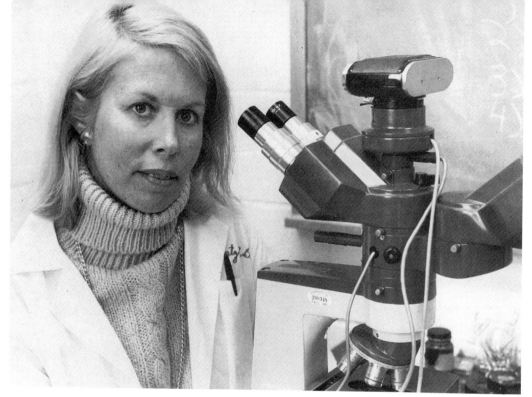

The presence of pigeons on the roof of the hotel set off a new line of inquiry. Some investigators wondered if the birds might be the key to this frustrating mystery: Could the pigeons have transmitted *psittacosis*, or parrot fever, to some of the hotel's guests? Psittacosis, caused by a type of rickettsia called *chlamydia* and carried by birds, indeed produces symptoms similar to those of Legionnaires' disease.

The psittacosis connection became even stronger at the end of September, when Sheila Moriber Katz, a pathologist at Hahnemann Medical College in Philadelphia, became ill with symptoms like those of Legionnaires' disease two weeks after examining a piece of lung tissue from a Legionnaire. In press interviews, Katz speculated that Legionnaires' disease was psittacosis, and a blood test showed that she had had the disease. Laboratory workers quickly set about testing the blood of Legionnaires' disease victims for chlamydia. But, once again, the tests were negative.

This appeared to be the last truly compelling lead. The epidemiologists and their computers had unearthed interesting evidence—pinpointing the source of the disease so convincingly that the Bellevue Stratford closed on November 18 because few people would risk staying there—but the laboratory scientists could not find the killer.

As the investigation stalled, thousands of citizens wrote to the Pennsylvania health department or called the hot line with their own diagnoses. Bachman received hundreds of letters from people who were sure they could solve the mystery. One

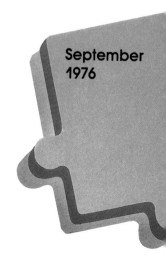

September 1976

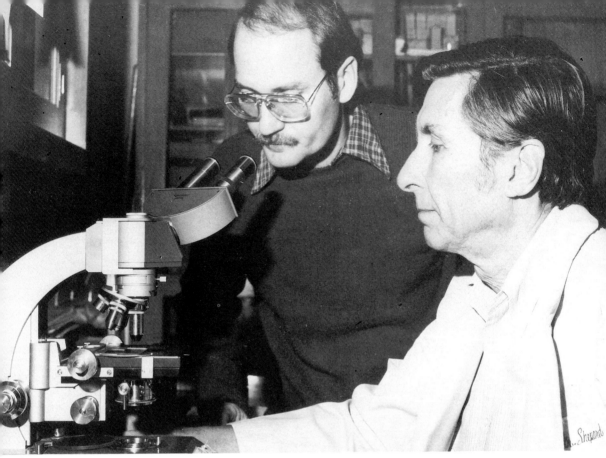

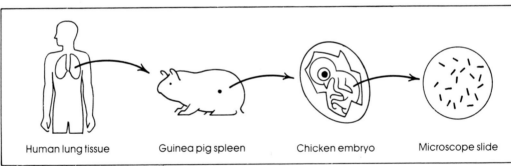

| Human lung tissue | Guinea pig spleen | Chicken embryo | Microscope slide |

The culprit tracked down at last

Researchers Joseph E. McDade and Charles C. Shepard, *top,* stumble across the cause of Legionnaires' disease using a procedure normally used to isolate microbes that grow only inside living cells. First, *above,* the researchers injected guinea pigs with a solution containing ground-up lung tissue from a victim of Legionnaires' disease. After the animals became ill, their spleens were removed and a bit of this tissue was injected into fertilized chicken eggs. After the chicken embryos died, the researchers placed pieces of the eggs' yolk-sac membranes on microscope slides and stained them. When viewed through a microscope, the membranes were found to contain clusters of a previously unknown rod-shaped bacterium, *right,* now called *Legionella pneumophila.*

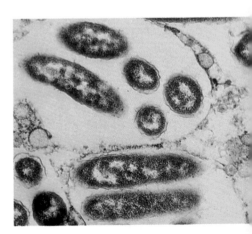

man claimed that by manipulating numbers after a "mystical experience," he had come to the conclusion that the disease originated in the African country of Zaire. Other citizens suspected that foreign terrorists had struck the American Legion using a secret, undetectable chemical or germ.

Few if any of these notions were plausible, and, by the end of the year, the investigators were dispirited at their lack of success. The epidemic, which had struck 221 people and killed 34, was now long over. The entire investigation had been under a media spotlight for months, with every false lead documented on television and in newspapers and magazines.

At a Christmas party, one of the CDC's laboratory scientists, Joseph E. McDade, listened to an acquaintance berating the CDC for its inability to solve the mystery. McDade, who had tried to find out whether the disease was caused by rickettsia, had eventually given up and gone on to other things.

During the post-holiday lull, McDade decided to take a closer look at the microscope slides from his Legionnaires' disease investigation. In August, he had ground up a piece of diseased lung tissue and injected it into the abdomens of guinea pigs, which soon developed fevers. But when he stained pieces of the guinea pigs' spleens and examined them under a microscope, he had found no evidence of rickettsia.

Now McDade brought out the same slides and began to examine them again, hoping to find a microorganism that had picked up the red stain. As he looked, he slowly moved a slide

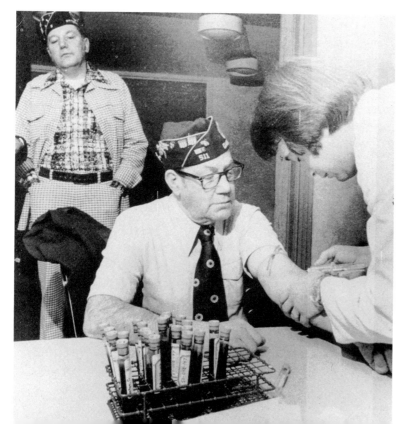

The last piece of the puzzle
A Legionnaire's blood is drawn so that it can be tested for the presence of antibodies to the newly discovered bacterium, *Legionella pneumophila.* Such testing proves conclusively that the bacterium caused the disease.

under his microscope, a process he compared to "searching for a missing contact lens on a basketball court with your eyes 4 inches away from the floor."

Suddenly a cluster of red rods appeared. "After looking for hours and seeing nothing but the blue-green background, the red cluster just jumped out at me," recalled McDade. He had never seen microbes that shape and size before. They were larger than rickettsia, and they had pointed ends rather than the round or square ends typical of rod-shaped bacteria.

Could this be the agent behind Legionnaires' disease, or was it just another false lead? First it would be necessary to culture the microbe. To accomplish this, McDade and his associate, Charles C. Shepard, injected a piece of guinea pig spleen, which had been kept frozen since August, into fertilized chicken eggs. The egg embryos died in a few days, and when McDade stained pieces of their yolk-sac membranes and then examined them under a microscope, he found more red rods.

Next, they had to show that the Legionnaires had been infected with this organism. McDade and Shepard tested a blood sample from a victim to see whether it contained antibodies—disease-fighting proteins formed by the body in response to an invader—for the new-found microbe. Good news at last: This test was positive. Blood from other victims also tested positive. And there were no such antibodies in blood samples from people who had not had the disease.

But this meant only that the Legionnaires had once come in contact with the organism. Determining whether this microbe had caused the particular illness that struck the victims the previous summer was another matter. To prove this, the scientists tested blood samples taken during various stages of the victims' convalescence. If the organism had caused the disease, the levels of antibodies would have risen during the course of the illness. Tests proved this was indeed the case.

They had found the killer.

Intrigued by the similarity of the Legionnaires' disease outbreak to other unexplained epidemics, the CDC tested blood samples from victims of the epidemics at St. Elizabeth's Hospital, the Pontiac health department, and the Odd Fellows convention. These samples also contained antibodies to the newly discovered microbe. This organism, eventually classified as a bacterium, had been killing people for years.

How had it eluded discovery for so long? No one can fault the laboratory investigators for failing to discover it sooner; the bacterium is like no other in many ways. Because the antibiotics usually given to patients with bacterial pneumonia had not helped the Legionnaires, the scientists were predisposed to think that a virus, rather than a bacterium, caused the illness. In addition, the bacterium (which was given the scientific name *Legionella pneumophila*) does not absorb the stains commonly used to detect bacteria. Nor does it grow in the media that scientists typically use for culturing bacteria.

After the bacterium was identified, scientists continued to study it and have developed methods of quickly diagnosing Legionnaires' disease. Although the bacteria are not vulnerable to penicillin, two other antibiotics, erythromycin and rifampin, are effective in treating it.

Scientists have discovered that these bacteria live in almost every lake and river, usually in numbers so small that they do not constitute a health threat. They can thrive, though, in fairly warm water—which can be found in cooling towers, humidifiers, reservoirs, even shower heads—and be spread through air-conditioning systems or any other mechanism that transports minute droplets of water through the air.

Although investigators were never able to recover *Legionella pneumophila* in the Bellevue Stratford, they nonetheless believe that the bacteria grew in the water in a rooftop cooling tower for the hotel's air-conditioning system and were spread throughout the hotel with the cooled air. They aren't sure why some people were infected and others weren't, but they suspect that many hotel employees had developed a natural immunity to the disease through previous exposure. Now it becomes apparent why the only employee to become ill was an air-conditioning repairman who did not work at the hotel consistently enough to have developed immunity, and who had close contact with the suspected source of infection.

Health experts believe that 25,000 to 50,000 of the 2.4 million cases of pneumonia diagnosed in the United States each year are actually cases of Legionnaires' disease, or, as it is sometimes called, *legionellosis*. Many physicians now suspect Legionnaires' disease when their patients develop a pneumonialike illness. Fatal outbreaks hit Burlington, Vt., in 1977 and Bloomington, Ind., in 1978. The worst epidemic since the bacterium was identified occurred in May 1985 in Stafford, England, where the disease struck 150 people, killing 34.

Although *Legionella pneumophila* probably never will be eradicated, the danger of future epidemics can be lessened by keeping cooling towers clean, health experts say. But they would prefer to find better methods to prevent outbreaks. Before they can do so they must determine exactly what set of circumstances causes the bacteria to multiply into a life-threatening force. That aspect of Legionnaires' disease remains a mystery.

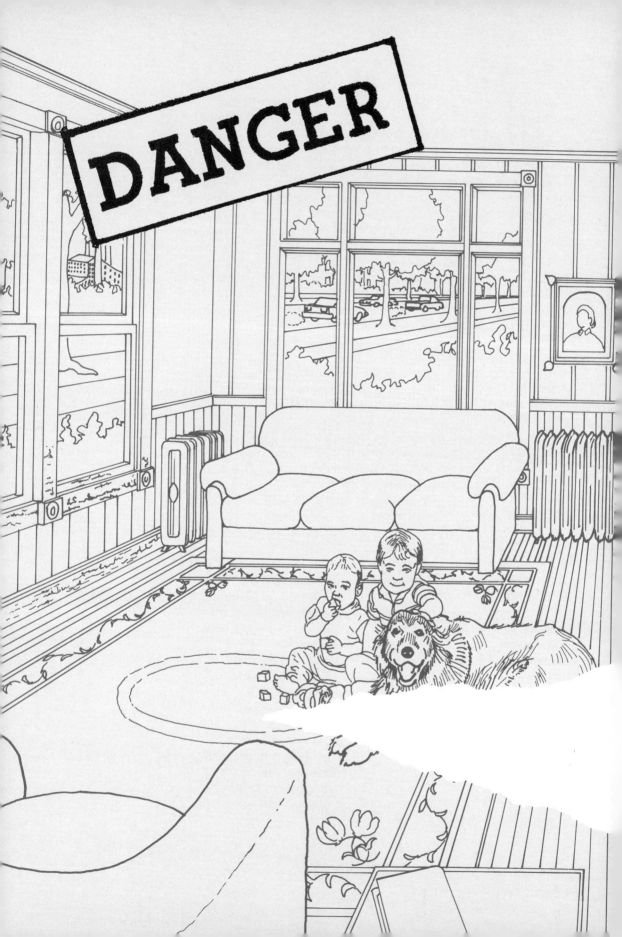

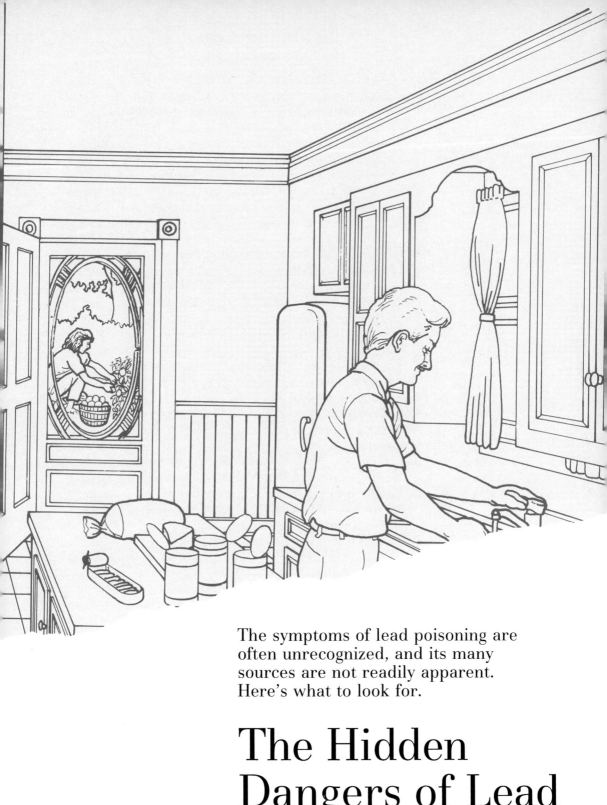

The symptoms of lead poisoning are often unrecognized, and its many sources are not readily apparent. Here's what to look for.

The Hidden Dangers of Lead

By Jan Ziegler

A 2-year-old Baltimore girl's toddling exploration of the world came to an abrupt halt in September 1987. She refused to walk or stand—unable, it seemed, to bear any weight on her legs at all. She also appeared to be in pain.

Doctors at a medical center clinic suspected her symptoms might be a reaction to an immunization for diphtheria that she had received five days earlier. They also knew that their young patient had a hereditary blood disorder called *sickle cell anemia*, an illness that sometimes makes joints and bones ache. Perhaps, they thought, the blood disorder might be playing a role in the child's condition.

But these suspected causes still did not fully explain the child's refusal to walk, and the doctors were puzzled. They decided to send her to another clinic for a series of X rays.

Meanwhile, in Jersey City, N.J., a man named Douglas was also experiencing some puzzling symptoms after spending several weekends restoring an 1840's row house. Starting in the morning and finishing up at midnight—wearing a dust mask that covered his mouth and nose—he had been burning off old interior paint with a device that resembled a hairdrier.

But soon he noticed that a day or two after his weekend restoration project, he'd feel as if he were coming down with the flu. After a few days, the symptoms—aching joints, upset stomach, and diarrhea—would disappear as quickly as they had appeared, only to return after another weekend of work in the old house. At first, his physician thought that Douglas had some sort of stomach or intestinal disorder. But when the doctor learned of his patient's weekend restoration work, he acted on a hunch and ordered a blood test.

The Baltimore child's X rays and the Jersey City man's blood test revealed that the two patients' misery had a common cause. Both had lead poisoning, a condition caused by excess lead or lead compounds in the body.

The toddler's X rays detected deposits of lead in her leg bones. They also revealed the source of the lead: Her abdomen was full of partially digested plaster and paint chips, which she had apparently devoured during a recent stay at her grandmother's house. And the results of Douglas' blood test—a procedure that measured the amount of lead circulating in his blood—confirmed the doctor's suspicion of lead poisoning. The face mask Douglas had worn during his restoration work did not protect him from the lead-laden fumes he created when burning off the house's old paint.

The author:

Jan Ziegler is a freelance writer based in Washington, D.C.

Harmful lead

Both patients were fortunate to have their illness correctly diagnosed. Lead poisoning is a serious disorder and one that can affect anyone. Lead is found everywhere—in the air, in soil and dust, in water, and in many manufactured products. Some people are poisoned by consuming lead-contaminated substances; others become ill after breathing lead-laden dust or fumes. Still others, such as artists who work with lead paints or people who work at shooting ranges and handle lead shot, can absorb toxic amounts of lead through the skin. In any case, if large enough amounts of lead are taken into the body over time, serious disability can result—ranging from brain and kidney damage to nervous system disorders.

Unfortunately, diagnosing lead poisoning is often difficult. Early symptoms are vague and often misleading because they are similar to those caused by other conditions. The warning signs of lead poisoning, for example, can resemble the effects of stress, heart disease, or the flu. Even in cases where a person shows no symptoms, lead may have already damaged vital organs. Furthermore, pregnant women who have too much lead in their bodies may not suffer ill effects themselves, but the lead may increase the chance of miscarriage or harm their fetuses. Early diagnosis is critical to preventing damage.

Among adults, lead poisoning is rare. When it does occur, it is most often caused by an occupation or hobby that brings the person into regular contact with high levels of lead. Working in a factory that makes products containing lead can be risky. So can restoring old houses.

It is among infants and young children that lead poisoning is the most prevalent—and dangerous. It takes less lead to harm the small, growing body of a child than that of an adult. Children may ingest lead simply by swallowing dirt or dust while playing or by putting dirty toys into their mouth.

Lead poisoning is one of the most common environmental diseases among children in the United States, according to an August 1988 report issued by the Centers for Disease Control (CDC) in Atlanta, Ga. The report said that about 17 per cent of the nation's children under the age of 5—nearly 2.4 million children—were being exposed to unacceptably high levels of lead. Of those, nearly 200,000 may need treatment.

Scientific data reported at a 1989 National Institute of Environmental Health Sciences lead research meeting in Research Triangle Park, N.C., indicate that low levels of lead that produce no obvious symptoms may stunt a child's growth and cause mild mental retardation, delayed motor development, hearing and balancing disorders, and other problems. And new studies suggest that older women may be at risk for lead poisoning because of changes that occur in their bones during menopause, the time when menstruation ceases.

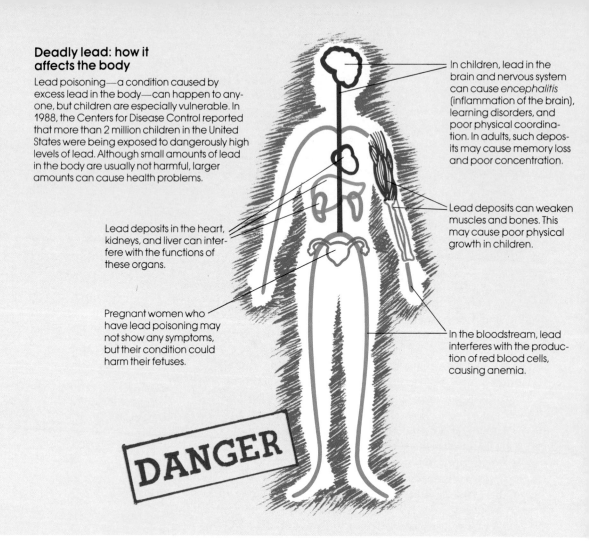

Deadly lead: how it affects the body

Lead poisoning—a condition caused by excess lead in the body—can happen to anyone, but children are especially vulnerable. In 1988, the Centers for Disease Control reported that more than 2 million children in the United States were being exposed to dangerously high levels of lead. Although small amounts of lead in the body are usually not harmful, larger amounts can cause health problems.

In children, lead in the brain and nervous system can cause *encephalitis* (inflammation of the brain), learning disorders, and poor physical coordination. In adults, such deposits may cause memory loss and poor concentration.

Lead deposits in the heart, kidneys, and liver can interfere with the functions of these organs.

Lead deposits can weaken muscles and bones. This may cause poor physical growth in children.

Pregnant women who have lead poisoning may not show any symptoms, but their condition could harm their fetuses.

In the bloodstream, lead interferes with the production of red blood cells, causing anemia.

DANGER

Few people die from lead poisoning, however. The National Center for Health Statistics (NCHS) in Hyattsville, Md., recorded only seven deaths from lead poisoning in the United States in 1986.

An ancient problem

People have been mining lead since at least 3,500 B.C. A soft, gray metal, lead is easily molded yet is also durable. The Romans called it *plumbum*—from which our word *plumbing* is derived—and they used it to line *aqueducts*, structures to carry water long distances. They also used it to line the inside of cookware and food containers, and valued it because it imparted a sweet taste to wine.

But even the ancients, with their scanty knowledge of the workings of the human body, soon realized that there was a price to be paid for using lead. In the 100's B.C., the Greek physician Nicander recognized that the stomach pain and constipation his patients experienced after consuming a wine-based syrup suffused with lead were symptoms of lead poisoning, or *plumbism*, to use the medical term.

A modern dilemma

Today, we realize that the health risks of lead poisoning can be far more serious than the complaints noted by Nicander. But although there has been considerable progress in reducing lead exposures in the United States in recent years, this ancient metal is still disconcertingly prevalent in our environment. At least 600,000 short tons (540,000 metric tons) of lead enter the air, water, and soil each year, says the National Academy of Sciences in Washington, D.C. For example, lead may be found in some artist and crafts supplies, in roofing materials, in ammunition, and in the lead-acid storage batteries that provide power for electrical systems of automobiles and other vehicles. It is also still used as *solder* (metal that joins metal surfaces or parts) for tin cans containing food, though its use for this purpose has tapered off in recent years. More common sources of exposure include leaded gasoline, lead-glazed pottery, lead-based paints, and lead-contaminated water.

Lead from gasoline. Thanks to the automobile, breathing lead-laden dust or fumes is the way most Americans come into contact with lead. A compound called *tetraethyl lead* was first added to gasoline in 1923 to improve engine performance. Unfortunately, it also contributed to lead pollution in the air.

Lead spewed into the air by cars (and other sources) settles onto dirt in playgrounds and yards. It enters homes through open doors and windows, covering furniture and pets. It is easy to see how small amounts of the metal makes its way onto fingers and toys that inevitably end up in children's mouths.

Fortunately, in 1972, federal regulations reduced the amount of lead permitted in gasoline, and 85 per cent of all gasoline sold in the United States today is lead-free. But as of

Types of lead poisoning

There are two types of lead poisoning: *acute* (quick) and *chronic* (long-term). Each has its own set of symptoms. Because symptoms often resemble those of other disorders, both acute and chronic lead poisoning may be difficult to diagnose.

Acute lead poisoning results from a single exposure to highly concentrated levels of lead. If the condition goes untreated, death may result. Symptoms usually appear within two or three days and may include—

- nausea and vomiting;
- convulsions; and
- coma.

Chronic lead poisoning results from repeated exposure to small amounts of lead that build up slowly in the body. Symptoms appear gradually, and some people may show no symptoms at all. Symptoms in children, which often differ from those found in adults, may include—

- crankiness;
- a refusal to eat, walk, or play;
- stomachaches, constipation, diarrhea, vomiting;
- unsteady walk;
- convulsions;
- encephalitis; and
- coma.

Symptoms of chronic lead poisoning in adults may include—

- memory loss;
- inability to concentrate;
- stomach and intestinal pain;
- weight loss;
- high blood pressure;
- heartbeat irregularities;
- congestive heart failure; and
- kidney damage.

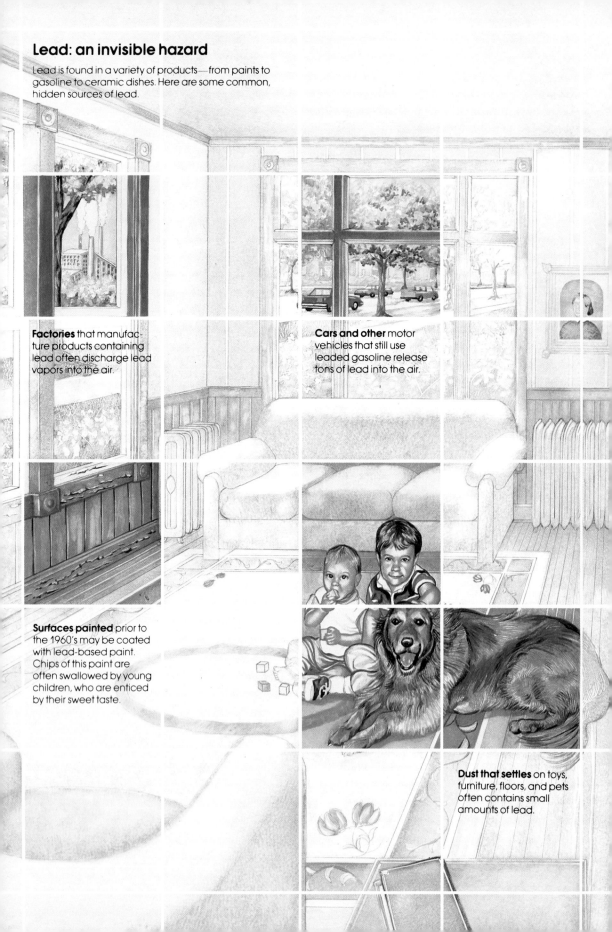

Lead: an invisible hazard

Lead is found in a variety of products—from paints to gasoline to ceramic dishes. Here are some common, hidden sources of lead.

Factories that manufacture products containing lead often discharge lead vapors into the air.

Cars and other motor vehicles that still use leaded gasoline release tons of lead into the air.

Surfaces painted prior to the 1960's may be coated with lead-based paint. Chips of this paint are often swallowed by young children, who are enticed by their sweet taste.

Dust that settles on toys, furniture, floors, and pets often contains small amounts of lead.

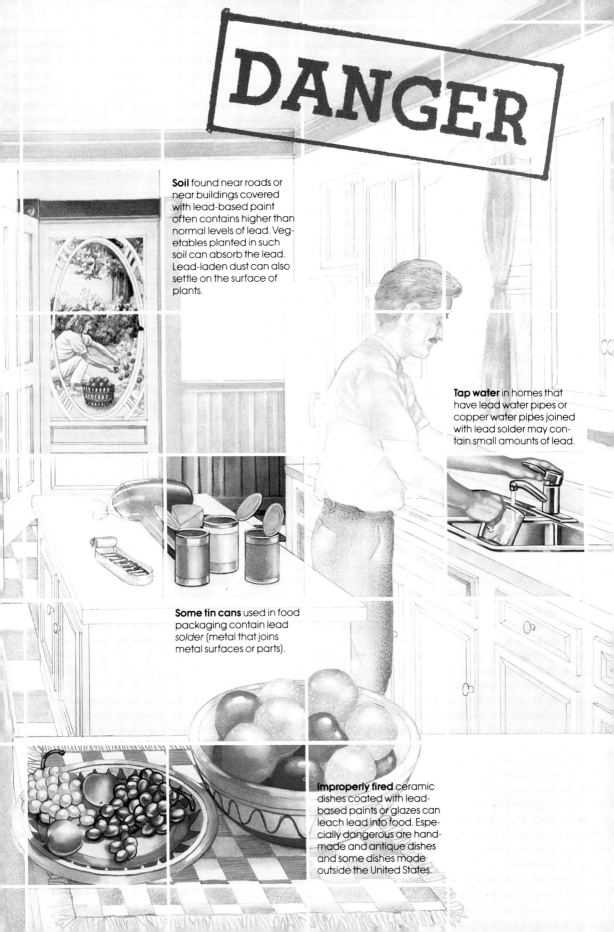

DANGER

Soil found near roads or near buildings covered with lead-based paint often contains higher than normal levels of lead. Vegetables planted in such soil can absorb the lead. Lead-laden dust can also settle on the surface of plants.

Tap water in homes that have lead water pipes or copper water pipes joined with lead solder may contain small amounts of lead.

Some tin cans used in food packaging contain lead *solder* (metal that joins metal surfaces or parts).

Improperly fired ceramic dishes coated with lead-based paints or glazes can leach lead into food. Especially dangerous are handmade and antique dishes and some dishes made outside the United States.

1985, about 22,000 short tons (20,000 metric tons) of lead were still entering the air from gasoline fumes each year.

Lead-glazed dishes. Another source of lead poisoning is food or beverages stored in pottery or ceramic dishes coated with an improperly fired lead glaze. Lead can *leach* or dissolve out of these dishes, contaminating foods. Imported pottery and ceramic dishes are most likely to leach lead.

Lead paint. Another dangerous source of lead are chips of lead-laden paint or plaster that are often swallowed by curious infants and toddlers who may be entranced by their sweet taste. Once ingested, these chips deliver a concentrated source of lead straight to the child's digestive tract, where it is easily absorbed into the bloodstream.

For this reason, the United States in 1978 banned the use of lead-based paint for housing, toys, and furniture. But older buildings, especially those built prior to the 1960's, may still wear their old, lead-saturated coats of paint.

Lead-contaminated water. Lead can also be ingested through water, though a person must consume a much more concentrated form of lead than that found in water for it to cause serious symptoms. In fact, public health authorities are unaware of any person who developed lead poisoning from drinking contaminated tap water. Nevertheless, lead in water can raise lead levels in the blood by small amounts—and such amounts can be dangerous as they build up over time, especially in children and pregnant women.

When water leaves a local water treatment plant it does not contain lead. But by the time it comes out of the kitchen faucet or office water cooler, it may no longer be lead-free because the plumbing systems of houses or buildings constructed before the 1930's have lead pipes. Houses built later contain copper pipes, but lead solder is usually used to join copper pipe sections. Tap water in older houses with lead-soldered copper pipes usually has lower lead levels because mineral deposits have built up along the pipe joints, coating the lead and preventing it from contaminating the water.

How does lead affect the body?

Medical experts have identified two types of lead poisoning—acute and chronic. Acute, or quick, lead poisoning occurs after a single exposure to highly concentrated levels of lead. Purposely sniffing leaded gasoline at close range or ingesting a large quantity of lead paint chips can cause this type of poisoning. Symptoms of acute lead poisoning appear over two to three days and include nausea, vomiting, convulsions, and, if severe enough, coma.

But public health experts consider chronic, or long-term, lead poisoning—the gradual accumulation in the body of small amounts of lead—as a more far-reaching and insidious problem. Chronic lead poisoning is particularly insidious because the body is unable to quickly eliminate the metal in body wastes. As a result, lead that enters the body in small amounts gradually accumulates in many tissues and bones, where it can begin to cause harm without producing any warning symptoms.

Once it enters the body, lead circulates in the bloodstream. There it interferes with the production of red blood cells, shortening their life span. It also reduces the amount of *hemoglobin* (an iron-containing protein that carries oxygen to tissues) in each cell. Thus, fatigue, pallor, loss of appetite, and other symptoms of anemia are often among the first signs of lead poisoning in adults.

The bloodstream carries lead to the muscles, to the brain and nervous system, and to the kidneys, liver, and other organs, where it forms deposits. Small deposits of lead are not dangerous, but as deposits grow, they cause a number of physical problems. Besides damaging the central nervous system, the liver, and the kidneys, lead slows down the body's production of *collagen*, the protein substance found in bones, ligaments, tendons, and connective tissue.

Eventually, lead reaches the bones and teeth, a process that appears to depend on a person's age and general health. Once lead has reached the bones, it stays there for many years. In fact, people who reach high lead levels may have some lead in their bones for the rest of their lives.

Misleading symptoms

How the body reacts to chronic lead poisoning—whether any symptoms develop or whether any permanent damage is done—depends on the amount of lead in the body and how long lead deposits have been accumulating in tissue and bones. The symptoms of lead poisoning also depend on the age of the victim.

In children, the early symptoms of chronic lead poisoning are ambiguous. A child may become cranky, cry for no reason, sleep poorly, and refuse to eat or play or walk.

If the exposure to lead continues, the symptoms get worse. The child often develops a stomachache and becomes constipated, though some children may develop diarrhea. The child may begin to vomit frequently, walk unsteadily, or develop a condition called *foot drop*, in which the muscles in the foot weaken, preventing the foot from flexing properly during walking. The brain and nervous system may be affected, causing convulsions, *encephalitis* (inflammation of the

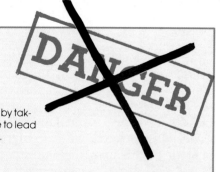

Minimizing your contact with lead

It is impossible to remove all the lead in the environment. But by taking a few simple precautions, you can reduce your exposure to lead and minimize your family's risk of developing lead poisoning.

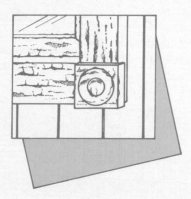

Getting the lead out...of tap water

The longer water sits in pipes that contain lead, the more lead it absorbs. For that reason, the U.S. Environmental Protection Agency (EPA) recommends that you run faucets that have been turned off six hours or longer until the water gets as cold as possible. The EPA also suggests not using hot tap water for cooking or drinking since lead dissolves more quickly in hot water. If you think your water contains lead, have it tested by a reputable laboratory. If necessary, you can install devices to remove lead from your tap water.

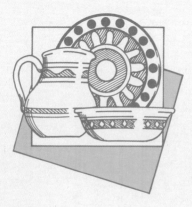

Removing the threat of leaded paint

To avoid having chips and dust from lead-based paint or plaster in your house, remove any paint that may have been applied before the 1960's. It is best to have experts handle the removal. But if you choose to do it yourself, wear a respirator that filters out lead fumes and dust, and cover any doors to the work area with plastic sheets to prevent lead vapors from spreading to other rooms. Experts also recommend sweeping up paint and plaster chips and dust, placing them in a sealable plastic trash bag, and washing down the entire room when the job is finished.

Steering clear of dangerous dishes

Although they are attractive, antique china, handmade pottery, and some ceramic dishes made outside the United States can be deadly if used to hold food or beverages. If improperly fired, the lead in the paint or glaze can leach into food, especially acidic foods such as juices, wine, tomatoes, or vinegar that can easily dissolve lead. If you are not sure if a dish contains lead, play it safe: Don't use the dish at all for cooking or serving food.

brain), coma, and even death. Luckily, most children are treated before these serious consequences occur.

The symptoms of chronic lead poisoning in adults are somewhat different from those in children. In the first months, adults may experience symptoms of anemia or may notice a deterioration in memory and an inability to concentrate or sleep. Whereas too much lead in the body may cause foot drop in children, in adults it often leads to wrist drop. Eventually, as an adult's exposure to lead continues over many years, any number of complications may appear, including high blood pressure, *congestive heart failure* (a condition in which the heart is weakened and unable to pump enough blood to keep the body functioning normally), and kidney damage.

Diagnosing lead poisoning

Medical authorities agree that a physician must never rely solely on a patient's symptoms and appearance to diagnose lead poisoning. The best way to confirm it is with a blood test.

Two different blood tests are used for lead poisoning. In one, a blood sample, taken with a syringe, is analyzed to determine the number of micrograms of lead per one deciliter of blood. In the other test, the patient's fingertip is pricked with a small needle to produce a drop of blood that is analyzed for *erythrocyte protoporphyrin* or *zinc protoporphyrin*, chemicals that play key roles in hemoglobin production. Because lead raises the amount of these substances in the blood, abnormally high levels show that the lead has interfered with hemoglobin production.

The protoporphyrin test is not as precise a measure of lead exposure as is calculating the amount of lead circulating in blood, but it does show whether lead has started to damage red blood cells. It also reveals long-term lead exposure, while lead blood levels indicate only that the patient has been in contact with lead recently.

How do physicians determine if a patient's lead level is excessive and should be treated? Unfortunately, there is no accepted standard for how much lead is too much for people of different ages. Guidelines issued in 1985 by the CDC to help physicians decide whether to treat their patients for lead poisoning state that a blood lead level under 25 micrograms per deciliter is acceptable. But new studies suggest that even this level is too high, particularly for children; some health experts are thus calling for new lead poisoning guidelines, citing lower acceptable levels.

New concern was raised in January 1989, when researchers at Albert Einstein College of Medicine in New York City released the results of a study that showed that measuring blood lead levels in children may not accurately reflect the amount of lead stored in the body. The researchers measured the level of lead in the blood and bones of 59 children who showed no symptoms of lead poisoning. They found that some children who had acceptable blood lead levels had bone lead levels three times higher than the accepted amount for healthy children.

Getting the lead out

Although it is difficult to diagnose, lead poisoning is easily treated. Patients are usually given drugs called *chelating agents*. These drugs attach to the lead and help carry it out of the body in the urine. Generally, these drugs are given by injection or intravenously. Iron supplements or a special diet may be prescribed if the patient has anemia.

A single course of treatment usually lasts three to five days and requires hospitalization. The patient is given the drug twice or more a day. Urine samples are analyzed every day to determine how much lead the body is eliminating.

One treatment course is usually all that is needed for someone with an acute case of lead poisoning. But a person who has been exposed to low levels of lead over many years may require two to three treatment courses to remove the lead that has built up in the body. In such cases, each course is usually followed by a week of observation so the doctor can monitor its effects before beginning the next course.

One of the most widely used drugs to remove lead is *calcium disodium edetate*. This drug, however, does not remove lead from the brain because the drug is unable to cross the *blood-brain barrier*, a protective arrangement of cells that prevents certain substances in the bloodstream from reaching the brain. The drug may cause a number of adverse side effects, including diarrhea and fever, and can deplete the body's supply of zinc.

Minimizing your contact with lead

The most important part of treatment is removing the lead from the patient's environment to prevent further accumulation of the chemical in the body. This may mean taking better precautions to reduce lead exposure while stripping off a home's lead-laden paint or avoiding lead-contaminated dishes and cookware.

The safest way to remove lead paint from your house, of course, is to have it done by experts. But if you decide to do the work yourself, safety experts suggest that you make sure the work area is well ventilated and that you wear a respirator that will filter out airborne lead. It is a good idea to cover any doors to the work area with plastic sheets to prevent lead dust and vapors from spreading to the rest of the house.

To avoid lead-contaminated dishes and cookware, stick to brand-name items. Avoid drinking from a mug a friend made in pottery class, eating from old ceramic ware purchased at a bazaar, or putting food on earthenware dishes imported into—or purchased outside of—the United States. If you have some questionable dishware, do not use it for acidic food or beverages, such as juices, wine, or tomatoes, which help to dissolve lead.

To reduce lead in tap water, the U.S. Environmental Protection Agency recommends flushing cold-water pipes by running every faucet in the house that has not been used for six hours or more until the water gets as cold as possible. Flushing faucets is important because the longer water sits in lead pipes or is exposed to lead solder, the more lead it contains. Since lead dissolves more quickly in hot water, do not use hot tap water for cooking or drinking.

The best way to determine the lead content of your tap water is to have it tested. Some local water utilities or health departments may do the testing for you or recommend a laboratory. The cost of such a test may run from $20 to $100.

You can reduce the amount of lead in your tap water by installing a treatment device. *Reverse osmosis devices* are treatment devices that filter water through a membrane to remove impurities. You can also purchase or rent *distillation units*, which boil water until it evaporates and then collect the pure water that condenses from the vapor.

Preventive measures clearly pay off. When the Jersey City man returned to his old row house to finish the job of removing the lead paint—this time wearing a respirator—he realized that he could have spared himself his illness had he taken proper precautions. And although the mother of the Baltimore girl who was poisoned from eating lead paint chips was thankful that her child was diagnosed and treated early enough to prevent serious illness, she also recognized the importance of protecting her daughter from further exposure to lead. We will never be able to remove all lead from our environment. But by being aware of lead's dangers and by taking steps to reduce its presence in our lives, we can help minimize its risks to our health.

For further information:

Wallace, Barbara, and Cooper, Kathy. *The Citizen's Guide to Lead.* NC Press, 1986.

Free pamphlets on lead are available from local U.S. Environmental Protection Agency offices or local health departments.

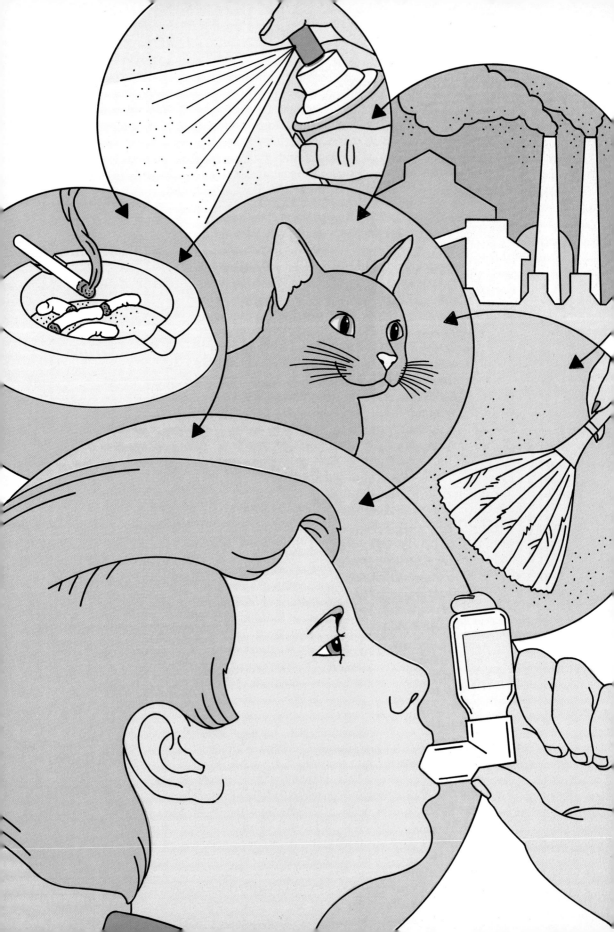

Many asthmatics live in fear of
the next attack of wheezing and
coughing. With education and
medication, they can take control
of their disease and their lives.

Living
with Asthma

By François Haas
and Sheila Sperber Haas

As soon as John entered the house, his lungs told him a cat
was around. He recognized the sudden tightening in his chest
as his airways constricted; the breathy wheeze as he exhaled;
the uncontrollable coughing. Then John couldn't breathe in
enough air. He was having an asthma attack.

But John didn't panic. He reached into his backpack and
pulled out his inhaler, a pocket-sized spray container of
medicine. Holding the device in front of his open mouth, he
breathed out hard, then sprayed the cool mist toward the
back of his throat as he inhaled. Medication-filled droplets
floated into John's lungs. He held his breath, counting to 10.
Then he repeated the process.

Almost immediately he felt his chest begin to relax. Breathing was easier. His cough died down. Even though it would be
hours or days before his lungs would fully recover, he knew
he was past the initial crisis.

John's asthma attacks years earlier had been different—
and frightening. He would struggle so hard to breathe that
his nostrils flared, his neck muscles bulged, and his heart
pounded. Sometimes he began to turn blue, a sign of lack of

oxygen. His terrified parents would rush him to a hospital emergency room, where a doctor would inject him with adrenaline, a powerful drug that dramatically eased his asthma symptoms. But this lifesaving drug scared him, because for a while it made his heart pound even more and intensified his feelings of anxiety.

Then he would miss school while he recuperated. And even when he was symptom-free, he was forbidden to run around, to play sports, or to go camping with his friends.

But asthma, and the fear of it, no longer control John's life. Instead, John and his parents have learned how to take control of his asthma—by working closely with his doctors and by educating themselves about what the problem is and how to cope with it.

What is asthma?

Asthma is a common lung disease defined mostly by its symptoms—recurring attacks of wheezing, breathlessness, and coughing. An attack occurs in response to some particular stimulus—perhaps a substance to which the person is allergic (such as pollen or mold) or a source of physical stress (such as exercise, cold air, or emotional pressure). Whatever the trigger, the airways in the lungs overreact by tightening up and filling with *mucus*, a slimy fluid produced by glands and cells in the airways. This leaves less room for air to flow into and out of the lungs.

Asthma is a major health problem in the United States and other industrialized countries. According to the National Center for Health Statistics (NCHS), 6.2 per cent of U.S. residents have been diagnosed as asthmatic. Among them are such well-known people as Olympic gold medalist Jackie Joyner-Kersee, former Vice President Walter F. Mondale, and movie director Martin Scorsese.

But experts suspect that many asthmatics never enter the records, either because they do not see a doctor for their breathing problems or because their condition is inaccurately diagnosed. The NCHS estimates the real figure as 10.5 per cent—or more than 20 million Americans.

The authors:

François Haas is director of the Pulmonary Function Laboratory at New York University Medical Center. He and Sheila Sperber Haas, a science writer, are authors of *The Essential Asthma Book: A Manual for Asthmatics of All Ages.*

Asthma takes a tremendous toll in money, time, and suffering. Medical treatment and lost productivity due to asthma add up to some $4 billion annually, according to the American Lung Association. Each year, asthma sufferers lose 9 million days of work.

And sometimes asthma kills. About 4,000 people died from asthma in 1986, the latest year for which figures are available. Strangely, although asthma usually can be controlled with the right treatment and precautions, the death rate has continued to rise, jumping an alarming 25 per cent in only four years.

The reasons for this rise are unknown, but investigators cite such problems as the failure to diagnose asthma; the failure to educate asthmatics about when to seek medical help; insufficient treatment, often because physicians fail to properly gauge the severity of attacks; the failure to monitor hospitalized patients correctly; and the inappropriate use of some medications. Perhaps most important, some experts suspect that these problems come in part from overconfidence. The very existence of new effective asthma medications may lead both patients and doctors to be careless in handling a potentially dangerous disease.

Who gets asthma?

Two damaging misconceptions have plagued asthmatics and their families for decades: that asthma is the physical expression of psychological problems, and that these problems stem from an abnormal relationship between child and mother. Scientists know now that asthma is not a psychiatric disorder, but these myths—and the needless stigma and guilt they create—persevere.

We still do not know exactly why some people get asthma, but scientific evidence overwhelmingly indicates that heredity plays a strong role. Eight hundred years ago, the famous Jewish physician and philosopher Maimonides noticed that asthma runs in families. Modern research has confirmed this. Compared with someone with no family history of asthma, a person whose brother, sister, or parent is asthmatic is 13 times more likely to develop asthma by age 49, and 33 times more likely to develop it by age 65.

Although heredity predisposes an individual to asthma, it is not the only factor. External conditions are apparently responsible for activating the disease. Asthma often first appears during or shortly after a viral respiratory infection, such as a cold. After that, respiratory viruses, allergies, stress, or other stimuli can trigger further attacks.

Asthma can develop at any age. Studies show that asthma in childhood appears up to about three times as often in boys as in girls, perhaps because boys are more susceptible to respiratory infections. That imbalance decreases somewhat after puberty—usually about age 14 in boys and age 12 in girls—because girls are more likely than boys to develop asthma at puberty. This is also the age at which childhood asthma, in both sexes, is most likely to disappear. Among the population as a whole, asthma affects slightly more males than females.

The prevalence of asthma also varies widely by race. Asthma is rare, for example, in certain tribes of American In-

How the airways normally work

The lungs have a branching network of airways that starts in the throat with the windpipe and, after many divisions, ends in millions of tiny air sacs. When you inhale, oxygen-rich air is carried through the airways to the air sacs. There, blood circulating around the air sacs picks up oxygen and gives up carbon dioxide. The air—now mostly carbon dioxide—retraces its route as you exhale.

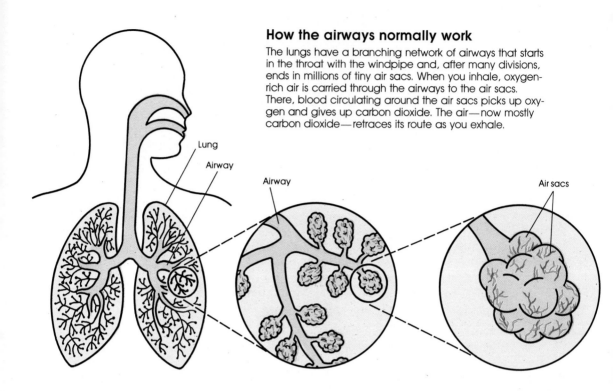

Lung

Airway

Airway

Air sacs

dians and Eskimos, and is generally more frequent among U.S. blacks and Hispanics than among whites. And research has turned up patterns that reflect income (asthma is more common below the poverty line than above) and region (with the highest rates in the South and the lowest in the Midwest). It's obvious that the relative influences of inherited factors and external ones—ranging from climate to life style—are not yet fully understood.

What happens during an asthma attack?

Scientists have not yet determined why some people get asthma. But they do know what happens when an asthmatic person has an attack. To understand what an asthma attack involves, we must first know how breathing normally works.

The lungs are made up primarily of airways and air sacs. The airways form a many-branching network that starts in the throat with the windpipe. The windpipe divides into two wide branches, each entering one lung. These air passages each divide into two branches, which in turn divide again and again, producing ever-narrower airways. After 23 divisions, the airways end at the 350 million tiny air sacs that are the lungs' working units.

The business of the respiratory system is to supply the body's tissues with oxygen and to carry away excess carbon

What happens in an asthma attack

Asthma attacks range in intensity from mild breathing difficulties to life-threatening suffocation. In a mild attack (1), the muscles surrounding the airway tighten, narrowing the breathing passage. In a more severe attack (2), cells lining the tightened airway produce mucus, restricting airflow further and causing coughing. In the most serious cases (3), the airway walls themselves swell, constricting the tightened, flooded air passage even more.

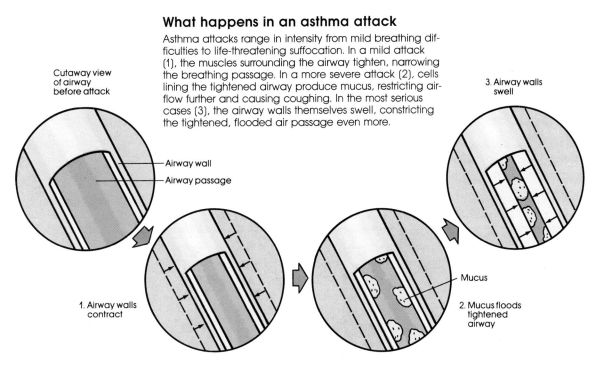

Cutaway view of airway before attack

Airway wall
Airway passage

1. Airway walls contract

2. Mucus floods tightened airway

Mucus

3. Airway walls swell

dioxide. When we inhale, oxygen-rich air passes into the throat and through the airways down to the air sacs. There, blood circulating around the sacs picks up oxygen and gives off carbon dioxide. The air—now mostly carbon dioxide—retraces its route as we exhale.

Breathing must overcome *resistance*, the frictionlike force created as air moves through the airways. Resistance is easily overcome during quiet breathing, but it increases if the air speed increases—for instance, when we breathe fast during exercise—or if the airways get narrower. (To get a feel for this, try breathing through a drinking straw—first open, and then with the straw pinched partly closed. Then try again while breathing faster.)

Although many different kinds of stimuli can provoke an asthma attack, the process that produces asthma symptoms is basically the same. In all attacks, the tiny muscles in the airway walls tighten up, which narrows the airways. That forces the breathing muscles—located in the chest, neck, shoulders, and back, as well as below the lungs—to work harder to overcome the greater resistance. In a mild attack, this may be all that occurs.

In more serious attacks, however, the airways also flood with mucus. Mucus normally serves to catch harmful matter, such as dust, as it enters the body. But excessive mucus further increases resistance. In addition, as mucus plugs some passages, it prevents oxygen from reaching the blood. Coughing begins as the lungs try to rid themselves of excess mucus.

In even more severe attacks, the airway walls themselves swell and narrow the airways even further. Swelling can become great enough to lift the cells lining the air passages temporarily away from the underlying airway walls.

In the most extreme attacks, the airways become completely obstructed from mucus plugs, detached airway cells, swelling, and constriction. Without immediate medical help, the patient may suffocate.

These stages of an attack—muscle constriction, mucus production, and swelling—may occur almost simultaneously, or they may take an hour or more to develop and subside. This period constitutes the *initial phase* of an attack.

Less obvious, but no less serious, is the *late-phase response* that occurs in some people. This peaks five or six hours after the initial symptoms pass and may last more than a day. During this phase, the irritated airways remain inflamed and are more susceptible to additional, more severe attacks. Some experts blame the increase in asthma deaths on failure to recognize the seriousness of the late-phase response. This may occur partly because drugs taken to relieve the initial symptoms work so well that asthmatics—and their doctors—do not realize that they are suddenly at high risk for a severe attack.

What triggers an asthma attack?

Asthma is often divided into two types, based on whether it is triggered by an easily identifiable *allergen* (a substance to which a person is allergic) or by some other type of stimulus. Although most asthmatic people react to both types of triggers, roughly half tend to respond most often and most strongly to obvious allergens, and the others respond predominantly to stimuli classed as nonallergenic. Recent research, however, suggests that most or all cases of asthma may ultimately reflect the same type of response, even if a particular trigger cannot be identified with standard tests.

Allergenic triggers travel as tiny particles in the air. The two most common triggers are pollen and mold. Problem pollens come from trees (which pollinate from late winter through spring), grasses (spring through summer), and weeds (late spring through fall). The major allergenic molds include those that grow on plants as well as the green mold that grows on old bread. Mold spores—the actual allergen—are not limited to one season, but they are most plentiful during dry, windy periods that follow rainy seasons. They appear in lower concentrations during freezing weather.

Animals are another common source of allergens. With some, such as cats and dogs, the allergen is their *dander* (skin particles). Cockroach feces are allergenic. So are the feathers used to stuff pillows, comforters, and coats.

House dust includes many allergenic materials, such as animal dander, molds, vegetable fibers, food particles, algae, dirt, and insect feces. Cockroach remnants, another allergen, are a major component of house dust in some areas. The worst allergen in house dust, however, seems to be the feces from microscopic mites that live in the dust.

Research suggests that the food we eat plays almost no role in asthma (except in very young allergic children). Still, because many patients report an asthmatic response when they eat certain foods, the issue is unresolved. (In some people, however, certain foods—such as shellfish or peanuts—can cause a life-threatening, bodywide allergic reaction called *anaphylaxis* that includes severe asthmalike symptoms.)

Nonallergenic triggers include substances that do not seem to be allergens but can still irritate oversensitive airways, as well as physical or emotional stresses. Asthma patients are particularly susceptible to air pollutants. These include ozone, cigarette smoke, and house dust (which in quantity is an irritant as well as an allergen). Even strong odors—particularly from insecticides, household cleaners, cooking, and perfume—can trigger asthma in some people.

Some asthmatics, mostly adults, are sensitive to aspirin. People who find that aspirin triggers their asthma should also avoid anti-inflammatory drugs similar to aspirin, such as ibuprofen, and should check with their physician or pharmacist before using any over-the-counter medication.

Viral respiratory infections, such as the common cold or influenza, are important asthma triggers, particularly in infants. Although it is not clear exactly how these infections provoke asthma, we do know that infections irritate and inflame the airways. This airway damage can take several weeks to heal; during that time, the airways are more sensitive than usual to various stimuli.

Many asthmatics experience wheezing and shortness of breath from vigorous exercise. This condition typically starts from 5 to 10 minutes after the activity ends and lasts about 30 to 60 minutes. Many theories exist as to why this happens; one suggests that the hard breathing exercise generates cools the airways and that this cooling may provoke an attack. This theory, which is debated, reflects the fact that cold air in itself can trigger asthma.

Although emotional stress does not cause asthma initially, it can act as a trigger for some asthmatics. For others, stress often increases susceptibility to their usual asthma triggers.

Occupational asthma triggers include both allergenic and non-allergenic substances, but they are classed separately because they are found primarily in specialized workplaces, where they provoke reactions from asthmatic workers. This problem has become worse as the number of asthma-provoking chemicals has grown in the industrial world.

Food particles can be allergenic if inhaled in quantity, and they are frequently linked with asthma in the workplace. "Baker's asthma," for example, is relatively common among people who work with flour. Other susceptible workers suffer from handling such foodstuffs as coffee, soybeans, and cottonseed. Eating or drinking these products, however, does not trigger asthma.

Diagnosing asthma

Asthma is not easy to diagnose. The three most common long-term respiratory diseases—asthma, emphysema, and chronic bronchitis—share a confusingly similar set of symptoms (though only asthma appears frequently in young people). To determine whether the problem is asthma, a physician depends on the patient's medical history, a physical examination, and laboratory tests.

Patient history often provides the key to asthma diagnosis. If the patient or family members have allergies, or if a relative has asthma, it is highly likely that the patient's symptoms stem from asthma. The physician also looks at such factors as the way the problem first developed and the times and places at which symptoms recur. Symptoms that come and go tend to point to asthma.

Physical findings can help confirm that a patient's airways are obstructed, whether by asthma or by another respiratory disease. The physician first listens with a stethoscope for wheezing—the sound of turbulence as air is forced around obstructions in the lungs. The doctor also watches to see which muscles the patient uses for breathing and how hard those muscles have to work.

Laboratory tests can then help the doctor decide which disease is causing the obstruction. A blood test might show a large quantity of certain white blood cells frequently seen in allergic asthma cases, as well as signs of underlying disease. Samples of *sputum*, the mucus coughed up from the lungs, can reveal both damaged cells and expelled mucus plugs. And chest X rays might show signs of complications.

But most important are the pulmonary function tests, which document the behavior of the patient's lungs. One procedure, in which the patient breathes through a mouthpiece into a machine, measures the volume of air in the lungs at different

Asthma-proofing your home

Help the asthmatic in your family breathe easier by clearing the air at home. These tips show ways to cut down on dust, mold, and other common asthma triggers; your routines will depend on the asthmatic person's particular sensitivities. To avoid missing anything important, write down a step-by-step asthma-proofing plan for each room. Start in the bedroom, since this is where people spend most of their household time. Clean properly rather than frequently. Use a damp cloth to avoid stirring up dust; when vacuuming is necessary, the asthmatic should stay away until the dust settles.

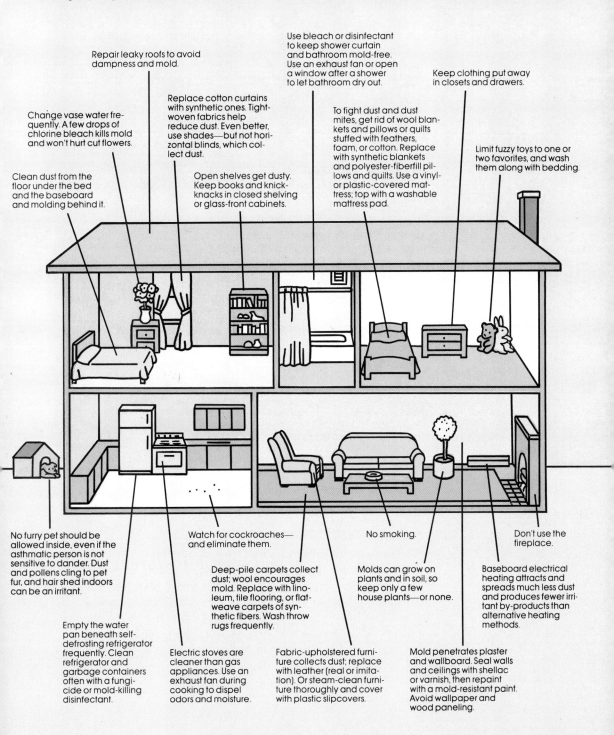

Repair leaky roofs to avoid dampness and mold.

Use bleach or disinfectant to keep shower curtain and bathroom mold-free. Use an exhaust fan or open a window after a shower to let bathroom dry out.

Keep clothing put away in closets and drawers.

Replace cotton curtains with synthetic ones. Tight-woven fabrics help reduce dust. Even better, use shades—but not horizontal blinds, which collect dust.

Change vase water frequently. A few drops of chlorine bleach kills mold and won't hurt cut flowers.

To fight dust and dust mites, get rid of wool blankets and pillows or quilts stuffed with feathers, foam, or cotton. Replace with synthetic blankets and polyester-fiberfill pillows and quilts. Use a vinyl- or plastic-covered mattress; top with a washable mattress pad.

Limit fuzzy toys to one or two favorites, and wash them along with bedding.

Clean dust from the floor under the bed and the baseboard and molding behind it.

Open shelves get dusty. Keep books and knick-knacks in closed shelving or glass-front cabinets.

No furry pet should be allowed inside, even if the asthmatic person is not sensitive to dander. Dust and pollens cling to pet fur, and hair shed indoors can be an irritant.

Watch for cockroaches—and eliminate them.

No smoking.

Don't use the fireplace.

Empty the water pan beneath self-defrosting refrigerator frequently. Clean refrigerator and garbage containers often with a fungicide or mold-killing disinfectant.

Electric stoves are cleaner than gas appliances. Use an exhaust fan during cooking to dispel odors and moisture.

Deep-pile carpets collect dust; wool encourages mold. Replace with linoleum, tile flooring, or flat-weave carpets of synthetic fibers. Wash throw rugs frequently.

Fabric-upholstered furniture collects dust; replace with leather (real or imitation). Or steam-clean furniture thoroughly and cover with plastic slipcovers.

Molds can grow on plants and in soil, so keep only a few house plants—or none.

Mold penetrates plaster and wallboard. Seal walls and ceilings with shellac or varnish, then repaint with a mold-resistant paint. Avoid wallpaper and wood paneling.

Baseboard electrical heating attracts and spreads much less dust and produces fewer irritant by-products than alternative heating methods.

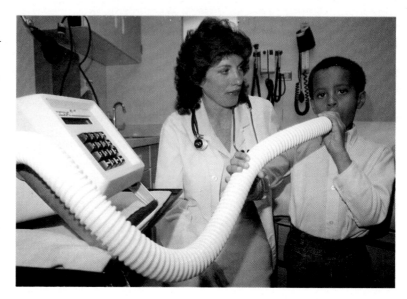

Pulmonary function tests (tests of the lung's abilities) are essential in diagnosing asthma. Here, a boy breathes into an instrument called a *spirometer,* which measures his lung capacity.

stages of the breathing cycle. Other devices monitor resistance and the rates of airflow into and out of the lungs.

A single set of tests verifies the presence of any airway obstruction and measures its severity. To identify asthma as the culprit, the physician must find out if the condition is reversible. This is what sets asthma apart from the other chronic lung diseases.

If the patient's breathing is impaired at the time of the examination, the doctor administers the pulmonary function tests before and after giving the patient medication to relax the airways. If the second set of tests shows that airflow has improved, the doctor can diagnose the problem as asthma.

If the patient is not having symptoms, the physician tries to provoke a brief, controlled asthma attack — either by asking the patient to inhale certain chemicals, by putting the patient through exercises, or by exposing the patient to cold air. If before-and-after tests show that a stimulus created airway obstruction, the doctor can diagnose asthma.

Asthma medication

Although asthma therapy involves many elements, its mainstay is medication to keep airways open and reduce their reactivity. This both relieves symptoms and prevents new attacks.

In an emergency that requires an immediate response, drugs can be given by injection. In general use, however, asthma drugs are either inhaled or taken orally. When the oral and inhaled versions of a drug are equally effective, the inhaled form is preferable. Inhaling takes medication directly to the lungs, so much smaller doses are needed than with oral medication, which must distribute a large dose throughout the body to ensure that the correct amount reaches the lungs. Because the inhaled dose is substantially less, inhalation minimizes side effects.

To inhale asthma medicine, older children and adults use a device called a *metered-dose inhaler*, a handheld container that administers a measured amount of the drug in spray form. Because using an inhaler requires coordinating breathing with spraying, it can prove difficult for small children. Children generally manage better with a *nebulizer*, a larger device that converts the medication into a mist, which is then inhaled through a tube or a mask.

Many drugs are available, and they work in different ways and at different points in the asthma process. Because every asthma patient responds differently, and because many of the drugs behave differently when used in combinations, individuals should work with their physicians to determine what mix of drugs and what dosages are safest and most effective.

The chart on page 195 describes some of the commonly prescribed antiasthma drugs. Most common are *bronchodilators*, which reduce the severity of attacks by opening up constricted airways. *Corticosteroids*, commonly called steroids, can relieve asthma symptoms dramatically, but because of their wide range of side effects, they are generally prescribed on a temporary basis and only in severe cases that do not respond to safer drugs. (Corticosteroids are different from anabolic steroids, drugs sometimes used by athletes to build muscle. See STEROID ABUSE: TURNING WINNERS INTO LOSERS, page 42, for information on anabolic steroids.)

Cromolyn sodium, which is meant for long-term, preventive use, reduces sensitivity to a broad range of triggers with few side effects. This drug, used successfully in Europe since the 1960's, was at first slow to gain acceptance after it was introduced to America in 1975. This was in part because, for many years, cromolyn could be inhaled only by using special equipment that many patients found awkward. Since 1986, cromolyn has been available for use in an inhaler, and it is now widely prescribed.

Asthmatics should avoid over-the-counter asthma drugs. For the most part, prescription drugs are more effective and cause fewer side effects. Perhaps more important, asthmatics who rely on over-the-counter drugs to ease their breathing problems may not be receiving the treatment and education they need for avoiding serious complications. People whose asthma is troublesome enough to require medication should consult a

Warning signs of an asthma emergency

These signs suggest that an asthma attack is becoming severe and that you should seek medical help immediately.

1. Your inhaled medicine fails to provide the usual relief, and you find yourself using it more frequently.

2. You have more and more trouble when you wake up, and the condition does not improve during the day.

3. You wheeze more, particularly at night.

4. You're short of breath more often and with less exertion than usual.

5. You cough more but find it harder to bring up mucus from the lungs. What does come up is extremely sticky.

6. You suffer from heightened anxiety, insomnia, and irritability.

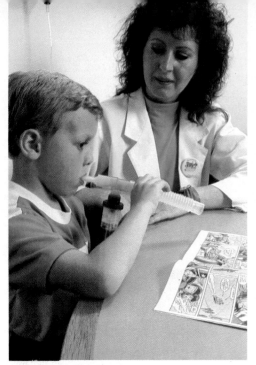

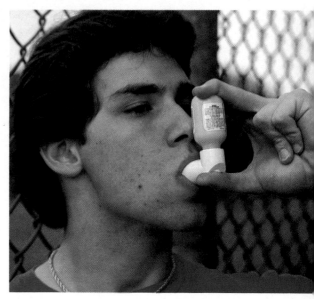

Many asthma medications can be inhaled. Young children typically take these drugs by breathing through a *nebulizer, above,* which converts the medicine into a mist. Older children and adults typically use an *inhaler, above right,* which delivers the medicine in spray form. This portable device is more convenient, but it requires coordinating breathing with hand motions— which can be difficult for young children.

physician—not only for prescriptions, but for the doctor's guidance on choosing and using an effective combination of drugs.

Other elements of asthma therapy

Asthma treatment focuses not only on easing physical discomfort but also on reducing the restrictions imposed upon the patient and the anger or anxiety that these restrictions can cause. Therapy may involve control of the environment, treatment to reduce allergic sensitivity, exercise to improve physical fitness, and stress management.

Allergen and irritant control. Often the best way to prevent asthma attacks is to stay away from the triggers that cause them. Together with a physician, the asthmatic must determine what his or her triggers are. If triggers aren't apparent, the patient might be able to identify them by keeping a diary of when and where attacks occur. The next step is to find ways to avoid or minimize exposure to triggers—or, if that is impossible, to decide, with a physician's help, when to use preventive medication.

Home is the easiest place to control triggers. Many common indoor allergens—such as house dust, feathers, animal dander, mold spores, and odors—can be reduced or removed. For more information on asthma-proofing the home, see the illustration on page 191.

Immunotherapy. If most of the patient's triggers are obvious

Drugs for breathing easier

Here are some of the most commonly prescribed antiasthma drugs. The many available medications work in different ways, and their effectiveness varies with the individual. Patients need to work closely with a physician to determine a safe, effective combination.

	Drug category and names	How the drugs work	Administration	Side effects and drawbacks
Bronchodilators	Specific beta-stimulators: *albuterol, metaproterenol, terbutaline*	Open up airways during or before attacks; mimic the chemistry by which the nervous system tells the airways to relax.	Taken orally, or inhaled for fewer side effects.	Side effects are minimal, including sleeplessness, nervousness, temporary muscle tremor, and quickening of the heart. Because these drugs relieve breathing without fighting airway inflammation, they can mask the patient's susceptibility to additional attacks.
	Nonspecific beta-stimulators: *adrenalin* is the only drug of this type in common use	Work like specific beta-stimulators to open up tight airways, but also affect other organs, particularly the heart and blood vessels.	Often injected in emergencies.	Side effects include headaches, increased blood pressure, disturbance of heart rhythm, and urine retention. Relief is short-lived. In most cases, adrenalin has been replaced by the newer specific beta-stimulators, whose effects focus on the airways.
	Theophylline	Relaxes airways and helps clear mucus during attacks; is a potent stimulant chemically related to caffeine.	Taken orally; dose size and frequency vary widely.	Side effects include sleeplessness, nervousness, and queasiness. The range between effective dose and poisonous overdose is narrow, so patient must have frequent blood tests to monitor drug levels.
Corticosteroids (called *steroids*): *Triamcinalone acetonide, flunisolide, beclomethasone*		Highly potent; dramatically relieve attacks by both reducing inflammation and relaxing airways.	Often inhaled; in severe cases, taken orally.	Side effects range from minor (yeast infections in the mouth, acne, facial bloating) to moderate (leg cramps, insomnia, mood changes) to serious (growth retardation, ulcers, high blood pressure, cataracts, psychosis). Steroids are typically prescribed only if safer drugs are ineffective.
Cromolyn sodium (called *cromolyn*)		Helps prevent asthma attacks by decreasing sensitivity to asthma triggers.	Inhaled; must be used daily over a long term.	Side effects are almost nonexistent. Although highly useful for preventing attacks, cromolyn does not relieve attacks in progress. Because it is relatively new, some physicians are unfamiliar with it.

allergens, the patient can try neutralizing them by *immunotherapy*, also called *desensitization*. This treatment, given by an allergist, involves a series of injections over the course of several years. The injections, which contain allergen extract, are meant to build up the patient's resistance to the allergen. But because immunotherapy is an inexact and controversial procedure, patients should not undertake it before thorough discussion with their primary physician and an allergist.

Exercise. Traditional asthma treatment bans vigorous physical activity. New drugs, however, enable most asthmatics to exercise without having attacks. In addition, studies suggest that regular exercise may reduce both the frequency and the severity of attacks triggered by other stimuli.

Certain types of exercise work best for asthmatics. Swimming and walking seem to be easier than running or cycling. A warm, humid environment—such as a swimming pool or a warm gym—is less likely to provoke an attack. Asthmatics who exercise outdoors on cold days should keep a scarf or a cold-weather mask over the nose and mouth. If these precautions fail to prevent attacks, the asthmatic should try taking preventive medication, as prescribed by a doctor, before the exercise. Some asthmatics need to do this routinely; others need to do so only under circumstances such as high air pollution, temperature or humidity changes, or a recent respiratory infection. The asthmatic exerciser should also develop a routine of medication, warm-up, and a cooling-down period. For a typical routine, see EXERCISE WITHOUT FEAR on this page.

Stress and anxiety management. Because stress, worry, and fear can worsen an asthma episode or even trigger one, techniques for controlling these feelings are useful elements of asthma therapy.

Although asthma is not a psychiatric problem, counseling can be helpful for asthmatics in two situations: if they suffer from anxiety or obsessive concern about their illness, or if they deny the reality of their condition and so refuse to cooperate in treating it. Group therapy, in the form of support groups of other asthmatics or parents of asthmatic children, can help counter isolation and frustration and also provide an invaluable educational network.

Studies indicate that regular muscle relaxation exercises may reduce the intensity of attacks. One well-known method involves tensing and relaxing all the major muscle groups one by one. Other research suggests that asthma patients may benefit from hypnosis, which induces a trancelike state through which the asthmatic may be able to learn how to relax and breathe easier. Similar help may come from *biofeedback*, a method of learning to control bodily responses that normally cannot be regulated voluntarily, such as heart rate and muscle tension.

What to do when an attack occurs

Despite the best preventive efforts, asthma attacks can still happen. Although emergency care can save an asthmatic's life in the case of a severe attack, it's far better never to need it. The asthmatic's best approach, then, is to minimize the chance that an attack will turn into an emergency.

Above all, this means working with a physician to develop a medication schedule—and then sticking to it. Medication should always be with the patient, not left at home or packed in a suitcase. And patient and doctor need to work out in advance how to modify drug use if asthma symptoms unexpectedly appear, if a trigger will be unavoidable, or if the patient will temporarily be far from medical help.

Successfully managing an asthma attack of any degree requires that the patient realize that an attack is beginning—typically by such signs as chest tightness, cough, wheeze, airway mucus, or breathing difficulty. Ideally, the patient stays calm and follows the routine planned earlier with a doctor. The mild asthmatic, who may not normally require medication, will need to use it at this time. An asthmatic who is already on maintenance medication may need to increase dosage or add a different drug.

Every asthma patient should learn the subtle signs that warn that an attack is becoming severe. A severe attack might take anywhere from a few hours to many days to develop. But the earlier the patient recognizes that the condition is getting worse, the easier it will be for medical professionals to treat the attack. An asthmatic noticing signs of an impending asthma emergency (see WARNING SIGNS OF AN ASTHMA EMERGENCY on page 193) should immediately call a doctor, who can help determine if the condition requires an office visit or emergency hospital care.

If an emergency room visit is necessary, the patient should already know which hospital to go to—typically the hospital with which the patient's doctor is affiliated. Asthma patients who travel should routinely check in advance with their doctors or the local branch of the American Lung Association to find out what hospital at their destination can provide the kind of care they might need.

Sometimes a patient will be unable to reach the doctor right away. If there is even the slightest doubt about whether treating the attack at home will be sufficient, the patient should go to the emergency room. If the attack turns out not to be an emergency after all, the patient will have lost a few hours and the cost of the visit. But if the emergency is real, a patient who stays home may lose his or her life.

Only a small number of asthmatics will ever have an attack severe enough to require a trip to the emergency room. What is important is that patients understand their condition—not only so that they know when there's a crisis but also to prevent a crisis from arising.

Asthmatics and their families need not be at the mercy of this disease. With education and motivation, they can prevent most attacks, minimize those that do occur, and live calmly and confidently without needless limitations.

Where to go for help

The American Lung Association offers educational programs and materials on asthma through more than 300 local offices. To find the branch nearest you, check the white pages of your telephone book. If none is listed, call the national office at (212) 315-8822, or write the American Lung Association, 1740 Broadway, New York, NY 10019.

The National Jewish Center for Immunology and Respiratory Medicine operates a telephone hot line for asthma information at (800) 222-5864; in Colorado, (303) 355-5864. Nurses are available to callers weekdays between 8 a.m. and 5 p.m. Mountain Standard Time. The center will also mail brochures on request.

Mothers of Asthmatics serves families with asthmatic children. Membership, which includes a monthly newsletter, costs $15 per year. For information and a sample newsletter, write Mothers of Asthmatics, 10875 Main St., Suite 210, Fairfax, VA 22030, or call (703) 385-4403.

The Asthma and Allergy Foundation of America provides pamphlets and other educational materials, some free. For ordering information, write AAFA, 1717 Massachusetts Ave., NW, Suite 305, Washington, DC 20036, or call (202) 265-0265.

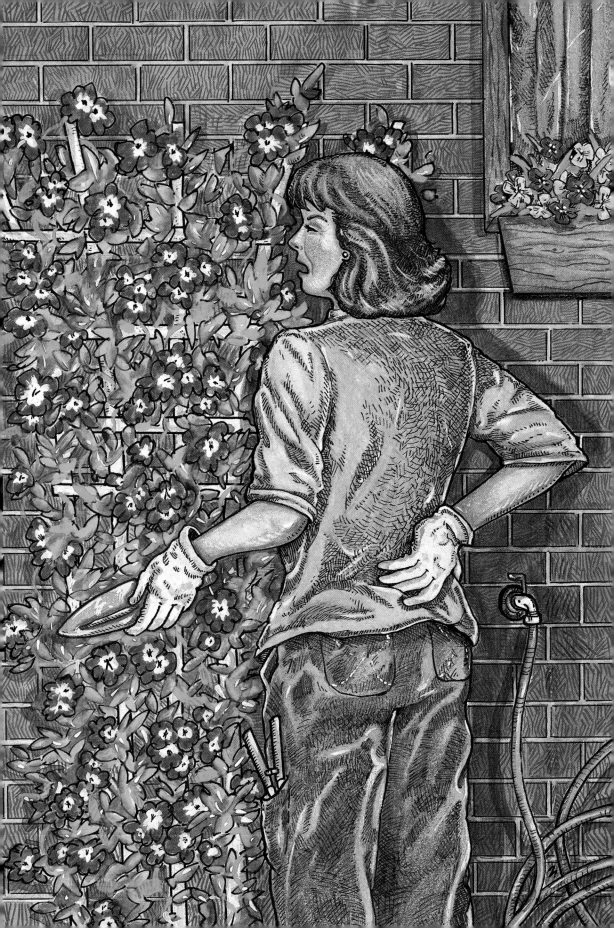

Four out of five Americans will have problems with their backs during their lives. And the causes of—and treatments for—back pain are almost as plentiful as its sufferers.

Oh, My Aching Back!

By Joseph Wallace

The most intense pain Laura had ever felt took her by surprise. "I was visiting friends and had just spent an hour sitting on an uncomfortable chair at the dinner table," she recalls. "After the meal, I pushed my chair back and tried to stand up. Suddenly I felt like I'd been stabbed in the lower back.

"By the time I limped home and fell into bed, I knew that somehow I'd badly hurt my back. But I didn't know why, or how, or what to do about it."

Laura was not alone—either in suffering a back injury or in not knowing how she got hurt, how to treat the problem, and how she might have prevented it. In fact, she was joining a club that welcomes millions of new members each year. The back-pain club encompasses those who merely feel an occasional twinge and those whose pain threatens their work, their social life, or even their day-to-day ability to function.

Figures vary on how many people suffer from back pain, but all the numbers are high. One medical journal, *American Family Physician*, reports that 6½ million Americans are under treatment for lower back pain on any given day. If you count other types of back pain—from mild muscle discomfort to severe injuries to the spine—estimates approach 8 million.

Back problems take a stunning toll in money and time. Various studies in the 1970's and 1980's estimated that medical bills, lost wages, and disability payments from back problems annually cost Americans between $16 billion and $20 billion, along with 93 million missed days of work every year. Orthopedic surgeon Robert G. Addison, who heads a back pain clinic at Northwestern University Medical School in Chicago, estimates that for every 25-cent postage stamp sold, one penny pays for back pain in a postal worker.

How the back works

Why do so many people have back trouble? To answer that, we must first know something about the spine and the structures that protect and support it.

The *spinal column*—the set of bones we call the spine or backbone—serves as the passageway for the *spinal cord*, the central channel of the body's nervous system. Your brain controls every move you make by sending commands through the spinal cord to a network of nerves that branches out to all the organs and muscles in your body.

The spine's second purpose, support for the body, is just as important. Not only must the spine hold the head and body upright and allow the neck and torso to bend, but it also must withstand constant strain. Your footsteps jolt and compress it, and even the lightest object you carry adds to the pressure.

The spine is composed mostly of 24 bones called *vertebrae*, piled in a flexible stack that runs from the lower back to the base of the skull. The sturdy drum-shaped front part of each vertebra is designed to bear weight. The back part is more complex: It includes an opening for the spinal cord, plus several projections called *processes*. Some processes on each vertebra hinge to the processes of the vertebrae above or below, forming *facet joints*. Each process is tipped with smooth cartilage to keep the bones from rubbing together.

The backbone is not just bones. Between the vertebrae are flat pads, or *disks*, about ¼ inch (6 millimeters) thick. Each disk consists of a protective shell of tough, flexible cartilage and an inner core of a watery gel—something like the soft inside of a gumdrop. The disks keep the vertebrae from rubbing against one another. They also act as shock absorbers, cushioning the vertebrae from the pounding of everyday life.

The spinal bones depend on ligaments and muscles for control and support. *Ligaments* are strong, flexible bands of tissue that stabilize joints and guide their motion. The spine's largest ligaments stretch from the top to the bottom of the spine and support the disks and the vertebrae. Smaller ligaments keep the facet joints from twisting out of place.

Muscles both control movement and provide support. The muscles around the spine have several functions. They move

The author:

Joseph Wallace is a New York-based writer specializing in medical and scientific topics.

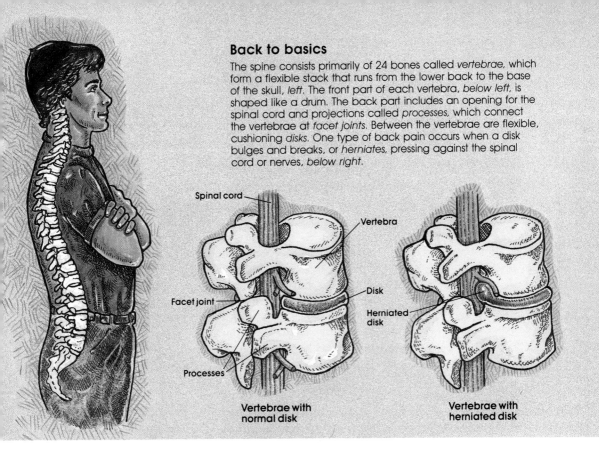

Back to basics

The spine consists primarily of 24 bones called *vertebrae,* which form a flexible stack that runs from the lower back to the base of the skull, *left.* The front part of each vertebra, *below left,* is shaped like a drum. The back part includes an opening for the spinal cord and projections called *processes,* which connect the vertebrae at *facet joints.* Between the vertebrae are flexible, cushioning *disks.* One type of back pain occurs when a disk bulges and breaks, or *herniates,* pressing against the spinal cord or nerves, *below right.*

Spinal cord

Vertebra

Facet joint

Disk

Herniated disk

Processes

**Vertebrae with
normal disk**

**Vertebrae with
herniated disk**

the spine—and therefore the entire torso—under orders from the brain. And they limit those motions to keep them from causing injury.

What causes back pain?

Physicians agree that one unstoppable force leaves everyone vulnerable to a bad back. That force is aging. Until you reach your mid- to late 20's, your bones—including your spinal bones—are still growing and developing. After that, they begin to degenerate slowly. The ligaments grow weaker, the facet joints begin to wear out, and the disks lose their fluidity and their shock-absorbing ability. When a person reaches age 60 or 70, some consequences of aging compensate for these disadvantages. By then, your spine becomes less flexible —so you are less likely to hurt it by twisting it out of position.

Back pain most commonly begins between the ages of 30 and 50. At any age, though, you can suffer from the wide variety of back ailments we know as *strains* or *sprains.* People usually use the word "strain" to describe a muscle problem and "sprain" to refer to a partially torn ligament, but the terms can mean almost anything; mostly, they simply mean your back hurts. Physicians, however, have pinpointed some types of back pain more precisely.

Muscle pain. One of the most common of all back problems is felt as pain in the muscle, because you have either stressed the back beyond its limit (by lifting a heavy object improperly or twisting the spine in an unnatural way) or used bad posture over a long period of time (such as sitting hunched in front of a computer or typewriter for hours at a time, day after day).

Such stress usually causes only vague discomfort in the lower back, the area where the vertebrae take the most pounding. Sometimes, however, one or more of the muscles suddenly contract and become rigid. This splinting action, called *spasm*, can follow an injury to the joints or ligaments, or it can result from poor posture, sitting too long in one position, or even emotional stress. Muscle spasm actually serves a protective function. By immobilizing both the muscles and the bones they support, spasm keeps them from further stress while they heal. Unfortunately, spasm itself is severely painful.

Laura's doctor explained her sudden after-dinner pain as muscle spasm—a symptom of underlying muscular fatigue. "I was an avid jogger, and the doctor told me I might have strained the muscle while running," she says. "Then, by sitting in one position for so long at the dinner table, I pushed it some more—and it went into spasm."

Disk problems. Laura was relieved to learn that she had not suffered the best-known back injury—the "slipped disk." The term is common but inaccurate. An injured disk doesn't slip out from between two vertebrae but instead begins to bulge outward, or *herniate*. In the most serious cases, the disk's cartilage shell ruptures and some of its internal gel oozes out.

You might not feel anything wrong until the bulge touches a nerve or ligament. Then you feel pain—either a sharp pain or a numbness or tingling that spreads down your arms or legs.

DON'T . . . lift using your back muscles or lift heavy objects above chest level. Don't reach to lift heavy objects or to put them down. Improper lifting and carrying is the most common cause of back injury.

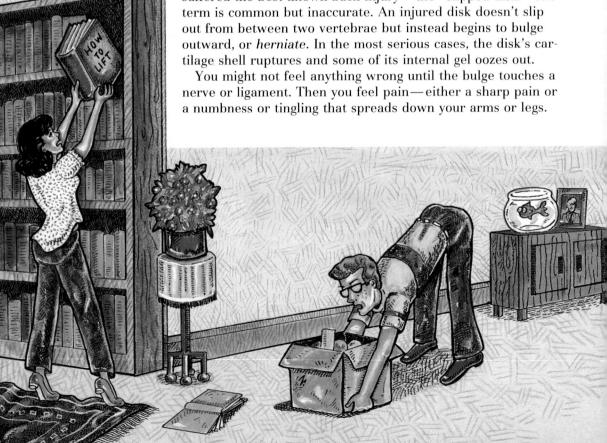

When the injured disk is in the lower back, the affected nerve is often the *sciatic* nerve, which carries the pain along the back of the hip and leg. This condition is called *sciatica*.

No one is exactly sure what percentage of back problems can be traced to disk injuries, but experts agree that the figure isn't very high. Estimates range from a low of 2 per cent to about 10 per cent. Many people who claim to have a "slipped disk" may actually be suffering from some other problem.

Stressed ligaments. Back pain may come from stretching a ligament too far. Ligaments are designed to stretch and twist, but they are not indestructible. Extreme stress—from a skiing accident or a car crash, for example—can strain any one of the spinal ligaments, causing moderate or severe pain.

More often, however, ligament strain results from poor posture, such as standing for a long time or sitting for hours bent over a keyboard. After years of such abuse, the ligaments may become stretched and less resilient—and painful.

Worn joints. Bulging disks, stressed ligaments, and the aging process can all contribute to another problem: the worn facet joint. Any of these conditions can bring the processes of two vertebrae closer together, so that the delicate bones scrape against each other. This pain, which may range from mild to severe, typically occurs when you arch your back.

Disease. Back pain can also be a sign of underlying disease. In general, back pain that is unrelieved by rest and that persists longer than one to three weeks should be checked to rule out a potentially serious disorder. Unusual symptoms—including sharp pains, persistent fever, vomiting, and bowel trouble—might signal a kidney infection or even cancer. In some people, especially women in their 50's or older, back pain may indicate bone damage from *osteoporosis*, a long-term disease that makes bones weak and brittle.

One common disease that affects the spine directly is *os-*

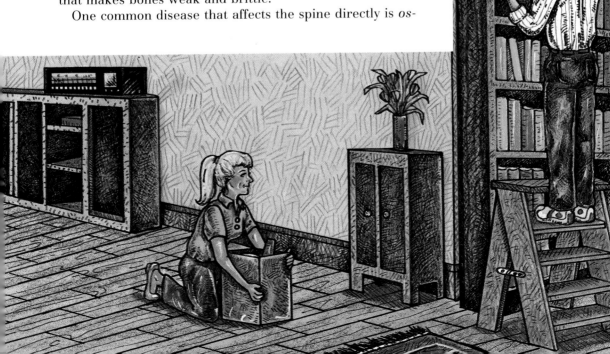

DO . . . bend your knees—not your back—when lifting, and let your legs support the weight. Keep the weight near your body. Use a sturdy stool or stepladder to reach high shelves—and be sure of your footing.

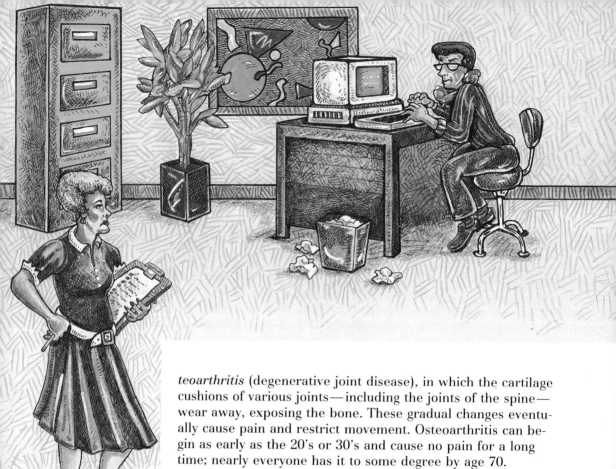

teoarthritis (degenerative joint disease), in which the cartilage cushions of various joints—including the joints of the spine—wear away, exposing the bone. These gradual changes eventually cause pain and restrict movement. Osteoarthritis can begin as early as the 20's or 30's and cause no pain for a long time; nearly everyone has it to some degree by age 70.

A rarer but more serious form of arthritis is *ankylosing spondylitis*, in which the joints in the back—usually the lower back—stiffen and swell, eventually fusing together. This disease afflicts mostly men and usually starts in the 20's or 30's.

Another spinal problem is *spondylolisthesis*, a shift of one vertebra over another. This condition, which occurs in 2 to 4 per cent of Americans, is not always painful. But pain may occur if the misplaced vertebra pushes against a nerve.

The most frightening—and most serious—source of back pain is cancer. It's also one of the rarest, causing fewer than 1 per cent of severe backaches. Few cancers begin in the spine; usually the spine is affected when cancer spreads from another part of the body. The likelihood that a case of back pain means cancer increases with such factors as age over 50, a history of cancer, long-term back pain that does not improve with standard treatments, and unexplained weight loss.

Diagnosing and treating back pain

More than four-fifths of all backaches have no obvious cause, and many go away on their own. So it's hard to be sure whether back pain merits a visit to a doctor. Some general pointers can help you determine how severe your problem is.

If the pain began after a fall or a blow, and you also feel

DON'T . . . stand or sit with your spine slumped or twisted—and don't stand or sit too long in one position. Avoid high heels; they throw the whole body off balance. When sitting, avoid leaning forward and arching your back—and don't slide down to the edge of the chair, either. Never cradle a telephone receiver between your ear and shoulder. Repeated poor posture can add up to chronic back pain.

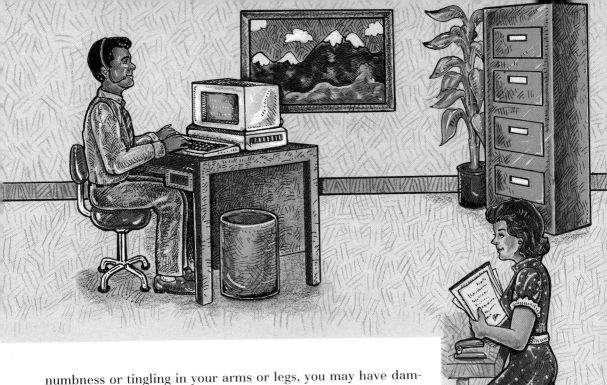

numbness or tingling in your arms or legs, you may have damaged a nerve or your spinal cord and should see a doctor immediately. But if you feel only mild ache or stiffness, it's likely that you overstressed your back and that rest alone will enable it to heal. If so, the best course might be simply to avoid putting strain on your back for a few days. Doctors often suggest taking an anti-inflammatory drug such as aspirin or ibuprofen to reduce swelling and pain. Chances are these simple steps will banish your backache, at least temporarily.

Still, the pain may grow worse—or simply not go away. This is what happened to Laura. "After two days, it didn't feel much better," she remembers. "I had visions of staying in bed for the rest of my life." Instead, she visited a doctor.

Most experts recommend that you first see the physician who knows you best. Even if you are sure of what caused your backache, the doctor will need to consider your complete medical history, including any previous back problems.

The physical examination will include a close look at the painful area for swelling, bruising, or other visible signs. The doctor may also take blood and urine samples and order other tests that may not seem to have much to do with your backache but which will help the doctor determine your general condition and spot a few unusual causes of back pain.

Perhaps most important, the doctor will ask specific questions about your pain: when and how it started, exactly where the worst ache is located, where the pain spread, and what activities you are unable to perform. At the same time, the doctor will evaluate your emotional state—because stress, anger, or depression can make a backache worse.

At this point, if the doctor has found nothing seriously

DO . . . stand with your spine relaxed but upright. When standing for long periods, put one foot up on a stool or step to ease strain on the lower back. Wear low, comfortable shoes, and change positions often. Sit straight, with feet flat and knees level with hips; you may need a footrest. Use the whole seat, and make sure it supports your lower back. And if you must talk on the phone while you work, use a headset.

wrong, he or she may still prescribe rest and painkillers or anti-inflammatory drugs. Laura's doctor told her to stop jogging for a while. "That was an easy order to obey," she says. "I could barely walk, so I had no intention of running." He also told her that as the injury healed, the pain would gradually ease—and it did. She was back at work the next week.

If your pain is particularly severe or persistent, your doctor may suggest a more thorough examination. This might be performed by an *orthopedist*, a specialist in bones and joints.

This second set of tests will probably include X rays of your back. But X rays show problems only of the bone itself; they miss muscle problems, most disk injuries, and even small cracks in the bone. Consequently, many doctors now use two powerful techniques, *computerized tomography* (CT) and *magnetic resonance imaging* (MRI), to get a closer look at the bone and the tissues that support it. A CT scan uses a series of X rays to scan cross-sections of the spine and other tissues a millimeter at a time. An MRI device uses magnetic energy and radio waves to scan the body and produce signals. In both procedures, a computer converts this information into detailed images. Both CT and MRI are particularly useful at detecting tiny fractures and disk disease as well as the rare tumor.

The orthopedist may also recommend a *myelogram*, a test in which a small quantity of dye is injected into the spinal canal. When X rays are taken, the dye highlights the disks, enabling the orthopedist to see any irregularities. A similar procedure, a *diskogram*, involves injecting dye directly into a disk. These techniques can be painful and are reserved most often for use in preparing for surgery. Doctors use them for diagnosis only when back pain is both mysterious and severe.

Still, in 85 per cent of backaches, the precise cause is never identified. If the doctor hasn't pinpointed a serious bone, disk, or ligament problem, he or she may simply recommend bed rest and drugs, followed by exercise as the pain eases.

Some recent studies, however, challenge the idea that long-

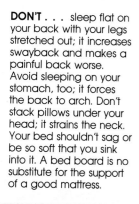

DON'T . . . sleep flat on your back with your legs stretched out; it increases swayback and makes a painful back worse. Avoid sleeping on your stomach, too; it forces the back to arch. Don't stack pillows under your head; it strains the neck. Your bed shouldn't sag or be so soft that you sink into it. A bed board is no substitute for the support of a good mattress.

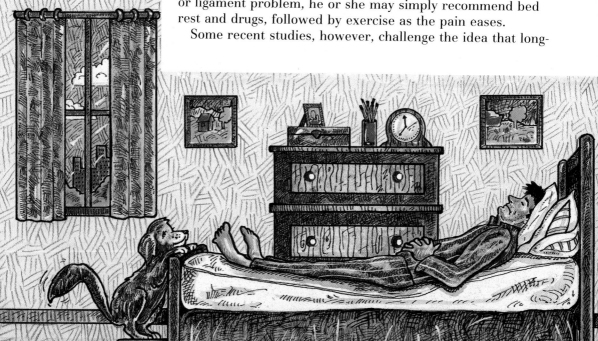

term rest is the best remedy. In 1988, orthopedist Alf Nach-emson of the University of Göteborg in Sweden announced results of a study of 106 automobile workers suffering from backaches. Half of the workers received the usual treatment, which included plenty of rest. The other half were asked to begin jogging, swimming, or doing other exercise almost im-mediately, even if their backs still hurt. On average, those who exercised returned to work seven weeks earlier than those who rested. After two years, the exercisers proved far less likely to miss work due to back pain or to retire because of back-related disability. Other studies have reached the same conclusions. Most of these researchers recommend a day or two of bed rest followed by a gradual increase in exercise.

Continuing therapy

Treating ongoing moderate back pain can be a long-term proc-ess. Thus, after making the initial diagnosis and recommend-ing immediate treatment, many doctors refer patients to physical therapists for continuing therapy. In addition, millions of people who suffer from recurring backaches seek help from many other types of practitioners. Treatment options vary greatly, and experts as well as patients disagree over the best approaches. Here are a few of the most common choices.

Physical therapy. Your doctor may refer you to a physical therapist (also called a physiotherapist). These licensed practi-tioners provide long-term therapy, both by treating existing pain and by suggesting ways to prevent recurrences.

Part of physical therapy involves easing the back pain you have right now. The therapist can call upon a wide range of techniques, such as heat or cold; *ultrasound*, which uses sound waves to stimulate and soothe damaged muscles; or *transcuta-neous electric nerve stimulation*— known as TENS—which uses electricity to interrupt pain signals to the brain.

Just as important, however, physical therapy involves chang-

DO . . . Sleep on your side, with hips and knees bent. Or lie on your back with a few pillows under your bent knees. One pil-low under your head will keep your neck straight. Buy a mattress that's firm but not uncomfortable. The best time to shop for one is when your back hurts—lie on a store mat-tress 20 minutes or more to see if it makes the pain better or worse.

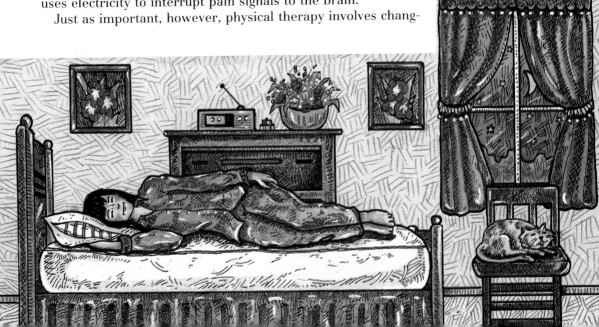

ing the patient's habits. A physical therapist will study you and your backache in detail to determine whether your job, your bed, your posture, or your habits are putting strain on your back. Since emotions can influence back pain, the therapist might also suggest stress-reducing techniques.

On the advice of her doctor, Laura visited a physical therapist, who prescribed back-strengthening exercises. "The therapist taught me how important it is to keep your abdominal and back muscles strong," says Laura.

A high proportion of physical therapy patients are equally pleased. According to a survey of 492 back-pain sufferers by market researcher Arthur C. Klein and science writer Dava Sobel—published in their 1985 book *Backache Relief*—65 per cent of those treated by physical therapists said they felt their condition had shown dramatic or moderate long-term improvement. This was one of the highest satisfaction rates reported among more than 100 types of therapy mentioned.

Osteopathy. Osteopaths, also known as doctors of osteopathy, are not medical doctors. But their training is nearly as extensive, involving four years of graduate study at an osteopathic college and an internship of at least a year at a hospital. Although they are licensed to perform surgery and prescribe drugs, osteopaths specialize in a technique called *manipulation*. This involves twisting and stretching the spine or other parts of the body to correct what the osteopath diagnoses as misalignment of the bones and muscles.

The back-pain patient may feel relief of pressure and stiffness from the movement and stretching of the spine. Klein and Sobel found, however, that unlike physical therapy, osteopathic treatment did not provide long-term relief to most of the patients surveyed. In fact, more than one-half of the 71 patients who had seen osteopaths said they thought the treatment was ineffective or actually made their pain worse.

Alternative therapies. Despite the good record of physical therapists, countless frustrated backache sufferers choose to visit therapists who are neither medical doctors nor recommended by one. The most popular alternative is to consult one of the 40,000 chiropractors licensed in the United States.

Chiropractic therapy almost always involves spinal manipulation. Of the 492 patients Klein and Sobel surveyed, 422 had consulted chiropractors; of these, 28 per cent said they experienced temporary relief of their backache. Another 28 per cent reported some long-term progress, but most of these people also received other therapy—such as stress reduction or exercise—in addition to manipulation. In general, the survey suggested that chiropractic therapy is effective over the long term only when combined with mainstays of physical therapy. Physicians also warn that in people with herniated disks, manipulation can make the injury—and the pain—worse.

Relaxation techniques offer another alternative approach for long-term management of back pain. One option is *yoga*, a regimen of stretching exercises designed to increase the flexibility of the spine and relax muscles. Many physicians have little respect for yoga as back therapy, but of the 45 back-pain sufferers in Klein and Sobel's survey who had tried yoga, 90 per cent reported dramatic or moderate long-term relief. Another relaxation technique used to relieve stress—and thus some chronic back pain—is *biofeedback*. People using this method learn to control bodily responses such as heart rate by monitoring their progress with machines.

Many other specialties offer solutions for back pain. For example, some people turn to *acupuncture*, a Chinese therapy that involves inserting thin needles into the skin. Others try *orthotics*, which uses shoe inserts to counter skeletal imbalances or leg-length differences. Because back pain can be as individual as its victims, each of the many alternative treatments may work for some people. But few studies have produced reliable data on how well various treatments work overall, and health professionals have mixed feelings on the effectiveness—and sometimes the safety—of these solutions.

Surgery. People with chronic, severely painful disk problems may consider surgery—perhaps the most debated treatment of all. Each year, more than 200,000 people have disk operations in the United States and Canada.

In the most frequent procedure, the surgeon removes part of the bulging disk. This may require *laminectomy*—the removal of a small piece of bone to allow access to the disk. In about a third of these operations, the surgeon also uses *spinal fusion* to stabilize the injured area. In this procedure, the doctor augments the injured vertebrae with strips of bone, often taken from the patient's hip. Within three or four months, the body's healing process fuses the new bone to the spine.

Disk surgery is sometimes essential. But surgery is not automatically the ideal solution to all disk problems. Orthopedic surgeons maintain that surgery succeeds in up to 90 per cent of cases if patients are selected properly. But the success rate falls if the source of the pain cannot be clearly determined, if more than one disk is involved, or if the patient's temperament or behavior contributes to the problem.

Surgery has other drawbacks, too: It is expensive, it requires a hospital stay, and it carries the risks associated with any operation that uses general anesthesia. Perhaps most im-

Back in shape

Many types of back-conditioning exercises exist to help people recover from back injuries and prevent new ones. Some, however, can be damaging if you are out of shape or already in pain. Consult a physician or therapist before beginning any exercise program; he or she can recommend exercises that are right for your abilities and your back. To avoid injury, exercise regularly and build up your endurance gradually. The following beginning exercises are safe for most backs.

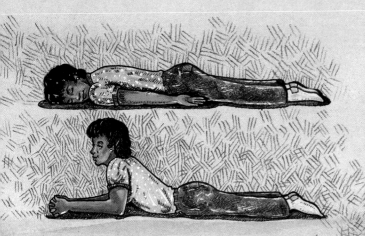

To maintain the normal curve in your lower back: Lie on your stomach as shown and relax for three to five minutes. Keeping your lower back relaxed, prop yourself up on your elbows for two to three minutes. Return to starting position and relax for one minute; repeat five times.

To loosen a stiff back: Start by lying flat with your knees bent and your feet flat on the floor. Without using your arms or hands, raise one knee to chest. Grasp and pull the knee to your body for five seconds. Return to first position; repeat five times. Then repeat with other leg, and then both legs.

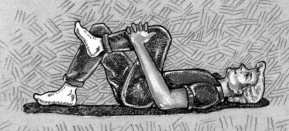

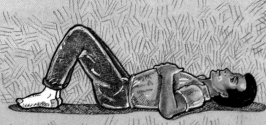

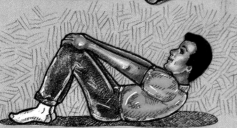

To strengthen abdomen: Start by lying flat with your knees bent and your feet flat on the floor. Slowly lift palms to knees, keeping head and neck aligned as you raise them. Hold for five seconds, and slowly return to starting position. Repeat five times.

portant, many doctors think less drastic treatments—such as injecting drugs into the spine—might work just as well. As one alternative to traditional disk surgery, some surgeons recommend an outpatient procedure called *percutaneous diskectomy*, which involves sucking out part of a bulging disk through a hollow needle. This procedure, however, is still new, and its long-term effectiveness is debated. And it is useful only in patients whose disks have not ruptured.

Preventing back pain

Fortunately, long-term treatment is not necessary for people whose pain is intermittent or moderate. A few simple rules can help the occasional sufferer—as well as those who have no back problems and want to keep it that way.

Although many types of activity can strain your back, the events that led to Laura's muscle spasm—jogging and sitting—are hardly the most common route to back injury. Typically, damage occurs from lifting or twisting. Almost everyone knows that lifting an object awkwardly can hurt your back; bend your knees, not your back, when lifting, and let your legs support the weight. And avoid twisting the spine unnaturally while lifting, carrying, bending, or reaching.

Good posture is probably the best bet to prevent or eliminate moderate backache. Stand with your back straight, not slouched. Just as important is your weight. If you're too heavy, you're putting undue stress on your back at all times.

Regular exercise can help you improve your posture, lose or redistribute weight, and strengthen stomach muscles. Be aware, however, that some forms of exercise—such as jogging and high-impact aerobics— carry risks of back injury. If you've ever had problems, it might be better to swim, walk, or use an exercise machine. A specialist can help you choose the exercise that is best for you.

Today, Laura follows these rules for back maintenance. She lost about 10 pounds (4.5 kilograms). She swims four or five times a week and does regular back-strengthening exercises. She's constantly checking to make sure that her posture is correct. And she's been virtually free of pain for five years.

"Even though I have to work hard to keep my back healthy, I feel very lucky," she says. "But if I had it all to do again, I would have started taking care of my back years ago."

For further reading:

Berland, Theodore, and Addison, Robert G. *Living with Your Bad Back*. St. Martin's Press, 1983.

Klein, Arthur C., and Sobel, Dava. *Backache Relief*. Times Books, 1985.

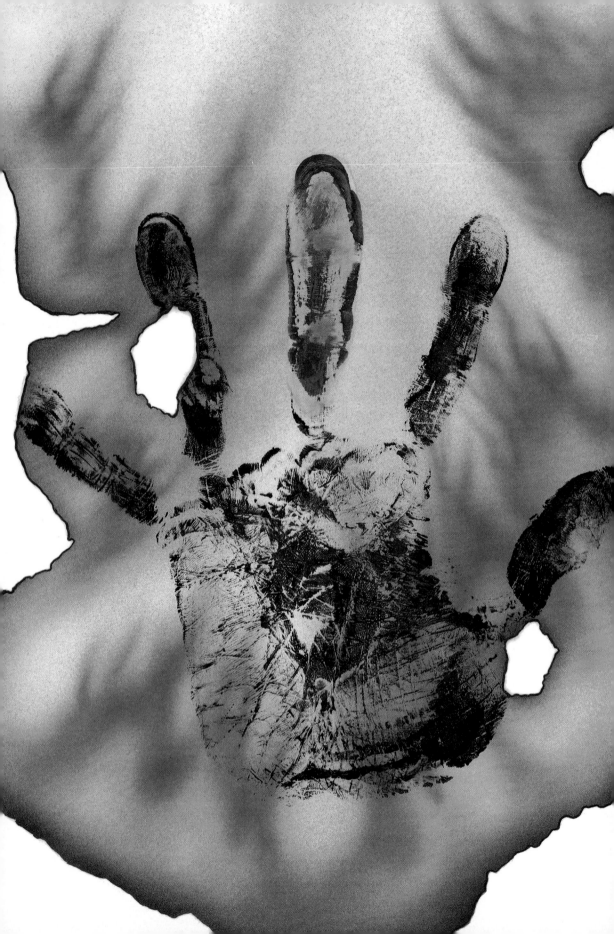

Severe burns destroy one of our most important defenses—the skin. Ever-better treatments are saving lives and helping patients heal.

Treating the Severely Burned

By Richard Trubo

The call came to the University of California Irvine Burn Center shortly after midnight. A boy about 6 years old, name unknown, had been severely burned in a motel fire and was being rushed by ambulance to the burn unit, located in the university's medical center in Orange.

Despite the late hour, the staff mobilized quickly, preparing for the arrival of the youngster. Although nurses and physicians are on duty around the clock, the late-night shift was too small to cope with so serious an emergency. Suzie Martinez, the burn unit's nurse manager, was awakened by a phone call and told of the imminent arrival of the young burn victim. As she rushed to the hospital, other staff personnel were summoned as well.

By the time the boy arrived at the center's emergency entrance, a team of burn specialists wearing blue sterile gowns, masks, and gloves was gathering. The six doctors and eight nurses knew they would battle through the night with one goal in mind—to save the boy's life.

The author:

Richard Trubo is a contributing editor for *Medical World News*.

As the ambulance pulled in front of the emergency room entrance, the youngster, covered with blankets, was already receiving fluids *intravenously*—through a *catheter* (slender tube) placed in a vein in his arm. He had been burned over 90 per cent of his body, and the burns clearly were severe. Within seconds, he was surrounded by an experienced staff and the most sophisticated medical equipment available.

The eight-bed burn facility of the University of California at Irvine (UCI) treats about 200 burn patients each year. But this youngster—doctors later learned his name was David—was one of the most seriously burned patients ever seen by the center's director, plastic surgeon Bruce M. Achauer, and the burn staff.

Even so, rather than focusing immediately upon the devastating burns, the doctors had to evaluate the boy's general condition—and it was very unstable. Without medical attention to help his body maintain such vital functions as breathing and fluid balance, David's life was in jeopardy.

First, the medical team had to ensure that David was able to continue breathing. Respiratory failure is the most common cause of death in the first few hours following a severe burn. Exposure to large amounts of smoke can cause carbon monoxide poisoning, which prevents the blood from supplying oxygen to the body. Also, the airways leading to the lungs may be swollen from inhaling very hot air. If this swelling obstructs the airways, the victim could die of asphyxiation.

Working quickly, doctors inserted a thin tube into David's *trachea* (windpipe) and began administering oxygen to assist the boy's breathing. Nurses began monitoring David's heartbeat and blood pressure.

Like all severely burned patients, David was experiencing a massive loss of body fluids through the large burned areas of his body. If a patient has severe burns covering more than 10 to 20 per cent of the body, doctors generally order a special fluid to be given intravenously. This fluid prevents the body from becoming dehydrated and also replaces essential nutrients that the body is losing. In David's case, with burns covering nearly all of his body, such treatment was essential.

The medical team then moved David from the center's emergency room to the burn unit itself. There they carefully submerged him in a special tub containing warm water. The tub's agitator swirled the water gently around him, loosening the dead skin, which can harbor and feed bacteria. Once the burns were cleaned, the staff could more closely evaluate them and decide how David's treatment should proceed.

Burns can happen to anyone. More than 2 million people in the United States—nearly 1 per cent of the population—suf-

Burns: the destruction of skin

One of the greatest dangers to skin is a burn. Burns are classified as first-degree, second-degree, or third-degree, depending on how deeply they penetrate the skin.

Skin has two layers; beneath them is a layer of tissue called *subcutaneous fat, below.* The outermost layer is a thin sheet of cells called the *epidermis.* Below the epidermis is a thicker layer of cells called the *dermis.* The dermis contains several structures, including sweat glands and hair follicles.

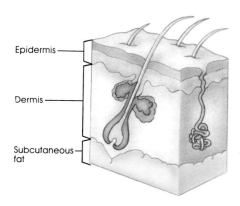

Epidermis

Dermis

Subcutaneous fat

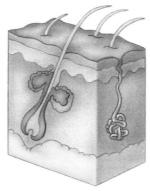

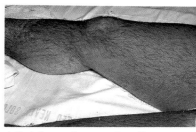

A *first-degree burn,* such as the sunburn shown above, damages only the epidermis. The skin is red and painful, but there are no blisters.

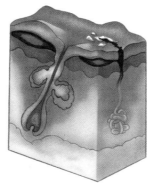

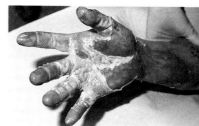

A *second-degree burn* damages the epidermis and part of the dermis. The skin—red, blistered, and oozing fluid—is very painful.

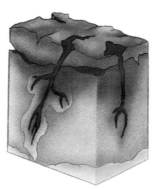

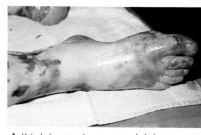

A *third-degree burn* completely destroys both the epidermis and the dermis. The skin may look leathery and be red, black, or pearly white in color. There is little pain because the nerves in the skin have been destroyed.

fer burns each year, according to the National Institute for Burn Medicine (NIBM) in Ann Arbor, Mich. Most of the burns are slight and can be treated safely at home (see TREATING MINOR BURNS AT HOME on page 224). But about 70,000 burn sufferers must be hospitalized. Burns are one of the leading causes of accidental death in America. Estimates vary, but burns are responsible for approximately 9,000 fatalities each year, according to the NIBM.

Serious burns are usually treated at one of the 150 burn centers in the United States. Thanks to these centers and to the increasingly sophisticated medical treatment for burns, the survival rate among seriously burned patients has greatly improved. Less than 30 years ago, most patients died if their burns covered 30 per cent of their bodies. Today, with proper care, nearly all of those patients survive. But recovery from a serious burn can be physically and psychologically agonizing. It often involves terrible pain, many operations, adjustment to scars, depression, anger, and anxiety over social rejection.

In burn centers, the staff inevitably focuses on that part of the body that suffers the greatest damage from burns—the skin. The skin is the body's largest organ. In an adult, the surface area of the skin is approximately 16 to 20 square feet (1.5 to 1.9 square meters). Flexible and elastic, the skin fits smoothly over every curve and crevice of the body.

The skin is composed essentially of two layers; below them is a layer of fat tissue called *subcutaneous fat*. The outermost layer, called the *epidermis*, is no thicker than a sheet of paper and is comprised of cells that form a protective covering. Below this layer is the *dermis*, which makes up most of our skin. The dermis is from 15 to 40 times thicker than the epidermis, and—unlike the outer layer—it contains blood vessels, sweat glands, nerve endings, and hair follicles.

Our skin, of course, is what we see when we look in the mirror, and it is critical to our appearance and self-esteem. Yet, except for an occasional pimple, bruise, or rash, few of us give much thought to the skin itself—even though it is vital to our survival. Like a space suit, the skin protects our bodies from bacteria, chemicals, harmful solar radiation, and excessive fluid loss and keeps the body's internal temperature at normal levels. Intact skin is one of our body's most important defense mechanisms, and breaching this defense can be life-threatening.

Burns can destroy the skin and thus threaten survival. They can be caused by dry heat, the moist heat of hot liquids and steam, corrosive chemicals, electricity, and radiation. Whatever the cause, the severity of burns depends partly on the extent of the area involved and partly on the depth of damage

Healing a
third-degree burn

Skin that has received a third-degree burn is so damaged it cannot heal on its own. To prevent infection and scarring and promote healing, a third-degree burn must be thoroughly cleaned and given a skin graft.

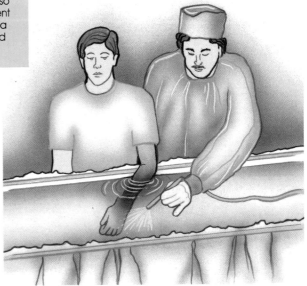

A person who has received a third-degree burn needs prompt medical attention. One of the first steps in treatment is to clean the wound. The burned area is submerged in warm water to loosen dead skin that can harbor bacteria.

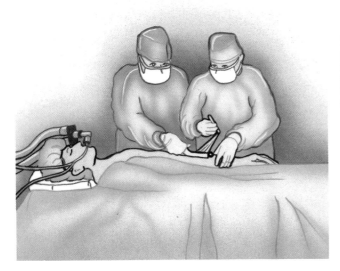

To prepare the wound to receive a skin graft, the patient undergoes a process called *debridement*. Using a special peeling device, the physician cuts off burned tissue until healthy tissue is exposed.

Whenever possible, the patient's own skin is used for the graft. In a procedure called an *autograft*, healthy skin is taken from an area of the patient's body—referred to as the *donor site*—and is sewn over the burn. When the patient does not have enough healthy skin for the needed grafts, skin from another source—usually a corpse—is sewn over the uncovered area until an autograft can be performed. This temporary graft is called an *allograft*.

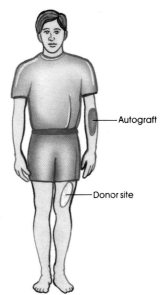

Autograft

Donor site

Artificial skin: New hope for the seriously burned

People with extensive third-degree burns often do not have enough healthy skin to graft onto all the burned areas on their bodies. In the past, the only immediate treatment for these patients was a temporary allograft using skin from a corpse. But scientists in the 1980's have developed a new option—artificial skin that can be grafted to burns until an autograft can be performed. Although it is in the experimental stage, results look promising.

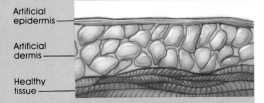

Artificial epidermis

Artificial dermis

Healthy tissue

Artificial skin is composed of two layers: an epidermis made of a special plastic and a dermis made of *collagen* (an animal protein) and a chemical derived from animal *cartilage* (tough, elastic tissue). Artificial skin is placed over the wound to prevent infection, hold in body fluids, and encourage the growth of new skin tissue.

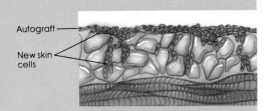

Autograft

New skin cells

When enough of the patient's own skin becomes available, the artificial epidermis is removed and replaced with an autograft. As skin cells grow out from the autograft and the healthy tissue, the artificial dermis eventually disintegrates.

---

to the skin. In *first-degree* burns, only the epidermis is affected. Although the skin is red and painful, there are no blisters. A sunburn is a first-degree burn. So is a *scald*—a burn caused by a splash of hot liquid to the skin or brief contact with steam. These burns usually heal within a week or two without scarring.

Burns that involve not only the epidermis but also some of the dermis are called *second-degree* burns. The skin is typically red and blistered, oozing fluid, and sensitive to the air. The pain can be severe. Once healed, the area may be scarred.

In *third-degree* burns, the epidermis and the dermis are completely destroyed. The burned skin has a dry, leathery appearance and has no blisters. The color of the burned area may vary from red to black to pearly-white. Because nerves in the skin have been destroyed, the patient is frequently without pain. Second- and third-degree burns occur when the skin is in prolonged contact with flames, chemicals, electricity, or hot objects or is immersed in hot liquids.

In the first few days after the injury, doctors often find it difficult to determine whether the patient has second- or third-degree burns. Sometimes, both types of burns have the same appearance. Also, the skin may be burned unevenly, so that a second-degree burn may occur next to a third-degree burn. Since third-degree burns usually require skin grafts for healing, accurate diagnosis is critically important.

A new device called a *laser Doppler blood profusion monitor* can help in this diagnostic process. This monitor can differentiate between second-degree and third-degree burns and can predict with 90 per cent accuracy which burns will need grafting and which are capable of healing on their own. The device uses a *laser* (a narrow and intense beam of light) to measure the speed at which blood flows through the injured area. Good blood flow indicates that the wound will probably heal without surgery. This monitor is used at more than a dozen U.S. burn units.

At the UCI burn unit, with David's condition finally stabilized and his burns cleaned, the staff could begin the long, laborious treatment that would ultimately return him to as normal a life as possible. In the initial phases of his treatment, nurses bathed his wounds daily and coated them with an antibiotic ointment to prevent infection. Without the ointment, microorganisms would accumulate on the burned area, contaminating the tissue within 48 hours of the injury.

For the severely burned patient who survives the first few days, infection is the primary cause of death. This is because the loss of skin allows harmful bacteria to enter the body. Also, in a process that is not yet fully understood, the body's disease-fighting immune system becomes suppressed a few hours after a serious burn has occurred. This makes a patient highly susceptible to infection. For these reasons, the patient is monitored continuously for the first few days. The staff is particularly alert for fever, which might indicate that an infection has occurred at the site of the burn. Besides keeping the burned area scrupulously clean and coated with antibiotic ointment, doctors may use oral or intravenous antibiotics to suppress bacterial invasion and growth.

The UCI burn staff also placed David on a special nutrition program to prevent malnutrition. As the bodies of burn patients attempt to heal themselves, they frequently require additional calories and protein. Calories supply the body with the energy necessary to sustain the healing process. Some patients with severe burns need as many as 5,000 calories a day. In comparison, the recommended caloric intake for most people, depending on their sex and age, ranges from 1,400 to 3,200 calories a day.

The body's supply of protein, which drops as a result of a loss of body fluids and the breakdown of protein in the injured area, must be replaced to promote wound healing. So burn patients are encouraged to consume several snacks a day in addition to regular meals. If they are unable to eat, they are fed through a tube that passes through the nose and into the stomach or are given nourishment intravenously.

Several days after arriving at the burn unit, David began to undergo the difficult procedure called *surgical excision* or *debridement*. This is the first step in preparing the burned area to receive a skin graft. It involves removing dead tissue to expose healthy tissue underneath. Without debridement, the skin graft would not take hold.

As burn patients lie on a bed under bright overhead lamps, the debridement process begins. Depending on the extent of

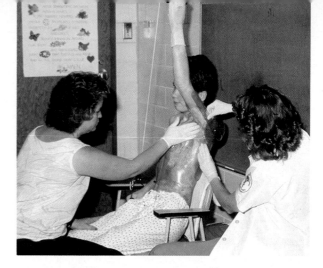

Physical therapists help a young burn patient to raise and lower his arm, *right*. Exercises such as this prevent scar tissue from restricting the movement of burned areas of the body. A social worker meets with a burn patient and his mother, *below*. Counseling to help severely burned people deal with the emotional trauma of painful and often disfiguring burns is another component in the healing process.

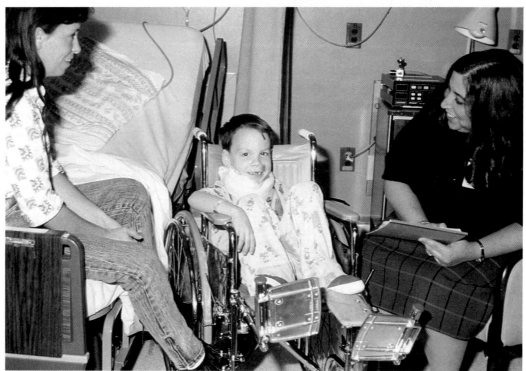

the burns, this can be a lengthy ordeal. A surgeon uses a surgeon's knife or a special peeling device called a *dermatome* to gently lift the dead tissue and cut it off the wound until healthy skin or fatty tissue is reached.

Depending on the size of the wound, the surgeon may take several days to debride all the burned areas. But, as doctors have become able to more effectively control blood loss during surgery, they can debride a larger section of skin each day, reducing the number of days it takes to complete the process. Debridement is also being started earlier than ever before— perhaps on the second or third day after the burn occurs.

Some patients have described the pain associated with debridement as the worst they've ever endured, and an anesthetic is often given to minimize the discomfort of the procedure. Doctors also must closely monitor the patient's temperature during debridement. Because severely burned patients have lost large areas of skin, their bodies are unable to regulate their internal temperature. Thus, cool air can cause chilling, resulting in rapid loss of body heat. To prevent this, both the surgical room and intravenous fluids are usually heated. A warming blanket is used as well.

Sometimes the debrided wound areas are covered with wound dressings and mesh gauze until skin grafts are performed. Each day, the staff checks the wounds through the semitransparent dressings for signs of infection. More likely, however, debridement is immediately followed by skin grafts. By promptly performing debridement and grafting, doctors have found that the length of the patient's hospital stay can be shortened, the number of graft surgeries the patient must undergo can often be reduced, the wounds generally heal better, and chances of survival from severe burns may be improved.

In minor burns, skin cells migrate into the wound from the surrounding area and produce a new layer of skin. But in serious burns, skin grafts are critical to the survival of the patient. Under ideal circumstances, the patient's own skin is used for grafting, since the body will not *reject* it. (Rejection is the work of the body's immune system, which is designed to rid the body of foreign substances, such as bacteria and viruses.) In this procedure, called an *autograft,* skin is removed from an unburned part of the patient's body—called a *donor site—* and placed upon the tissue that has been exposed by debridement. Healthy skin might be stripped from a buttock or a thigh, for example.

Donor sites are usually quite painful for a day or two, and may take a week to 10 days to fully heal. The skin taken from these areas is stretched so that it will cover a larger area than it originally did, permitting maximum use of the skin available for grafting. The surgeon then carefully sews the skin over the burn. Nylon netting or bandages placed on the graft exert a small amount of pressure on the wound. This encourages the transplanted skin to "take" as new cells growing out of the grafted skin and the tissue attach to each other.

In many cases, several grafting operations must be performed. Each of them can be extremely painful and accompanied by significant blood loss. But the finished result is usually cosmetically acceptable, even though it falls short of recreating a perfectly normal appearance.

In some patients, particularly those who are extensively burned, the body does not have enough healthy skin for all the necessary grafts. In these cases, *allografts* are performed using skin from other sources—most commonly from human *cadavers* (corpses). Allografts provide the body with temporary protection from bacterial invasion and fluid loss, buying time until more of the patient's own donor skin is available. Unfortunately, the body often rejects the cadaver skin, but by then, more of the patient's own donor sites may have healed, and new skin can be taken from them for permanent grafts. Although cadaver skin was once in short supply, it can now be donated—just as hearts and other organs can—and kept in organ banks for future use.

Researchers are studying ways to effectively counter the rejection of cadaver skin in burn patients. The body's immune system rejects skin from other sources when it detects unfamiliar protein molecules—called *antigens*—on the skin's surface. To counteract rejection of cadaver skin grafts in extensively burned patients, some researchers have administered the drug cyclosporine, which suppresses the action of the immune system.

Scientists at the New York Hospital-Cornell Medical Center in New York City have spearheaded research in another direction—growing cadaver skin in the laboratory and then transplanting it to a burn patient. In this experimental process, cells taken from cadaver skin are placed in a *culture* (a specially prepared medium), where they multiply, forming a sheet of skin. In about three weeks, the skin is grafted onto the burned area.

This process looks promising as a treatment for some severe burns. In 1986, immunologist John Hefton at New York Hospital-Cornell Medical Center reported that cultured cadaver skin produced rapid healing in 11 of 12 patients with second-degree burns. But 14 patients with third-degree burns who received such grafts did not fare as well. Apparently, when wounds are so serious that no dermis remains, cultured skin grafts contribute little to healing.

Hefton noticed that in the laboratory, cultured cadaver skin seems to lose the antigens that cause a patient's immune system to reject the foreign tissue. Thus, the cultured cadaver skin apparently could be used without the risk of rejection.

Physiologist Howard Green of Harvard Medical School in Boston used a similar technology to grow a burn patient's own skin in the laboratory, clearly eliminating the problem of rejection. In just three weeks, a specimen of skin cells—collectively the size of a postage stamp—can multiply to form sheets of skin cells, enough to cover an entire body.

Doctors hope to have an additional option for covering severe burn wounds until enough of the patient's skin is available for grafting. Throughout the 1980's, researchers have been working to perfect artificial skin made from a combination of animal substances, such as *collagen* (a protein found in the fibers of connective tissue, bones, and cartilage), and manufactured materials, such as plastic membranes. At Massachusetts General Hospital, surgeon John F. Burke has treated burn wounds with an artificial skin developed by mechanical engineer Ioannis V. Yannas of the Massachusetts Institute of Technology in Cambridge.

The artificial skin has two layers that correspond to the epidermis and dermis of human skin. In the artificial skin, however, the epidermis is a temporary, removable layer made of a special rubberlike plastic, while the dermis combines two materials—collagen and a chemical derived from animal cartilage.

The artificial skin is placed over the wounds, usually in sheets measuring about 4 by 6 inches (10 by 15 centimeters). When patches of the patient's own skin become available, very thin layers of it are used to replace sections of the outer plastic epidermis. Until that happens, the artificial skin helps prevent bacterial infection and fluid loss, while also encouraging cells and blood vessels in the patient's tissue below it to produce a new dermis. Eventually, the artificial dermis, which supports the new skin, is absorbed by the body. Thus, the artificial skin is finally replaced by the patient's own newly formed skin.

Artificial skin has some theoretical advantages over transplanted cadaver skin. It can be mass-produced and its shelf life is indefinite. Artificial skin does not, however, eliminate the need for skin grafts, and it can become infected. Most burn experts agree that though tests on artificial skin are quite promising, more research is needed.

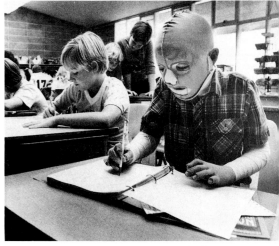

With his head and body encased in elastic pressure garments that help minimize the scars of his skin grafts, a boy who nearly lost his life in a gas explosion returns to school to resume his studies and be with his friends.

The average length of stay in a burn center ranges from one to three months. But for severely burned patients, the recovery process is not over upon discharge. For example, some patients wear form-fitting elastic pressure garments—gloves, face masks, vests, and leotards custom-tailored to fit the injured area—for a year or more in an attempt to minimize scarring. As skin grafts heal, the skin contracts, frequently causing red and raised scars. But the elastic garments apply pressure to counter the contraction of the grafted skin and thus minimize this problem.

These pressure garments are uncomfortable, and some patients are embarrassed to wear them. But if they are worn nearly 24 hours a day until the scar tissue becomes flat and pliable, they can provide long-term cosmetic benefits.

Physical therapy, which is often started in the first few days after the burn injury, also can reduce scarring, as well as ensure that a patient's full range of motion will be maintained. Because it is not very flexible, scar tissue often limits the motion of parts of the body or causes pain with movement. Doctors may prescribe exercises designed to stretch the scar tissue. The patient usually performs these daily exercises, which can be painful, for months after leaving the burn unit.

In many cases, the rehabilitation process includes cosmetic and reconstructive surgery. Because every serious burn heals with scar tissue, these burned patients will never look exactly like they did before. The cosmetic surgeon's scalpel, however, can help them regain as normal an appearance as possible. While skin grafts are the most common reconstructive surgical procedure undergone by burn patients, other techniques are sometimes used. Plastic surgery is often done to correct disfiguring scars, though this is usually delayed until about a year after the initial injury, when the outcome of reconstructive surgery seems to be more satisfactory. Repeated surgeries are often needed to rebuild ears, eyelids, the nose, and the mouth.

Treating minor burns at home

Burns no more than 2 to 3 inches (5 to 8 centimeters) in diameter and affecting only the *epidermis* or outer layer of skin, are considered minor. These burns may be red and painful and sometimes cause minor swelling. They usually can be safely treated at home, though you should see a doctor if the victim is under 2 years old.

■ Immediately flush the burned area with cool water for 10 to 15 minutes or until the pain ebbs. If you can't place the burn under running water, apply cold compresses to the affected area. This will reduce pain and prevent further damage to the skin tissue. Do not put ice on the injury, since it can damage the tissue.

■ Cleanse the burn gently with water and mild soap.

■ Keep the burned area away from heat or dirt.

■ Don't burst blisters since they help to protect the wound.

■ Don't place butter or grease on the burn. These substances will retain heat and can promote infections.

■ A bandage or other covering is not necessary, unless the burn is likely to become rubbed or bumped because of its location.

There are times when a burn requires medical attention. See your physician if the burn:

■ Covers more than a few square inches.

■ Increases in redness or pain or starts to discharge pus, or if you develop a fever. These symptoms may indicate an infection.

If you have any doubt about what to do, call your family doctor or go to the nearest emergency room. [R. T.]

Psychological counseling is another important component of the burn patient's therapy. Immediately after their accident, burn patients sometimes seem very calm, typically because psychological processes, such as denial, allow them to distance themselves from the reality of their injuries. But with time, the psychological impact of their wounds becomes more apparent. Anxiety and agitation may surface, giving way to depression and, sometimes, to suicidal thoughts. Many patients experience anger, hostility, and a loss of self-esteem, often corresponding with their degree of disfigurement. Some may suffer from insomnia, nightmares, or a loss of their sexual drive (sometimes due to their physical pain). Before going home, they may feel unable to return to work or participate in social life. If such fears are not dealt with, these individuals risk becoming recluses, rarely venturing out in public.

To accelerate "inner healing," most burn centers offer individual counseling, as well as support groups comprised of both current and former burn patients. At these group sessions, anxieties and insecurities are shared and relieved.

The families of burn patients, too, are usually offered psychological counseling. Family members may be overwhelmed by their loved one's tragedy and may develop feelings of guilt. ("If only I had helped him light the barbecue. . . .") They may feel anxiety over mounting medical bills or resentment over the burden of taking care of an injured family member. Therapy can help them deal with their anxieties.

Although the recovery process is slow and painful, the overwhelming majority of burn patients return to a normal life. They pull through the ordeal, and some become stronger for having endured this experience. After more than 50 plastic surgeries over the past five years, David's treatment is finally ended. Although he still carries physical and emotional scars from his terrible injuries, his life is getting back to normal. The stories of burn patients like David may be filled with suffering and long-term rehabilitation. But thanks to modern medicine, almost all begin leading productive lives again.

For information about burn support groups, contact:

Phoenix Society, Inc.
National Organization for Burn Victims
11 Rust Hill Road
Levittown, PA 19056
(215)946-4788 or (800)946-BURN

National Burn Victim Foundation
308 Main Street
Orange, NJ 07050
(201)731-3112

Health & Medical File

In 41 alphabetically arranged articles, *Health & Medical* contributors report on the year's major developments in health and medicine.

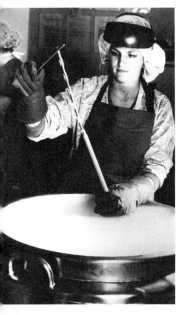

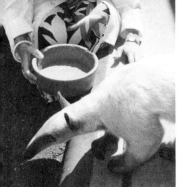

Aging 228
Brain research
Fitness

AIDS 230
Drugs, vaccine research
Testing

Alcohol and Drug Abuse 233
Student drug use
Substance abuse research

Allergies & Immunology 236
Immune system research
Food allergies
Close-Up:
   Ultrasonic humidifiers

**Arthritis and
Connective Tissue Disorders** 240
Arthritis research
Exercise benefits

Birth Control 243
Abortion drug
Contraceptive vaccines

Blood 244
New treatments

Bone Disorders 246
Osteoporosis
Bone healing

Books of Health and Medicine 248

Brain and Nervous System 250
Brain research
Memory loss
Immunity

Cancer 254
New treatments
Cancer research

Child development 257
Media violence
Infant intelligence test
Self-control, shyness, deceit

Dentistry 261
Tooth restoration
Gum disease

Diabetes 262
Predictive test
Diabetes research

Digestive System 264
Diagnostic tests
Gallstone treatments

Drugs 267
New drugs
Close-Up:
   Antibiotic resistance

Ear & Hearing 271
Hearing loss

Emergency Medicine 273
Long distance heart treatment
Air travel

Environmental Health 275
Agent orange
Toxic pollutants

Exercise and Fitness 277
Health benefits of exercise
Close-Up:
   Low-impact exercise

Eye and Vision 281
Contact lenses
Cataracts and sun

Financing Medical Care 284
The uninsured
Catastrophic care

Genetics 286
Genetics research
Prenatal diagnosis

Glands and Hormones 289
Hormone research
Kidney stones

Health Care Facilities 290
Medical waste
Hospitals and AIDS

Health Policy 294
Human fetal tissue
Needles for drug addicts
Speeding drug approval
Race and health care

Heart and Blood Vessels 296
Treatments
Diagnosis

Infectious Diseases 300
Common cold
Hepatitis test
Measles outbreak

Kidney 303
Anemia drug
Drugs linked to kidney disease

**Mental and
Behavioral Disorders** 304
Research on mental disorders
Violence

Nutrition and Food 308
Nutrition research
Close-Up:
    Lactose intolerance

Pregnancy and Childbirth 313
Caesarean sections
Circumcision benefits?

Respiratory System 316
Asthma
Cigarette smoking
Diagnosis of lung diseases

Safety 318
Accident prevention
Air safety
Close-Up:
    Pesticides in foods

**Sexually
Transmitted Diseases** 324
Genital herpes
Human papilloma virus
New chlamydia test

Skin 326
Faster wound healing
New treatments

Smoking 328
Health risks
Breaking the habit

Stroke 330
Preventive treatments

Urology 331
Prostate gland
Incontinence

Veterinary Medicine 332
Medical research
Flea control

Weight Control 335
Weight control research
Who is overweight?
Close-Up:
    Liquid protein diets

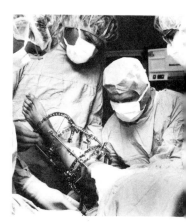

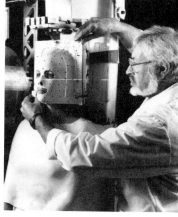

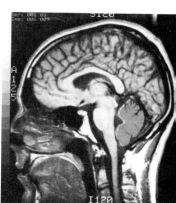

Aging

Researchers in 1988 and 1989 significantly advanced their understanding of two types of health problems that affect older people. The first type, disorders involving degeneration of nerve cells in the brain, includes Alzheimer's disease. There is still no cure for this ailment, but scientists are working on a treatment that may one day enable the body to regrow nerve tissues as well as a drug that may slow the progress of the disease.

The second type of problem involves falls and their consequences—such as broken bones. Researchers are studying why elderly people frequently fall, determining how to prevent falls, and developing treatments for patients who have fallen.

Nerve regrowth. Severely damaged areas of the brains of laboratory rats regrew nerve tissue after a transplant treatment, according to a December 1988 report. The researchers who performed the transplant were led by Fred Gage, a neuroscientist at the School of Medicine of the University of California at San Diego.

Ordinarily, damaged brain tissue cannot regrow. Previous research had suggested, however, that damaged or diseased areas might be induced to grow by increasing their supply of small protein molecules known as *nerve growth factors* (NGF's).

Normally, certain brain cells produce NGF's. When transmitted to other nearby nerve cells, NGF's stimulate the growth of *dendrites* (extensions of nerve cells), which receive input from other nerve cells.

First, Gage and his colleagues used genetic engineering techniques to modify rat cells grown in laboratory culture dishes so that these cells would synthesize NGF's. The researchers then transplanted the modified cells into damaged areas of the brains of rats that belonged to the same strain as the rats that were the source of the cultured cells. The transplanted cells grew and produced NGF's, which, in turn, stimulated the regrowth of nerve cells and dendrites in the damaged area.

Testing a drug for Alzheimer's. A clinical trial that began in August 1987 continued to generate data about the safety and effectiveness of the drug tetrahydroaminoacridine (THA) in treating patients who have Alzheimer's disease. The brain tissues of Alzheimer's victims lack a brain chemical called *acetylcholine;* THA blocks the action of an enzyme that destroys acetylcholine.

Researchers have theorized that

Balance tester
A balance platform tests an individual's equilibrium and the strength of his muscles. Nursing home patients were tested with such a device for a study to determine why elderly people frequently fall.

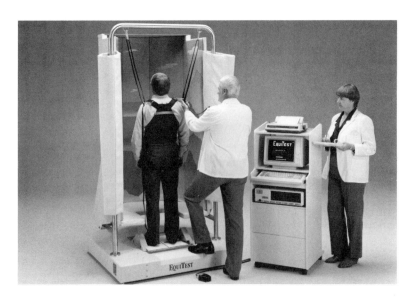

Symptoms of depression that are often undetected in the elderly

Signs often mistaken as symptoms of a medical disorder or a side effect of a drug	Signs that are missed if the patient does not mention them or the physician ignores them
Change in appetite, or gain or loss of more than 5 per cent of weight in one month	Irritability or sadness
	Marked loss of interest or pleasure in normally favorite activities
Insomnia or sleeping much longer than usual	Feelings of worthlessness or guilt
Fidgeting, agitation, or extremely slow movements or speech	Inability to concentrate or make everyday decisions
Fatigue	Recurring thoughts of suicide or death

Source: Stephen R. Rapp, *The Journal of Consulting and Clinical Psychology.*

Aging (cont.)

THA might bolster the level of this chemical in Alzheimer's victims and alleviate some of the symptoms. The committee in charge of the trial completed an evaluation of THA in July 1989 and decided to continue the trial to completion in 1990.

Problems of falling. About 30 per cent of people 65 years and older fall one or more times every year, making falls one of the major factors responsible for the admission of individuals to nursing homes. Mary E. Tinetti, a specialist in geriatric medicine at the Yale University School of Medicine in New Haven, Conn., reported in December 1988 that besides producing severe fractures of the hip and other bones, falls in older people also are often so frightening that a person who falls may sharply cut back on usual activities.

Most falls occur in the home. Causes of falls include chronic disabling conditions affecting vision, strength, and balance; and environmental hazards. Almost every fall can be traced to a combination of risks taken by the victim; many of these can be minimized while maintaining normal activities.

Body building. A loss of muscular strength is widespread in older people, especially in individuals who are more than 80 years old. Many elderly people are caught in a vicious circle of inactivity. Becoming more sedentary decreases the strength of their muscles. This loss of strength, in turn, makes these people even less active. Muscular weakness can hinder balance and gait, increasing the risk of falling.

Two groups of researchers reported that exercising the legs of elderly individuals can improve dramatically both the size of muscles and their strength and function. A team of researchers headed by Maria A. Fiatarone, a specialist in internal medicine in Cambridge, Mass., announced in April 1989 that a program of resistance training improved leg muscles of nine men aged 90 and over. These men exercised their *quadriceps* (the large muscle of the front of the thigh).

After eight weeks of this training, these muscles gained an average of 170 per cent in strength and 10 per cent in mass. Similar gains were reported by researchers led by Walter R. Frontera, a specialist in physical medicine in Brookline, Mass. Physical medicine deals with curing disorders by physical means, especially physical therapy. During a 12-week strength-training program, 12 men aged 60 to 72 exercised the muscles that bend and straighten the legs at the knees and hips.

□ T. Franklin Williams

In WORLD BOOK, see AGING; ALZHEIMER'S DISEASE; NERVOUS SYSTEM; OLD AGE.

AIDS

AIDS testing
In 1989, officials continued to urge people to undergo voluntary testing for the AIDS virus so that those infected could be given appropriate therapy as soon as possible.

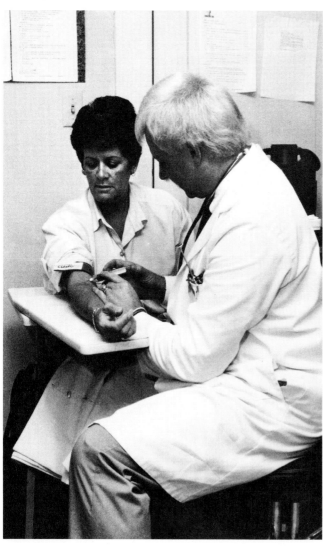

The number of cases of AIDS continued to increase in 1988 and 1989. Although researchers still had not found a cure for the disease, they could point to positive developments, particularly related to drug therapy, that might eventually contribute to control of the epidemic.

AIDS statistics. As of July 31, 1989, 102,621 people had contracted AIDS and 59,391 of them had died of the disease in the United States, according to the Centers for Disease Control (CDC) in Atlanta, Ga. Among white homosexual and bisexual males, how-

ever, the number of new cases increased at a slower rate than noted previously. The reported number of new cases among these high-risk groups was lower in 1987 and early 1988 than in previous years, according to the CDC, even in the metropolitan areas with the most AIDS cases—New York City, San Francisco, and Los Angeles.

The proportion of AIDS cases among white males dipped from 64 per cent of the total number of cases in 1987 to 57 per cent in 1988. Black and Hispanic males accounted for 25 per cent and 16 per cent of all AIDS patients in 1988, respectively—an increase from 22 per cent and 12 per cent the previous year.

AIDS spread particularly rapidly among intravenous drug users, who, if infected, can transmit the AIDS virus to people they share needles with, as well as to sexual partners. In May 1989, the CDC estimated that between 5 per cent and 33 per cent of intravenous drug abusers in the United States were infected with HIV, the virus that causes AIDS.

In the population at large, from 1 million to 1.5 million people in the United States are believed to be infected, according to federal health officials. U.S. officials also reported that, as of December 1988, AIDS was the seventh leading cause of death among people age 15 to 24.

AIDS experts also expected a growth in the epidemic worldwide. The World Health Organization in Geneva, Switzerland, projected that the number of cases of full-blown AIDS (cases in which the infected individuals experience characteristic complications of the disease, including *Pneumocystis carinii* pneumonia [PCP], a life-threatening respiratory infection) would rise from 500,000 in June 1989 to more than 6 million by the year 2000.

AIDS drug news. Preliminary tests in a small number of patients of a promising new AIDS drug—dideoxyinosine (DDI), a compound chemically related to zidovudine (AZT)—showed that the drug improved the

AIDS (cont.)

functioning of the immune system and lowered the levels of HIV in the bloodstream. Researchers at the National Institutes of Health (NIH) in Bethesda, Md., detected only minimal side effects associated with the drug. In late July 1989, NIH officials announced that, because DDI appeared so promising, expanded trials using nearly 2,000 volunteers would begin as soon as possible.

Human studies began in May 1989 on another promising new drug called GLQ223, which is a highly purified preparation of *trichosanthin*, a protein obtained from the root of a Chinese cucumber plant. In laboratory tests, GLQ223 killed HIV-infected cells while leaving noninfected cells unharmed.

Several other drugs were being examined in 1988 and 1989 for their therapeutic value against AIDS. An artificially produced protein called CD4 was found to prevent HIV from infecting cells in monkeys, according to a February 1989 report. Studies of the protein's safety for use in human beings began in August 1988, and preliminary results were encouraging.

AZT, which was approved for use in March 1987, remained the primary drug for people with AIDS, however. The medication has been shown to prolong the lives of some patients, apparently because it pre-

vents HIV from multiplying. In August 1989, U.S. health officials announced the findings of a new study showing that AZT can delay the onset of AIDS in HIV-infected people whose immune systems are impaired but who have not yet developed AIDS symptoms. The officials said that these findings underscore the need for people at risk for AIDS to undergo voluntary testing so that they can benefit from AZT.

In March 1989, however, scientists at the University of California, San Diego, Medical Center reported that a small number of patients who took AZT for more than six months showed signs that the HIV had become resistant to AZT. See Drugs (Close-Up).

FDA actions. The U.S. Food and Drug Administration (FDA) relaxed some regulations and adopted new procedures to help physicians cope with the AIDS crisis. In August 1988, for example, FDA officials said they would permit individuals to import medications not approved for use in the United States. Such importation is permissible only if small quantities of the drugs are imported for personal use.

In October 1988, the FDA also announced that new procedures would be adopted for the approval of AIDS drugs. The procedures would streamline human research

The chart below shows the number of AIDS cases diagnosed in the United States in each six-month period since the early 1980's and the number of those cases that had resulted in death by June 1989.

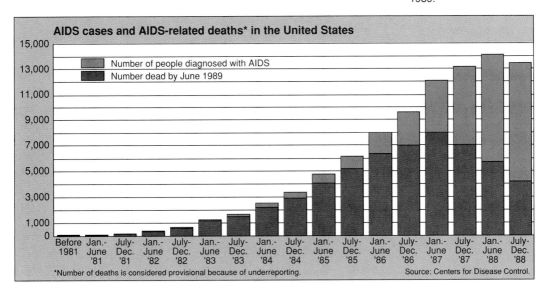

AIDS cases and AIDS-related deaths* in the United States

- Number of people diagnosed with AIDS
- Number dead by June 1989

*Number of deaths is considered provisional because of underreporting.

Source: Centers for Disease Control.

AIDS (cont.)

and make new AIDS drugs available more quickly. The approval time for new medicines was expected to be cut by one-third to one-half.

In November 1988, a protein substance called alpha interferon was approved by the FDA for treatment of Kaposi's sarcoma, a form of cancer seen most commonly in AIDS patients. Studies had shown that large doses of alpha interferon reduced the size of Kaposi's sarcoma tumors in many patients.

In February 1989, the FDA assigned special status to the *aerosol* (spray) form of pentamidine. Although an intravenous form of pentamidine has been approved to treat PCP, doctors had begun prescribing the aerosol form of the drug to try to prevent the pneumonia. Because the FDA assigned special status to the aerosol form, physicians can legally prescribe it while researchers continue to study its effectiveness and safety.

In May 1989, an FDA advisory committee recommended approval of ganciclovir, a drug shown to be effective in treating an AIDS-related eye condition called cytomegalovirus retinitis, which can cause blindness. Research showed that the drug halted the condition.

AIDS testing. Several new AIDS screening tests won FDA approval

or were under development during 1988 and 1989. In December 1988, the FDA approved the Recombigen HIV-1 Latex Agglutination Test. The test, which is inexpensive, is expected to be utilized primarily in remote areas—where other AIDS tests are not available or are considered too costly for use in widespread screening programs. The new test is not as accurate as other AIDS tests, but it produces findings much more quickly—in only minutes rather than hours.

AIDS tests for home use were also being developed, but many health experts opposed them. A major objection to home testing is that people using such tests will not receive the counseling typically given when people are informed of AIDS test results.

HIV update. Evidence continued to mount that years may pass before a person infected with HIV develops full-blown AIDS. In March 1989, San Francisco researchers reported that 9.8 years after a group of homosexual men were infected, only half had any AIDS symptoms.

A variant of the AIDS virus, HIV-2, which is common in west Africa, was reported to be spreading quickly in Brazil, too, according to a study published in April 1989. HIV-2 was also detected in patients in Europe, and isolated cases of HIV-2

AIDS education

Students learn about AIDS at the University of California at Berkeley, one of many schools whose administrators were concerned in 1988 and 1989 about the spread of AIDS among sexually active young people.

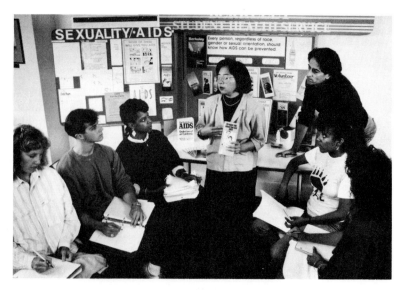

AIDS (cont.)

infection were found elsewhere.

Researchers at the University of California at San Francisco detected both HIV-1 (the virus responsible for nearly all U.S. AIDS cases) and HIV-2 in a west African AIDS patient. The researchers' article, published in the British journal *Lancet* in December 1988, provided the first definitive evidence that both viruses can infect the same person.

Vaccine research continued at research centers in 1989. In June, Jonas E. Salk—the first person to develop an effective polio vaccine and now head of the Salk Institute for Biological Studies in La Jolla, Calif.—reported that he had developed a vaccine that eliminated HIV in two infected chimpanzees.

Studies of the safety and effectiveness of this vaccine in humans have been underway since November 1987. The vaccine has been found to improve the function of the immune system in some patients and appears to have no significant toxic side effects.

☐ Richard Trubo

In the Special Reports section, see MEDICAL ETHICS AND THE AIDS EPIDEMIC. In WORLD BOOK, see AIDS.

Drug abuse in the United States declined by about 25 per cent from 1985 to 1988, according to a national survey released by the National Institute on Drug Abuse on July 31, 1989. The number of Americans who smoke marijuana dropped 28 per cent, and—though the number of people addicted to cocaine increased—occasional use of cocaine declined more than 33 per cent. Officials credited drug abuse prevention campaigns with the encouraging trend.

Student drug use continued to decline in 1988, according to survey results published in February 1989 by the University of Michigan Institute for Social Research in Ann Arbor. The institute, which has conducted national surveys of high school drug use since 1975, found in 1988 the lowest drug-use rates since beginning the surveys.

While this overall decrease is occurring, however, it appears that a subgroup of teen-agers—adolescents who drop out of school—abuse drugs more compulsively than students do. Drug abuse rates are 50 to 65 per cent higher among dropouts than among those who complete school. This may become a significant problem because some metropolitan areas report dropout rates of 40 to 50 per cent. Other groups found to be especially prone to substance abuse include children of substance abusers, those with psychiatric disorders, and abused or neglected children.

Genetic link to alcoholism. Convincing data indicating that a predisposition toward alcoholism may be an inherited trait have been available now for at least a decade. Research reported in October 1988 by psychiatrist C. Robert Cloninger of the Washington University School of Medicine in St. Louis, Mo., suggests that there are at least two types of alcoholics who have inherited a tendency toward the disease from alcoholic parents. These two types are distinguished by certain personality traits and the age at which they become alcoholic.

Cloninger labeled as *Type I alcoholics* males or females who become alcoholic after age 25 and have little need for novelty and a great desire to avoid harm. *Type II alcoholics* are males who become alcoholic before age 25, are aggressive when drinking, and have a great need for novelty and little desire to avoid harm.

People who inherit the personality traits of Type II's appear to have an especially strong tendency toward alcoholism. They are nine times more likely to become alcoholic than people who are not the children of alcoholics. According to

Alcohol and Drug Abuse

Alcohol and Drug Abuse (cont.)

Cloninger, Type II's represent about 25 per cent of all alcoholics.

A biological marker for alcoholism may soon be found. Such a marker could conceivably be used to test people for the tendency to become alcoholic—just as blood pressure tests are now used to detect people who may be at risk for cardiovascular disease. Scientists at the University of Wisconsin in Madison reported in early 1989 that when samples of white blood cells from a group of alcoholics were mixed with certain chemicals, they produced roughly twice the amount of *phosphatidylethanol*, a fatty by-product, than would be expected. These results were achieved in only 50 per cent of the tests, however. A more promising potential marker, according to an October 1988 report, may be cortisol, a hormone secreted by the adrenal glands. A researcher at the University of California at San Diego School of Medicine found that cortisol levels are unusually low in some alcoholics.

At the present time, however, the only way to predict if a person may have a predisposition to alcoholism is by examining the person's experiences with drinking. According to a report at the Second Conference on Alcohol Abuse and Alcoholism held in San Diego in October 1988, people at risk for alcoholism often have a particularly large capacity for alcohol when they first drink and suffer few hangovers and other adverse effects. Both symptoms may be related to an inherited trait governing the production of certain enzymes in the liver, the organ that metabolizes alcohol.

Those at risk for alcoholism may also experience euphoria when they drink—perhaps due to a deficiency of certain brain chemicals that govern mood. In other words, people who are susceptible to alcoholism tend to experience more positive than negative effects of drinking.

Substance abuse and fetal health.
A federal law requiring that all beer, wine, and liquor containers be labeled with warnings that alcohol can cause health problems and birth defects was scheduled to take effect in November 1989. More than 5,000 babies born in the United States suffer from the full effects of *fetal alcohol syndrome*, a disorder that results from heavy maternal drinking during pregnancy, according to estimates by U.S. officials. The syndrome's full effects include mental retardation, developmental stunting, facial malformations, and defects of major organs, such as the heart. Perhaps as many as 50,000 babies born each year show some signs of deformity or impairment associated with fetal alcohol syndrome.

Other drugs ingested during pregnancy cause problems for the fetus as well. A Boston City Hospital study published in the *New England Journal of Medicine* in March 1989 found that babies born to women who used cocaine or marijuana were smaller than those born to women who did not use these drugs. Another finding of the study was that women who abuse drugs are more likely than other women to smoke cigarettes and have inadequate nutrition while pregnant. This produces an even larger decrease in birth weight—an average of 1 pound (0.45 kilogram) less than the weight of babies born to well-nourished women who do not abuse drugs.

Because the AIDS epidemic has increased the urgency for enrolling heroin-addicted people in methadone maintenance programs, researchers have begun to compare the amount of fetal damage caused by heroin abuse with that associated with methadone use. Both drugs produce handicaps related to slower growth and development, as well as withdrawal symptoms, according to a report published in late 1988 by researchers at the Howard University Hospital in Washington, D.C. More severe withdrawal symptoms were found in babies of mothers on methadone, however.

A 1988 study by obstetrician Kenneth C. Edelin at the Boston University School of Medicine found that babies born to women who took

Alcohol and Drug Abuse (cont.)

large doses of methadone suffered more profound and prolonged withdrawal symptoms than those born to women who took smaller doses of methadone. Unfortunately, women who took the smaller doses were more likely to abuse other drugs. Although pregnant women in methadone maintenance programs tend to receive better prenatal care than heroin addicts, methadone seems worse for their babies than heroin.

Understanding drug craving.

Recent research has focused on examining brain chemistry to understand why some people crave alcohol and other drugs. One theory involves *neurotransmitters*, chemicals that occur naturally in the brain and transmit impulses between nerve cells. Inadequate amounts of neurotransmitters can cause insomnia and tremulousness and influence feelings such as craving, anxiety, and depression. Of the many types of neurotransmitters, a few are associated with the development and continuation of alcohol and drug dependence, probably because an occasional dose of these drugs can increase neurotransmitter levels, producing euphoria and a sense of well-being. People who are predisposed to addiction may have been born with a deficiency of neurotransmitters, making them crave drugs once use has begun.

According to the work of several researchers, including a study reported in 1988 by pharmacologist Kenneth Blum of the University of Texas in San Antonio, chronic use of alcohol and other drugs depletes neurotransmitter levels. This can lead to a dependence on drugs to maintain a feeling of well-being. A preliminary study reported by Blum and his colleagues in 1989 suggested that cravings could be reduced if patients being treated for substance abuse were given a mixture containing vitamins and amino acids that are necessary for producing neurotransmitters.

Eating disorders. Two studies published in late 1988 suggest that up to 50 per cent of people with eating

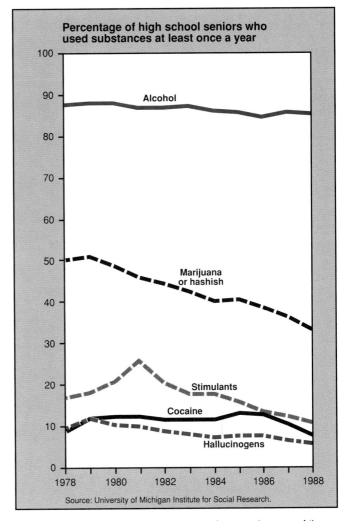

Percentage of high school seniors who used substances at least once a year

Source: University of Michigan Institute for Social Research.

disorders also have problems with alcohol and drug use. Just as addicts compulsively use drugs, people with food disorders often report that they feel driven to overeat by forces beyond their control and that much of their lives are centered on eating, fasting, and purging. Some experts now assume that there may be a common genetic trait that predisposes people to both eating disorders and substance abuse. Several research groups have noted an unusually high incidence of alcoholism and drug addiction among close relatives of people who have eating disorders, for example.

In 1988, researchers at the Eating

An annual survey of the use of alcohol and drugs among high school seniors shows that—although the level of alcohol use remains high—use of other substances continued to decline in 1988.

Fetal hazard
The problem of drug abuse among women has garnered attention as researchers continue to amass evidence that women who abuse cocaine or other drugs during pregnancy can seriously harm their babies.

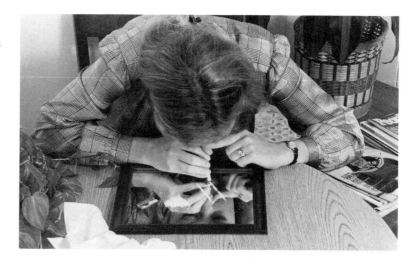

Alcohol and Drug Abuse (cont.)
Disorders Program and Research Facilities at Fair Oaks Hospital in Summit, N.J., found that 70 per cent of a group of adult children of alcoholics reported that they had had binge episodes in which they consumed at least 2,000 calories, and 44 per cent reported binging at least once per week.

There is also some evidence that eating disorders—like drug and alcohol addiction—may be linked to a chemical imbalance in the brain. The chemicals involved are *opioids*, which can slow the metabolism to conserve energy and can cause a feeling of elation. According to the

Fair Oaks Hospital researchers, when patients with a food disorder were given drugs to prevent the breakdown of opioids, they decreased their binge eating.

Such findings have implications for diagnosis and treatment of addicted people. When both substance abuse and eating disorders are present, diagnosis may be difficult because one problem can mask the other. Experts suggest that both problems may need to be treated at the same time.

☐ Gayle R. Hamilton
In WORLD BOOK, see ALCOHOLISM; DRUG ABUSE.

Allergies and Immunology

Scientists' basic understanding of how allergic attacks are initiated in the body received a boost in 1989 as a result of research at the National Institutes of Health (NIH) in Bethesda, Md. Investigators at the NIH reported in April that they had worked out the structure of a molecule on the surface of certain cells of the immune system that plays a central role in the production of allergic symptoms.

The molecule is a *receptor* on immune-system cells called mast cells. A receptor is a sort of lock into which another kind of molecule—the "key"—fits to gain access to the cell. In this case, the key is *immunoglobulin E* (IgE), one

of a class of immune-system molecules called antibodies. Most antibodies protect us against dangerous invaders, such as viruses and bacteria, but IgE is involved primarily in allergies. Why the body manufactures IgE, which serves no apparent purpose, is not known. In allergic individuals, IgE causes reactions against otherwise harmless substances such as dust particles and pollen.

The IgE molecules sit on the surface of mast cells and function as a trigger. When an *allergen*—a substance to which an individual is allergic—enters the body, it joins with the IgE molecules that have been

How safe are ultrasonic humidifiers?

In recent years, many consumers have embraced the ultrasonic humidifier as the high-tech remedy for the problem of dry indoor air, considering the device preferable to conventional humidifiers. Researchers reported in September 1988, however, that ultrasonic humidifiers may present a greater danger to human health than their low-tech predecessors.

The ultrasonic humidifiers, which use sound waves to break up water into tiny droplets and in the process pulverize microorganisms, had been regarded by many as safer to use than other types of humidifiers. The old-fashioned vaporizer, which boils water to produce steam, can present a scalding hazard. The "cool-mist" impeller humidifiers, in which a fan forces room-temperature air through a filter, can send disease- and allergy-causing microorganisms into the air along with the mist.

But scientists working for the United States Environmental Protection Agency (EPA) and a private engineering firm stumbled onto a discovery that ultrasonic humidifiers may produce hazards of their own. While researching the indoor air quality in homes heated by wood-burning stoves, the researchers were surprised to find that one of the homes studied had unusually high concentrations of fine particles in the air. After reexamining the data and visiting the house, they discovered the source of the particles—an ultrasonic humidifier in a child's bedroom.

Further testing showed that the sound waves that break up water in these humidifiers also pulverize minerals dissolved in the water into minute particles fine enough to be inhaled into the lungs, where they may cause respiratory problems. In tap water, these minerals may include such known toxic agents as aluminum, asbestos, and lead. Gases dissolved in water—radon, for example—can also be released. About 90 per cent of the minerals and gases dissolved in the water eventually are dispersed in a breathable form.

The problem is worse if tap water is used instead of the distilled water typically recommended by manufacturers of the appliances. Tap water can produce particulate levels that exceed the EPA's air-quality standard by 50 per cent. Even distilled water can produce abnormally high particulate levels.

In December, the Consumer Product Safety Commission urged consumers to use only distilled water in their ultrasonic humidifiers, and recommended cleaning the water container frequently to discourage the growth of microorganisms. Although the units' sound waves kill microbes by pulverizing them, breathing fragments of microorganisms can cause allergic reactions in some people.

If the expense of using distilled water and the bother of frequent cleaning seem too great, the solution may be to switch back to the steam vaporizer, which proved safer than either the ultrasonic or the impeller humidifiers in EPA tests. New models of vaporizers are sturdier than the old-fashioned kind, minimizing the risk of accidental scalding.

Some consumers may also consider simply living with dry indoor air. While moist air is good for plants and furniture and may feel more comfortable in cold weather, there is little scientific evidence to indicate that healthy people benefit from using humidifiers of any type.   □ Jinger Hoop

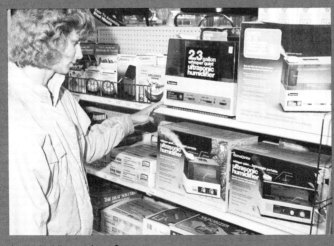
A worthwhile purchase?

Allergies and Immunology (cont.)

produced to "recognize" that allergen. The IgE molecules then signal the mast cells to release powerful chemicals known as *mediators*, which produce the symptoms of an allergic reaction.

The discovery of the IgE receptor's structure may make it possible to block allergic reactions. Researchers will now work on developing drugs that keep IgE molecules from attaching to mast-cell receptors. It may even prove possible to stop the immune system from manufacturing IgE.

New light on food allergies.

Dermatitis (inflammations of the skin) caused by allergies to particular foods results from the action of a chemical called *histamine releasing factor*. That finding was reported in July 1989 by scientists at the Johns Hopkins University School of Medicine in Baltimore.

The scientists studied 63 patients with food allergies that produced dermatitis. Tests of the patients' blood revealed that the foods to which the individuals were sensitive stimulated mast cells to secrete histamine releasing factor. The chemical then interacted with IgE bound to the surface of *basophils*—white blood cells that are similar to mast cells—causing them to discharge histamine, an important mediator.

That in turn caused the skin to become inflamed.

The findings showed that food allergies are more complex than scientists had thought. Allergists think this new knowledge will lead within a few years to more-accurate tests for food allergies. Improved treatments may also result.

Cure for the common cold?

A long-sought goal—protecting people against the common cold—may be a step closer as the result of a discovery announced in March 1989. Scientists at the Center for Blood Research and at Harvard University Medical School, both in Boston, reported that a molecule on human white blood cells is the major receptor for *rhinoviruses*, the cause of about half of all colds.

Because there are more than 100 varieties of rhinoviruses, each with a slightly different structure, researchers have been unable to develop a vaccine against them. But the discovery of the cell receptor, designated ICAM-1, simplifies the problem immensely. Because 90 per cent of rhinoviruses invade human cells by way of that one receptor, strategies against rhinovirus infections can now be directed at the receptor rather than the viruses.

It should be possible to develop drugs that will inhibit white blood cells from producing the ICAM-1

Hot air for colds

The Viralizer, a device aimed at easing cold symptoms, was introduced in late 1988. The manufacturer—Viral Response Systems, Incorporated, of Greenwich, Conn.— claims that the instrument, which blows hot air and medication into the nose, creates a hostile environment for viruses. Some doctors, however, have questioned the Viralizer's effectiveness.

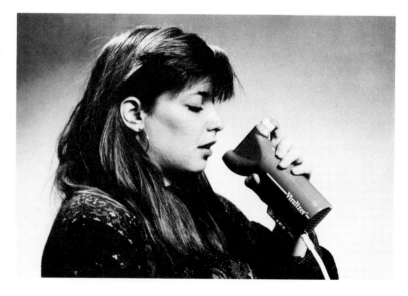

Allergies and Immunology (cont.)

molecule or that mimic the receptor and act as substitute targets for the viruses. As significant as that achievement would be, however, the remaining few rhinoviruses that do not interact with the ICAM-1 receptor—not to mention the dozens of additional viruses that cause the other 50 per cent of colds—would still have to be reckoned with.

A better test for AIDS. A recently developed technique called the *polymerase chain reaction* (PCR) has made it possible for physicians to diagnose AIDS (acquired immune deficiency syndrome) infections faster and with a higher degree of certainty. The technique is a laboratory method for creating thousands or millions of copies of a segment of *deoxyribonucleic acid* (DNA), the molecule that genes are composed of. With such a greatly increased quantity of DNA, it becomes much easier to identify particular genetic sequences, including genes from the AIDS virus that the virus has inserted into a cell's DNA.

One of the first uses of this procedure, to test people at risk for developing AIDS, was reported by researchers in France in September 1988. The scientists used PCR to look for AIDS infections in infants born to women with the virus. AIDS-virus DNA was detected in 6 of the 14 newborns tested. That outcome was in accord with previous findings that 30 to 40 per cent of AIDS-infected pregnant women pass the virus on to their offspring.

Warning on "clinical ecology." A new form of practice being taken up by some allergists, known as "clinical ecology" or "environmental medicine," is based on an unproven theory and should be regarded warily by both doctors and patients. That warning was issued in July 1989 by the American College of Physicians, the largest society of internists in the United States.

Clinical ecologists hold that some people are affected by very small amounts of synthetic chemicals in the environment and suffer damage to their immune systems. The symp-

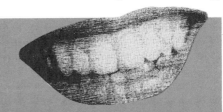

Upbeat attitude seems to boost immunity
Having a positive attitude may give a lift to the body's disease-fighting immune system, researchers at the Pittsburgh Cancer Institute reported in April 1989. The scientists said that people who tend to look on the bright side of things have more "natural killer" (NK) cells, immune-system cells that help protect us against cancers and infections.

In a six-month study of 120 men and women, the investigators found that subjects who had an upbeat attitude had greater numbers of NK cells and suffered fewer colds and other viral infections than the more pessimistic members of the group. Moreover, when the happier individuals did get sick, their illnesses lasted a shorter length of time.

The researchers also studied 30 people who were being treated for colon cancer or malignant melanoma, a severe form of skin cancer. All the patients' tumors had been surgically removed before reaching an advanced stage, but the patients still lived with uncertainty about the final outcome of their disease.

Eighteen of the people received counseling for eight weeks on how to cope with their condition and avoid depression. The other 12 patients received standard medical care with no counseling. At the end of the eight-week period, the individuals who had undergone counseling reported less depression and anger and had significantly higher levels of NK cells than the patients who had not undergone counseling. But whether the upbeat patients would fare better in the long term remained to be seen.

toms of this alleged condition are said to include nausea, constipation, headaches, anxiety, depression, and a variety of others.

The College of Physicians said that because the symptoms are so many and varied, it is unlikely they have a single cause. Furthermore, it said, the diagnostic methods and treatments used by clinical ecologists are costly and without scientific foundation.

Mice with human immunity. The search for a cure for AIDS may be helped along by an achievement reported in September 1988 by two California research groups: the creation of laboratory mice with a func-

Transplanted immunity
A mouse—one of a strain born with no immunity to disease—was given a human immune system in 1988 by scientists at Stanford University in California. Human tissues implanted in the mouse produced *lymphocytes,* cells that fight infection. Transplanting components of the human immune system into mice will make it easier for researchers to test drugs and vaccines and study how the body fights disease.

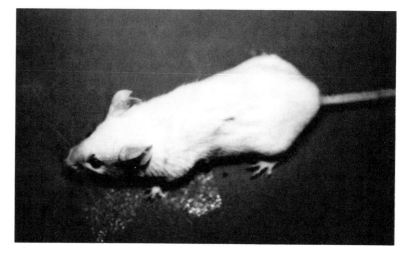

Allergies and Immunology (cont.)
tioning version of the human immune system. In addition to making it easier for scientists to study the effects of the AIDS virus on the immune system, the mice are expected to serve as a "model" for testing drugs and vaccines.

The research was carried out at the Medical Biology Institute in La Jolla and at Stanford University. Although the two teams of scientists took different approaches, both started with a strain of mice that are born with no immune system.

The La Jolla researchers injected the mice with two kinds of human white blood cells, *B cells* and *T*

cells, two of the body's major defenses against infection. Within the animals' bodies, the cells multiplied and developed into a working immune system.

The Stanford scientists implanted into the mice human fetal liver tissue, thymus-gland tissue, and lymph nodes. The liver tissue produced *stem cells,* the precursors of B and T cells. The lymph nodes and thymus tissue converted the stem cells into T cells and B cells.

☐ Robert A. Goldstein

In the Special Reports section, see LIVING WITH ASTHMA. In WORLD BOOK, see ALLERGY; IMMUNITY.

Arthritis and Connective Tissue Disorders

In December 1988, rheumatologists Peter Gregerson and colleagues at the Hospital for Joint Diseases in New York City reported new evidence that *rheumatoid arthritis* (RA), a crippling inflammation of the tissue around joints, has a genetic component.

Genes, the basic unit of heredity, are composed of deoxyribonucleic acid (DNA) and are arranged on structures in the cell called chromosomes. Gregerson and his colleagues reported that people with a particular *genetic marker* are statistically more likely to develop RA than people without the marker. A genetic marker is a piece of DNA that indicates the approximate loca-

tion on a chromosome of a gene or genes that may be responsible for a particular disorder. The researchers suggest that the marker may be a useful tool in helping to determine the risk of developing RA.

Juvenile rheumatoid arthritis.
Genetic studies reported in December 1988 confirmed earlier suspicions that different forms of *juvenile RA*—a condition with symptoms similar to those of adult RA—are distinctly different from the adult disease. Previously, rheumatologist Walter Maksymowych and colleagues at the Children's Hospital

Arthritis (cont.)

in Cincinnati, Ohio, determined, based on observations of patients, that juvenile RA is actually four diseases; these diseases differ in the number and type of joints affected. In their latest study, Maksymowych and his colleagues conducted genetic studies and found different genetic markers associated with each of the four forms of juvenile RA.

Rheumatoid arthritis and the pill.
Taking oral contraceptive pills may halt the development of RA or lessen its symptoms, according to a study reported in April 1989 by rheumatologists Tim Spector of St. Bartholomew's Hospital in London and Marc Hochberg of Johns Hopkins Hospital in Baltimore. Because RA occurs more frequently in women than in men, rheumatologists have long suspected that female hormones may influence the development of the disease or intensify its symptoms. As a result, some rheumatologists have argued that women should not take contraceptive pills if they have or develop RA. (Oral contraceptive pills contain female sex hormones.)

The researchers analyzed nine major studies of the relationship between oral contraceptives and RA. They found that the pill actually slowed the development of RA.

Women with RA who were taking the pill also suffered fewer and less intense symptoms of the disease than did RA patients who did not take the pill.

Education and arthritis. A link between education level and the severity of symptoms in RA patients was reported in November 1988 by rheumatologists Lynn Callahan and Theodore Pincus of Vanderbilt University in Nashville, Tenn. The researchers tested 385 RA patients to determine the severity of their symptoms and then related that information to the level of formal education completed by the patients.

Callahan and Pincus found that patients who had not completed high school had a greater number of and more intense symptoms than patients with a high school diploma. The more education up to college level the patients had, the better they did. The researchers said the most logical explanation was that patients with better education seek medical attention earlier, when RA symptoms are milder and easier to treat.

Reactive arthritis. The discovery of the first evidence directly linking *reactive arthritis* with a bacterial infection was reported in September 1989 by researchers at the University of Birmingham in Great Britain

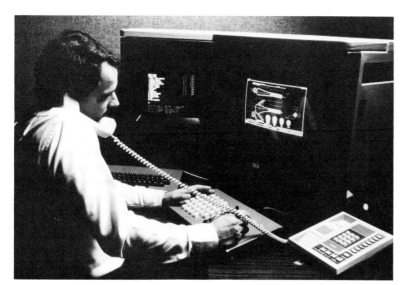

Customized implants
A technician uses a computerized design and manufacturing system to create a customized shoulder implant for a patient with arthritis. Because such implants fit precisely into the joint, they reportedly cause less pain, last longer, and allow greater movement than standardized implants.

Behavioral Disorders
See Mental and Behavioral Disorders

Arthritis (cont.)

and the University of Turku in Finland. Reactive arthritis is an inflammation of the joints that follows a bacterial infection of the genitourinary or gastrointestinal tracts. Researchers have long suspected that this type of arthritis is triggered by the bacteria involved in these infections. But they had been unable to find the bacteria themselves in the fluid from the inflamed joints.

Instead of directly searching for the bacteria, the researchers looked for the immune system "footprints" they would have left behind. They theorized that if bacteria had been in the joints, certain white blood cells called *lymphocytes* would "remember" that such an infection had occurred.

When bacteria or some other microbe invades the body, certain types of lymphocytes produce proteins called antibodies specifically designed to neutralize or destroy that microbe. At the same time, other lymphocytes are primed to recognize and respond quickly to any future invasion of the microbe. This ability to respond can be measured in the laboratory.

For their study, the researchers extracted lymphocytes from fluid removed from the joints of people who had suffered from reactive arthritis. When they exposed the lymphocytes to the bacteria suspected of triggering the disease, they found that the lymphocytes recognized them, indicating that the lymphocytes had been exposed to these bacteria previously.

The researchers also found that most of the people in the study had a protein called HLA-B27 on the surface of each body cell. They suggested that doctors could identify those people who are susceptible to reactive arthritis by testing for HLA-B27. Such knowledge would enable people with HLA-B27 to receive prompt treatment with antibiotics in case of bacterial infection and so perhaps prevent the development of reactive arthritis.

Exercise benefits. Contrary to common belief, exercise can help overcome the effects of *inflammatory joint disease* (a term used to describe a family of different diseases that cause joint inflammation), according to research published in September 1988 by researchers at Copenhagen Community Hospital in Denmark. The researchers studied the effect of a twice-weekly aerobic exercise program on volunteers with moderately active joint disease. The researchers found that, compared with patients who did not exercise, the patients in the program had significantly fewer swollen joints.

□ John Baum

In WORLD BOOK, see ARTHRITIS.

The poison palette
In his later years, French impressionist artist Pierre Auguste Renoir became so crippled by rheumatoid arthritis (RA) that he could paint only if brushes were tied to his hands. In 1988—nearly 100 years later—two Danish researchers proposed a link between Renoir's disease and the vivid colors he favored in his work.

Their study is the first to suggest that toxic materials—in this case, heavy metals in the paints—help trigger RA. Many of the brightest colors on the artist's palette were once commonly made with toxic metals. Bright red and bright orange were made with mercury. Cobalt blue contained cobalt and aluminum.

Internists Henrik Permin and Lisbet Milling Pedersen of University Hospital in Copenhagen, Denmark, compared the color preferences of several famous artists, including Renoir, who had suffered from RA with those of healthy contemporaries. They found that the artists with RA were much more likely to have used brighter, more toxic colors. About 60 per cent of the colors used by Renoir, for example, were made with heavy metals. Next, the researchers hope to explore whether toxic metals play a role in modern cases of RA.

Amid much controversy, a revolutionary drug that ends pregnancy at an early stage was introduced, withdrawn, and then returned to market in late 1988. The drug, RU 486, is likely safer than surgical abortion. It was approved for marketing in China and France in September.

On October 26, about one month later, Groupe Roussel Uclaf, the French distributor of RU 486, announced it was discontinuing distribution because of opposition by antiabortion groups in France and the United States. Two days later, however, the French minister of health intervened, declaring that the drug was an important health benefit. He ordered the firm to resume distribution. Roussel Uclaf complied but limited the drug to France and China.

RU 486 is administered as a one-dose pill within the first six weeks of pregnancy. The drug stops the development of a pregnancy by interfering with the action of progesterone, a hormone that is essential for *implantation* (the process by which the fertilized egg embeds itself in the lining of the uterus). Progesterone also is crucial for the continued growth of an embryo. Two days after taking RU 486, the patient usually receives an injection of drugs that cause the uterus to contract and expel the lining.

The potential for future distribution of RU 486 in the United States is uncertain. In addition to intense opposition by antiabortion groups, barriers include high research costs, low projected profits, and the high cost of liability insurance.

Contraceptive vaccines. Two studies reported in 1988 reflect growing scientific interest in contraceptive vaccines. The first phase of clinical trials of a vaccine designed to prevent the implantation of the fertilized egg into the lining of the uterus was reported by a team of researchers from Ohio State University's College of Medicine in Columbus. The vaccine triggers the production of antibodies to human chorionic gonadotropin (HCG), a hormone produced by the cells that form the *placenta* (afterbirth), and that is essential in the implantation process.

The researchers administered the vaccine to 30 women who had been surgically sterilized. They found that all 30 women developed significant levels of HCG antibodies. The women experienced no side effects. Future studies will determine whether the vaccine actually prevents pregnancy.

Interrupting fertilization. A vaccine that seems to disrupt the process by which sperm fertilize eggs was

Birth Control

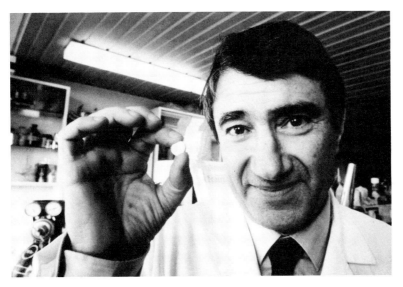

Abortion drug
French researcher Etienne Beaulieu holds a tablet of RU 486, an abortion drug approved for marketing in France and China in 1988. Discovered by Beaulieu in 1982, the drug ends pregnancy at a very early stage by interfering with the action of a hormone that is necessary for the fertilized egg to implant in the uterus.

Birth Defects

See Genetics

Birth Control (cont.)

100 per cent effective in laboratory tests with both male and female guinea pigs. Those results were reported in October 1988 by cell biologists at the University of Connecticut Health Center in Farmington. The vaccine consists of a protein called PH-20 found on the surface of guinea pig sperm cells. Although the researchers have not discovered the exact role PH-20 plays in fertilization, they do know that the protein is crucial in helping the sperm bind to the egg.

The researchers administered the vaccine to 25 female and 6 male guinea pigs. None of the females became pregnant. In addition, none of the males were able to impregnate female guinea pigs.

The researchers also found that the vaccine apparently is reversible. Fifteen months after receiving the vaccine, all the female guinea pigs produced litters.

The study was valuable in demonstrating that a vaccine against sperm is possible. Researchers have not yet, however, found a protein on human sperm cells that plays the same role as PH-20.

□ Louise B. Tyrer

In WORLD BOOK, see BIRTH CONTROL.

Blood

Researchers from the University College and Middlesex Hospital School of Medicine in London reported in early 1989 on a new technique that eliminates symptoms of a type of cancer called *Hodgkin's disease* in some patients who do not respond to more traditional therapies. Hodgkin's disease is usually characterized by painless enlargement of *lymph nodes*, small bean-shaped structures that form part of the *lymphatic system*—a network of vessels that drain fluid (lymph) from body cells into the bloodstream. The new technique eliminated all evidence of the disease in 22 of a group of 44 patients with Hodgkin's disease who did not respond to traditional treatments—radiation therapy, treatment with anticancer drugs, or a combination of the two.

The new treatment involves three steps. First, some of the patient's own *bone marrow* (the soft tissue that fills the center of most bones and produces both red and white blood cells) is removed and frozen. Then the patient receives large doses of anticancer drugs. Finally, after the drugs have passed out of the body, the marrow is thawed and returned to the patient through a needle inserted into a vein.

Growth in the rate of transfusion of red blood cells leveled off in 1983, according to a survey of 103 United States hospitals. Indications that AIDS could be transmitted by transfusion began to appear in 1982 and may have slowed the demand. By contrast, the rate of transfusion of *platelets* (structures involved in clotting) continued to grow, due in part to the fact that most platelet recipients are chemotherapy patients who urgently require large quantities of platelets.

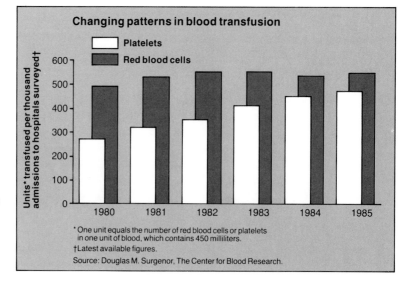

Changing patterns in blood transfusion

- ☐ Platelets
- ■ Red blood cells

Units* transfused per thousand admissions to hospitals surveyed†

1980 1981 1982 1983 1984 1985

* One unit equals the number of red blood cells or platelets in one unit of blood, which contains 450 milliliters.

†Latest available figures.

Source: Douglas M. Surgenor, The Center for Blood Research.

Blood (cont.)

The replacement of marrow compensates in part for the use of drug doses that are so large that they not only destroy cancer cells but also—unavoidably—make the patient's marrow unable to produce blood cells. The use of the patient's own marrow, rather than marrow donated by another individual, minimizes the risks of *graft-versus-host disease*, in which donated cells attack the recipient's body. This disease occurs because certain protein molecules in donated cells do not match the corresponding molecules of the recipient's cells.

Help for hemophiliacs.
Researchers in the United States, Italy, and Sweden in 1988 and 1989 investigated the use of a genetically engineered protein called *clotting factor number 8* to treat *hemophilia*, a hereditary disease in which the blood does not clot normally. In genetic engineering, organisms such as bacteria, yeast cells, or animal cells are used as "biological factories" to produce large quantities of a protein. The "factories" for clotting factor number 8 were laboratory-grown descendants of cells removed from the ovaries of hamsters.

People with hemophilia bleed excessively when injured and can even bleed when they are not injured. Sometimes this bleeding threatens their lives.

About 85 per cent of hemophiliacs lack natural clotting factor number 8. Doctors treat patients who have this form of hemophilia by giving them concentrations of the factor. Until 1987, all this concentrate was prepared from blood plasma collected from many donors. As a result, hemophiliac patients had a risk of catching AIDS (acquired immune deficiency syndrome), because the virus that causes this disease is carried in the blood.

In 1986, however, hematologist Randal Kaufman and his colleagues at Genetics Institute, a biotechnology company in Cambridge, Mass., reported that they had used genetic engineering techniques to produce clotting factor number 8, setting the stage for the elimination of plasma

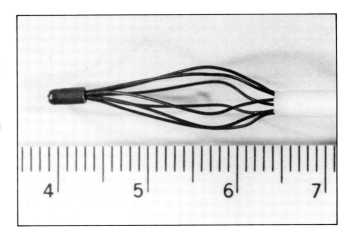

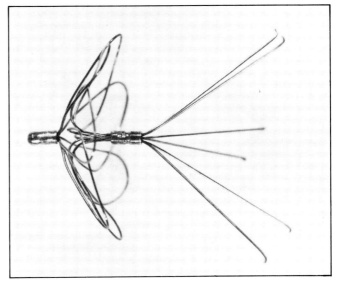

as the source of the concentrate. Researchers at the University of North Carolina in Chapel Hill began to treat patients with laboratory-produced factor number 8 in March 1987. Such treatments also have begun with patients in Los Angeles; Milan, Italy; and Stockholm, Sweden. The artificial factor 8 has worked as well as factor 8 taken from blood plasma.

Anemia drug approved.
On June 1, 1989, the United States Food and Drug Administration, an agency of the federal government, approved the use of genetically engineered *erythropoietin* (EPO) to treat anemia

Blood clot catcher
A substance that holds one shape at a low temperature and another when warmed is being used in a filter designed to prevent potentially fatal blood clots from reaching the heart and lungs. A flexible tube containing a narrow set of wires is threaded into a large vein; as the wires are pushed out of the tube, body heat causes them to expand, *top*. When completely open, *above,* the wires form a filter about 2.5 centimeters (1 inch) across.

Blood (cont.)

in kidney patients. EPO is a hormone that regulates the production of red blood cells and is normally produced by the kidneys.

Hematologist John W. Adamson and his colleagues at the University of Washington in Seattle showed in 1987 that laboratory-produced EPO can correct anemia in patients who have severe kidney diseases. This success led to the use of artificial EPO to treat various other diseases and clinical conditions.

In 1988 and 1989, for example, researchers used EPO to increase red blood cell production in patients who want to store their own blood before they have surgery. The use of a patient's own blood—an *autologous blood transfusion*—eliminates the risk of *incompatibility* (poor matching of blood, leading to harmful reactions) and the risk of infection by viruses in donated blood. Normally, to avoid depleting the supply of red blood cells to an unhealthy level, the typical autologous donor can safely give only 3 to 4 pints (1.4 to 1.9 liters) of blood during the five to six weeks that the blood can be stored.

☐ G. David Roodman

In WORLD BOOK, see BLOOD; BLOOD TRANSFUSION.

Bone Disorders

Subjecting bones to a weak electric current or an electromagnetic field may help reverse or prevent osteoporosis, a chronic disease that involves a loss of bony tissue and results in bones that are thin and brittle. That possibility, based on research with animals, was reported in early 1989 by two groups of scientists in the United States.

In February 1989, *orthopedist* (bone specialist) Carl T. Brighton of the University of Pennsylvania School of Medicine in Philadelphia reported that osteoporosis in rats' spines can be reversed with electricity. Brighton and his colleagues placed small electrodes under the skin of male rats with osteoporosis. After stimulating the rats with an electric current for six to eight weeks, the researchers examined the animals' spines. They found that the density of the bones had been restored to near-normal levels.

In March, orthopedist Clinton T. Rubin of the State University of New York in Stony Brook announced similar findings. Rubin and his associates operated on turkeys to make one of their wing bones inoperative. They then attached battery-powered coils that produced an electromagnetic field to the birds' wings.

Stretching leg bones
Surgeons at the University of Texas Southwestern Medical Center in Dallas fit a bone-lengthening brace—developed in the 1940's by a Soviet physician, but not introduced in the West until the 1980's—on a patient's leg. By pulling along the length of a bone—which has been cut around its perimeter to create a region for new growth—the brace can cause the bone to grow.

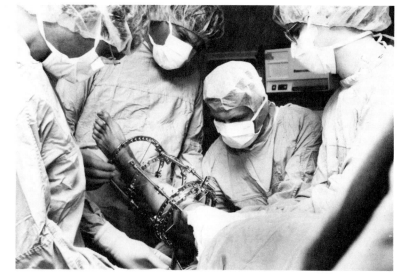

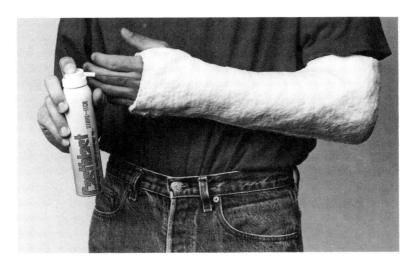

Relieving cast itch
Cast wearers may get relief from itching with Castblast, introduced in 1989. Consisting of talcum powder mixed with alcohol, Castblast is sprayed under the cast through a narrow tube. The alcohol dries quickly, leaving the talc on the skin to absorb moisture and inhibit the growth of bacteria, which can cause odor as well as itching.

Bone Disorders (cont.)

The researchers found that the electromagnetic stimulation of the bones actually increased their density. In contrast, the inactivated wing bones of untreated turkeys became porous and weak.

Leg-bone stretcher. A "new" technique for lengthening or straightening the long bones of the leg was evaluated in April 1989 by orthopedists in Italy and at Children's Hospital in New Orleans. The procedure was pioneered in the 1940's by a Soviet physician, Gavriel A. Ilizarov, but was not introduced in the West until the 1980's. The American and Italian investigators found that the technique seems safe and effective and merits further study.

In the traditional method of correcting a bone that is crooked or short, the bone is cut in two and then augmented with a piece of bone from another part of the body or from a donor. Sometimes, the leg does not heal properly, necessitating a second operation to add more bone grafts.

The Ilizarov technique employs a metal brace, consisting of two or more metal rings connected by adjustable rods, that exerts tension on the bone. The surgeon inserts several long pins through the upper and lower parts of the leg bone and perpendicular to the bone. The pins extend outward through the skin and are attached to the rings, which encircle the leg. The surgeon then makes a shallow cut around the circumference of the bone to make the two halves of the bone separate slightly.

Every few days, the rods are adjusted to increase the tension on the rings. The bone, responding to the pulling force, gradually lengthens. New bone is created at the site of the cut to make this "stretching" possible.

Improved bone healing. Because broken bones and bone grafts do not always heal, scientists are always looking for ways to aid bone growth and healing. In October 1988, orthopedist Jeffrey J. Tiedeman of Creighton University in Omaha, Nebr., reported that bone marrow and powdered bone are effective in stimulating the healing of bones.

Tiedeman and his associates treated dogs whose leg bones had been surgically severed and then seared with an electric current to prevent them from knitting back together. The researchers injected the dogs' legs with either bone marrow or a combination of marrow and demineralized bone powder. The investigators found that marrow alone stimulated bone growth significantly, but the marrow-powder combination was even more effective. □ John J. Gartland

In WORLD BOOK, see BONE.

Books of Health and Medicine

Here are 25 outstanding new health and medical books suitable for the general reader. They have been selected from books published in 1988 and 1989.

Drugs. *Drug Information for the Consumer, 1989 Edition*. This guide to more than 5,000 prescription and over-the-counter drugs gives the uses and side effects of each. (Consumer Reports Books, 1989. 1,504 pp. $25)

Drugs & the Body. Robert M. Julien, a pharmacologist, explains in nontechnical language how drugs work. The book covers all major classes of drugs except mind-altering drugs. (Freeman, 1988. 287 pp. $19.95)

The experience of illness. *After the Stroke: A Journal*. May Sarton, a novelist and poet, recounts her struggle to regain her health and strength after suffering a stroke. (Norton, 1988. 280 pp. $16.95)

A Bomb in the Brain: A Journalist's True Story of His Brain Disease and the Surgery and Science That Saved Him. Steve Fishman gives an engaging personal account of the discovery and treatment of a potentially fatal blood-vessel abnormality, an arteriovenous malformation, in his brain. (Scribner, 1988. 352 pp. $19.95)

Borrowed Time: An AIDS Memoir. Paul Monette, a novelist and screenwriter, records the 19 months prior to his lover's death from AIDS. Monette's narrative describes the two men's commitment to each other and the hatred and ignorance they endured. (Harcourt Brace Jovanovich, 1988. 400 pp. $19.95)

Loving Rachel: A Family's Journey from Grief. Novelist Jane Bernstein gives a vivid account of her family's experience with a disabled child. (Little, Brown, 1988. 279 pp. $17.95)

Illness Narratives: Suffering, Healing and the Human Condition. Arthur Kleinman, a physician, relates the personal trials of seriously ill individuals and tells how patients sometimes find new meaning in their lives. (Basic Books, 1988. 274 pp. $19.95)

Healers and healing. *Medicine and Culture: Varieties of Treatment in the United States, England, West Germany, and France*. The author, medical journalist Lynn Payer, compares medical practices in the above countries and concludes that there is a need to establish objective international criteria for medical care. (Holt, 1988. 204 pp. $18.95)

Other Healers: Unorthodox Medicine in America, edited by Norman Gevitz. This collection of scholarly perspectives covers all the major forms of alternative medicine, including homeopathy, osteopathy, chiropractic, botanical medicine, folk medicine, and faith healing. (Johns Hopkins University Press, 1988. 293 pp. $12.95)

A Piece of My Mind: A Collection of Essays from the Journal of the American Medical Association, edited by Bruce B. Dan and Roxanne K. Young. America's doctors share their most memorable, dramatic, and inspiring experiences. (Feeling Fine, 1988. 256 pp. 18.95)

Health policy. *Caring for the Disabled Elderly: Who Will Pay?*, by Alice M. Rivlin and Joshua M. Wiener with Raymond J. Hanley and Denise A. Spence. The authors analyze the major options for reforming the financing of long-term care for the disabled elderly and recommend an expanded role for private insurers and a new public insurance program. (Brookings Institution, 1988. 318 pp. $11.95)

Competition in the Health Care Sector: Ten Years Later, edited by Warren Greenberg. Seven participants in a 1977 conference on competition in the health-care industry debate why health-care costs have continued to escalate through the 1980's despite increased competition. (Duke University Press, 1988. 141 pp. $24.95)

Science and the Unborn: Choosing Human Futures. Author Clifford Grobstein examines the new technologies of reproduction and the painful ethical dilemmas that sometimes result. (Basic Books, 1988. 208 pp., illus. $18.95)

Books (cont.)

Worse than the Disease: Pitfalls of Medical Progress, by Diana B. Dutton with Thomas A. Preston and Nancy E. Pfund. Using four case studies—involving the synthetic hormone diethylstilbestrol (DES), the artificial heart, swine flu immunizations, and genetic engineering—the authors show that advances in medical science often contain hidden dangers and thus must be adopted with caution by the health-care establishment. (Cambridge University Press, 1988. 511 pp. $29.95)

Mind and body. *Fasting Girls: The Emergence of Anorexia Nervosa as a Modern Disease*. Joan Jacobs Brunberg, the director of women's studies at Cornell University, explores various facets of this eating disorder. (Harvard University Press, 1988. 368 pp. $25)

The Mind. Richard M. Restak, a neurologist, presents a brisk and readable account of current research on the human brain and how it influences behavior. Restak's topics include aging, addiction, pain, healing, depression, mood, and language. (Bantam, 1988. 384 pp. $29.95)

Worried Sick: Our Troubled Quest for Wellness. Arthur J. Barsky, an associate professor of psychiatry at Harvard, argues that the pursuit of good health can be self-defeating when it becomes an obsession. (Little, Brown, 1988. 255 pp. $17.95)

Self-care and nutrition. *Columbia Encyclopedia of Nutrition,* edited by Myron Winick. Staff of the Institute of Human Nutrition at Columbia University's College of Physicians and Surgeons present information on nutrition and related topics. (Putnam, 1988. 352 pp. $22.95)

Health and Fitness Excellence: The Scientific Action Plan. Author Robert K. Cooper translates the latest scientific findings on human health into concrete guidelines for achieving optimal well-being in body, mind, and spirit. (Houghton Mifflin, 1989. 516 pp. $19.95)

Lower Your Blood Pressure and Live Longer. Marvin Moser, a consultant to the National High Blood Pressure Education Program, tells how to avoid hypertension and enjoy prolonged good health. (Villard, 1989. 291 pp. $18.95)

Osteoporosis: A Guide to Prevention & Treatment. John F. Aloia, a leading researcher and clinician, answers questions about this bone-thinning disease that affects many older people, especially women. (Leisure Press, 1989. 215 pp. $12.95)

Symptoms. Physician Isadore Rosenfeld tells how to interpret possible warning signals of disease and advises when to consult a phy-

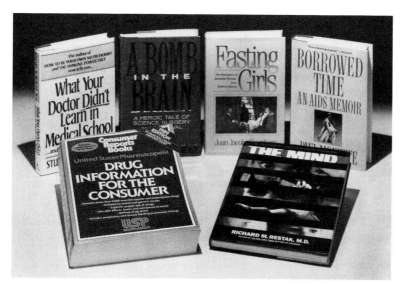

Books of interest
Books on health and medical topics published in 1988 and 1989 included *What Your Doctor Didn't Learn in Medical School,* advice on getting the most from the health-care system; *A Bomb in the Brain,* a man's account of his ordeal with a brain abnormality; *Fasting Girls,* a look at an eating disorder; *Borrowed Time,* a writer's memoir of his lover's battle with AIDS; *Drug Information for the Consumer,* data on more than 5,000 drugs; and *The Mind,* an examination of the brain's influence on behavior.

Books (cont.)
sician. (Simon & Schuster, 1989. 366 pp. $19.95)

Using the health-care system.
Medicare Made Easy, by Charles B. Inlander and Charles K. MacKay. The authors cover a number of topics relating to Medicare, including the rights of hospital patients, supplemental health insurance, and how to negotiate doctors' fees. (Addison-Wesley, 1989. 336 pp. $10.95)

Taking Charge of Your Medical Fate, by Lawrence C. Horowitz. In this informative and unsettling indictment of modern medicine,

Horowitz, a former staff director of the U.S. Senate Health Subcommittee, tells how to put yourself "in the driver's seat" when receiving medical care. (Random House, 1988. 307 pp. $18.95)

What Your Doctor Didn't Learn in Medical School, and What You Can Do About It!, by Stuart Berger with Pat Golbitz. Berger, a physician, advises patients on how they can make the health-care system work to their greatest advantage. (Morrow, 1988. 384 pp. $18.95)

☐ Margaret Moore Ovitsky

Brain and Nervous System

Many of the behavioral differences between males and females may result from differences in their brains, scientists reported in 1989. The researchers found male/female differences in two regions of the brain.

In February, scientists at the University of California at Los Angeles (UCLA) reported on their studies of a portion of the brain called the *preoptic anterior hyphothalamic area* (PO-AHA), which has long been known to influence the secretion of sex hormones. *Neurons* (nerve cells) in the PO-AHA are organized into clusters called nuclei.

The UCLA researchers counted the neurons in the PO-AHA nuclei of 22 male and female brains. They found that while some nuclei had similar numbers of neurons in the brains of both sexes, two nuclei contained three to four times as many neurons in the male brains as in the female brains.

In March, neuroscientist Sandra F. Witelson of McMaster University in Hamilton, Canada, announced the discovery of a male/female difference in the *corpus callosum*. The corpus callosum is a thick band of tissue, containing millions of individual nerve fibers, that links the left and right *hemispheres*, or halves, of the brain. Nerve impulses originating in one hemisphere are transmitted via the corpus callosum to the other hemisphere, permitting a

smooth exchange of information between the two halves of the brain.

Witelson and her colleagues studied the brains of 15 men and 35 women. They found that two parts of the corpus callosum, called the *splenium* and the *isthmus*, were significantly larger in the female brains than in the male brains. These bundles of fibers link regions of the hemisphere involved with speech and the perception of space.

But how might these anatomical differences relate to the mental and behavioral differences between the sexes? Women, for example, are credited with strong nurturing instincts and on the average, tend to be superior to men in verbal abilities. But men, on the average, are usually better than women at tasks involving spatial relationships, such as problems dealing with geometric patterns. Whether such differences are due mostly to brain anatomy, hormonal differences, variations in upbringing, or a combination of such factors, is unknown.

The nose and Alzheimer's. It may be possible to diagnose Alzheimer's disease by noting changes in nerve cells inside the nose. That finding was reported in February 1989 by neuroscientist Barbara R. Talamo of Tufts University's New England Medical Center in Boston.

Alzheimer's disease, a severe

Brain and Nervous System (cont.)

brain disorder of unknown cause in which neurons degenerate and die, becomes more frequent with advancing age. The first sign of Alzheimer's is memory loss, but as the victim's condition worsens, speech, movement, and thought all deteriorate until the patient's entire mind is destroyed.

Alzheimer's disease is difficult to diagnose. The physician must first exclude other possible causes of the patient's mental decline, such as brain tumors, strokes, and hormonal disturbances. Even under the best of circumstances, the disease is correctly diagnosed prior to death in only about two-thirds of cases.

Usually, Alzheimer's can be diagnosed with certainty only after the patient's death, when tissues from various parts of the brain can be examined under the microscope for telltale abnormalities. Those abnormalities include clumps of filaments called *neurofibrillary tangles* and patches of degenerating nerve fibers called *neuritic plaques*.

Talamo and her colleagues studied neurons in the *olfactory epithelium*, a part of the membrane lining the inside of the nose. They decided to examine those tissues because a common symptom of Alzheimer's disease is a deteriorating sense of smell.

The researchers analyzed olfactory epithelium neurons from nine people who had died of Alzheimer's disease. They discovered that the cells of eight of the nine individuals contained the same sorts of tangles and plaques that are characteristic of Alzheimer's disease (and that autopsies had revealed in those people's brain tissues). In contrast, the olfactory neurons of only 2 of 14 other people, whose brains showed no evidence of Alzheimer's disease, contained those abnormalities.

If the scientists' findings are confirmed by other investigators, examination of the olfactory epithelium may provide a simple way to help diagnose Alzheimer's disease while a patient is still alive.

Calcium in the aging brain. One cause of memory loss in old age may be excessive amounts of calcium in brain cells, according to a February 1989 report by neuroscientist Robert A. Deyo and his colleagues at the Northwestern University School of Medicine in Chicago. The researchers reported that nimodipine, a drug given to many heart disease and stroke patients, may help neurons achieve a more-normal level of calcium.

Neurons undergo a number of changes as they age, including a reduced ability to control calcium levels. Calcium can thus accumulate in and harm older neurons.

Fetal tissue recipient
Don Nelson of Denver, *below left,* a Parkinson's disease patient, tests his manual dexterity and reflex time in May 1989, six months after becoming the first person in the United States to receive a fetal-tissue implant. Doctors implanted fetal cells into two parts of the man's brain—the *putamen* and the *caudate nucleus, below*—in an attempt to relieve symptoms of the disease. It was hoped that the cells would produce a needed brain chemical, *dopamine.*

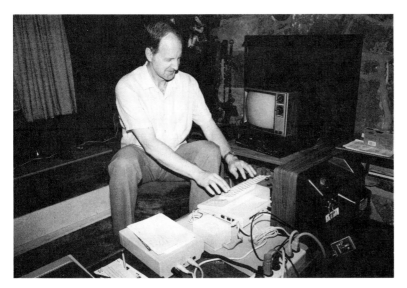

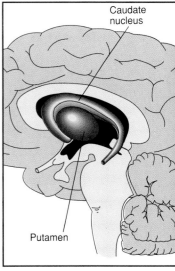

Caudate nucleus

Putamen

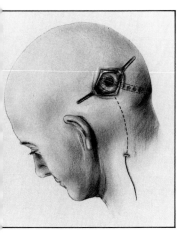

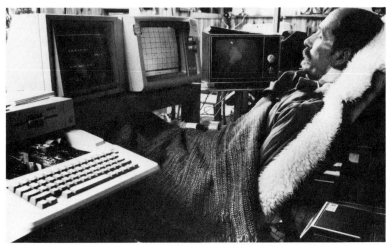

Eye contact

A system developed by California researchers enables severely disabled individuals to communicate using just their eyes. The user gazes at any of 64 squares, each containing a word or letter, on a video screen, *above right*. Each square flashes at a specific frequency, and that frequency is transmitted through the brain to electrodes implanted under the skull, *above*. The signal is then relayed to a computer, which displays the desired word or letter on a word processor.

Brain and Nervous System (cont.)

Calcium enters neurons through specialized openings in the cell membrane known as calcium channels. During the past 10 years, medical scientists have developed drugs called *calcium channel blockers* that prevent calcium from entering cells. Nimodipine is one such drug.

Deyo and his associates tested the effects of nimodipine on the ability of rabbits to learn to associate a particular reflex, eye blinking, with a stimulus (an audible tone) other than the one that first produced it (a puff of air). The rabbits were exposed to an audible tone followed quickly by a puff of air in their eyes, which caused them to blink. After an average of about 450 trials, young rabbits (3 months of age) learned to associate the tone with the puff of air, and thereafter they blinked their eyes as soon as they heard the sound. Aged rabbits (at least 3 years old) did much worse. Four rabbits failed to learn the response, and two others required nearly 1,000 trials to learn it.

Older rabbits treated with nimodipine did significantly better than the other rabbits their age—and even slightly better than the young rabbits; they could be taught the eye-blink response in less than 400 trials. While the exact mechanism for this enhanced learning ability is not known, it suggests that changes in calcium use by brain cells are

important in the learning process and that elevated levels of calcium in aging neurons inhibit learning.

Link with immune system. Evidence for strong interactions between the body's nervous system and the disease-fighting immune system was reported in January 1989 by psychologist Glenda Mac-Queen of McMaster University. In experiments with rats, MacQueen and her colleagues found that stimulating the *central nervous system* (the brain and spinal cord) induced a response by the immune system.

Researchers have realized for some time that there are some similarities between the immune and nervous systems, including the way each system's cells use chemicals to communicate with one another. In the nervous system, these chemicals are called *neurotransmitters*; in the immune system, they are called *monokines* and *lymphokines*, depending on which cells produce them. In addition, cells from each system can produce, and respond to, the chemical transmitters utilized by the other system.

Among the clinical evidence for the interaction of the immune and nervous systems is the observation that stress can produce effects on the immune system. Such effects can include a decreased ability to fight disease and even the eruption of hives or other skin conditions.

Brain and Nervous System (cont.)

One response of the immune system is *anaphylaxis*, a potentially life-threatening allergic reaction that causes the contraction of muscles lining the air passages in the lungs. Anaphylaxis results in the release of a chemical called *histamine* from immune-system cells known as mast cells. These cells also produce a substance known as *mast cell protease II*, which acts to break down proteins in the body.

The researchers studied interactions between the nervous system and the immune system in rats that had been sensitized to egg *albumin*, a protein found in eggs and many other animal and plant substances. (A sensitized animal has been previously exposed to a substance, like albumin; the substance will cause an allergic reaction when the animal next encounters it.)

The rats were divided into several groups. One group was given injections of albumin at the same time that it was exposed to an audio-visual stimulus—that is, to lights or sounds that stimulated their nervous systems. Other rats either were exposed to the stimuli but received no albumin injections or received the stimuli and the injections at different times. In all the rats receiving injections, mast cell protease II was released into the bloodstream. These procedures were repeated several

times for each group of rats over a period of about one month.

At the end of that time, the researchers exposed all the rats to the audio-visual stimulus, but did not inject any of them with albumin. They also tested the rats' blood for mast cell protease II to determine whether the rats' immune systems were reacting.

Only the rats that had earlier received simultaneous albumin injections and audio-visual stimulation had elevated levels of protease II in their blood. In other words, in rats that had come to associate a light and sound stimulus with an albumin injection, the audio-visual stimulus alone was enough to cause an immune response.

It seems likely that there is a similar interplay between the nervous and immune systems in human beings—one that can lead to undesirable immune reactions triggered by nervous-system stimuli such as stress, fear, and depression. If so, it may be possible to mentally suppress such responses. Similarly, it may be within the power of patients to increase their immune response to infections, thereby enhancing the effects of antibiotics or other treatments. □ Gary Birnbaum

In the Special Reports section, see WHAT EVERYONE NEEDS TO KNOW ABOUT STROKE. In WORLD BOOK, see BRAIN; NERVOUS SYSTEM.

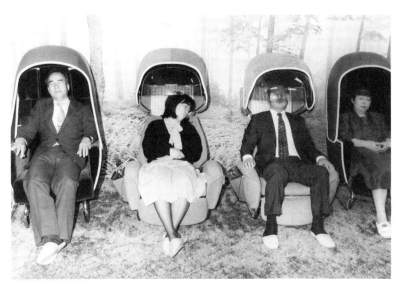

Clearing the circuits
Taking a break from the stresses of everyday life, people at a Tokyo relaxation salon unwind for an hour in Refresh Capsules. Floor-to-ceiling photographs of a tranquil forest and the recorded sound of twittering birds are intended to lull a salon visitor into a relaxed mental state.

Cancer

Scientists at the National Institutes of Health in Bethesda, Md., launched a new era in medicine on May 22, 1989, when cancer researchers injected special cancer-fighting cells containing a nonhuman gene into a patient with advanced *melanoma* (skin cancer). The first approved experiment using a nonhuman gene transferred into a human cell was performed by researchers Steven A. Rosenberg and R. Michael Blaese of the National Cancer Institute (NCI) and W. French Anderson of the National Heart, Lung, and Blood Institute.

The gene transfer was not in itself intended to treat the cancer. Instead, it served as a "marker" gene—a way to trace the whereabouts of cancer-fighting *lymphocytes* (white blood cells) in order to show where the cells end up in the patient's body and what progress has been made against the disease.

The experiment is an extension of Rosenberg's previous studies using cancer-fighting cells called *tumor-infiltrating lymphocytes* (TIL). In those studies, Rosenberg and his colleagues reported striking improvement in some patients, especially patients with advanced melanoma or *renal cell cancer* (a type of kidney cancer), who had not responded to any other treatment.

In December 1988, Rosenberg and his co-workers reported that TIL therapy resulted in *remission* (a halt in tumor growth) in 11 of 20 patients with advanced melanoma. In April 1989, independent investigators confirmed the effectiveness of TIL therapy in patients at six other centers around the United States.

Scientists, however, still do not understand why some patients respond to the treatment while others do not. The gene transfer experiment was designed partly to find out why some patients do not respond. In the experiment, the scientists removed TIL cells from a patient's tumor. The cells were then grown in a laboratory for several weeks with interleukin-2 (IL-2), a substance that stimulates the immune system. The marker gene, which is a gene from a bacteria that is resistant to the antibiotic neomycin, was then transferred to the cells. These gene-altered TIL cells were then returned to the patient. Later, the researchers will remove a small part of tissue from the tumor and expose the tumor cells to neomycin. Those cells with the marker gene that is resistant to neomycin will survive the exposure, thus telling scientists if the TIL cells successfully infiltrated the tumor.

Initially, the scientists will test the usefulness of the marker gene in only 10 patients with advanced mel-

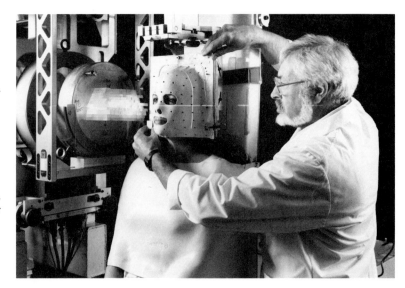

Targeting a tumor
A technician adjusts a device that holds a patient's head rigid so that a beam of charged particles from a particle accelerator can accurately target a cancerous tumor. Scientists at the Lawrence Berkeley Laboratory in California pioneered in the use of accelerators—first used for research in high-energy physics—to destroy cancerous cells. Due to their success, some hospitals are now installing their own accelerators.

How IL-2 fights cancer

T-cells

IL-2

Receptors

TIL's

Tumor

New cancer treatment
Surgical oncologist Steven A. Rosenberg, *above,* reported in December 1988 results of a promising experimental cancer treatment. The treatment uses a natural body substance called *interleukin-2* (IL-2), to stimulate *T-cells* (a type of lymphocyte, or white blood cell) that have infiltrated the patient's tumor. The treatment, *above left,* involves removing pieces of a patient's tumor and mixing them with IL-2, which binds to proteins called receptors on T-cells. The IL-2 encourages these T-cells—called *tumor-infiltrating lymphocytes* (TIL's)—to multiply rapidly. The TIL's are then reinjected into the patient, where they attack and destroy cancer cells.

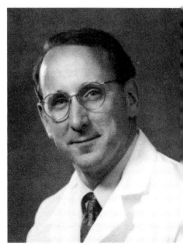

Cancer (cont.)
anoma. "Ultimately," said NIH Director James B. Wyngaarden, "this new technique could open the door to studies that will use gene insertion to produce therapeutic results in a wide range of diseases."

Genes and cancer risk. Scientists made increasingly rapid progress in 1988 and 1989 in identifying the location on human chromosomes of genes that play a role in cancer. (In human beings, each body cell contains 46 chromosomes, tiny thread-like structures that occur in pairs. The chromosomes carry genes, which contain the information for hereditary traits.) The risk of cancer may be increased when such a gene is altered or accidentally *deleted* (removed) from a chromosome. Previous studies focused on rare, inherited cancers. Now, however, new studies are shedding light on common cancers.

In September 1988, researchers at the Johns Hopkins University School of Medicine in Baltimore and the University of Utah School of Medicine in Salt Lake City looked at alterations of chromosomes in *adenomas* (benign tumors) of the large intestine. Many scientists believe these benign tumors are the precursors of colon cancer. Working also with scientists from the State University of Leiden in the Netherlands, the scientists found evidence that multiple genetic changes occur in

colon cells when cancer develops. The scientists found that in colon cancer cells, chromosomes 5, 17, and 18 appeared to be missing certain genes more frequently than other chromosomes, suggesting that those genes are important in blocking the development of cancer.

In April and June 1989, many of the same investigators looked more closely at these chromosome changes. In 56 tissue samples from colon cancers and adjacent normal tissue, the scientists often found genetic material (*deoxyribonucleic acid* [DNA], the molecule that makes up the genetic substance of the chromosomes) missing from the cancer cell's chromosome. Patients whose cancer cells showed more deletions of genetic material were more likely to develop recurrent disease and their cancers were more likely to spread.

Also in April 1989, many of the same scientists involved in these studies reported on research concerning one of the most common genetic alterations in colon cancer, the deletion of part of chromosome 17, which occurs in more than 75 per cent of colon cancer cases. The research showed that the deletion is associated with a mutation in a gene that normally functions to suppress cell growth in colon cells. In animals, the mutated gene is associated with cancer development.

Cancer (cont.)

Despite the remarkable progress made in understanding colon cancer during 1988 and 1989, scientists cautioned physicians not to overinterpret the predictive value of individual genetic abnormalities.

Hereditary melanoma. Researchers reported in May 1989 that they had found a gene for a hereditary form of skin cancer, *familial malignant melanoma*, on chromosome 1. Scientists from the NCI, the Massachusetts Institute of Technology (M.I.T.) in Cambridge, and the University of Pennsylvania in Philadelphia tracked down the gene by studying the DNA of 125 members of six melanoma-prone families.

Locating the gene for malignant melanoma means that scientists will be able to determine those who are most susceptible to the disease. Thus, for a melanoma-prone family, "we can give parents a pretty good idea about whether their child has inherited the melanoma gene and to have them protect the child from burning sunrays, even as an infant," said geneticist Sherri Bale of the NCI. Ultraviolet radiation from the sun can cause skin cancer.

Twenty-six *DNA probes*—molecules tailored to detect cancer genes—were used to analyze the chromosome 1 region thought to contain the melanoma gene. In the study, 99 relatives and 26 spouses in the melanoma-prone families were examined for malignant melanoma or abnormal moles that often precede it.

Skin *biopsies* (tissue samples) of moles and melanomas were evaluated by researcher Wallace Clark, Jr., an expert on skin cancer at the University of Pennsylvania School of Medicine in Philadelphia. Then, molecular biologist Nicholas Dracopoki and his colleagues at M.I.T. tested the DNA from the study participants.

Using laboratory and statistical techniques, the scientists found that the gene is located within a particular region of chromosome 1. The next step is to analyze the gene in order to understand the cause of hereditary melanoma. "It's even possible that study of this gene may help us understand the effects of ultraviolet light and other exposures that can cause nonhereditary melanomas," said Bale.

Treatment progress. Experimental drugs made from *growth factors*—protein molecules that enhance cell growth—emerged as powerful new tools in cancer treatment during 1988 and 1989. The most clinically effective growth factor to date is granulocyte-colony stimulating factor (G-CSF).

G-CSF is part of a network of substances that regulates the growth

Boron "bomb"
A computer graphic displays the structure of a boron "bomb," a compound that has been used experimentally to kill tumor cells. By using computer graphics to study the structure of these boron compounds, scientists hope to understand what makes some compounds more effective than others at destroying cancer cells.

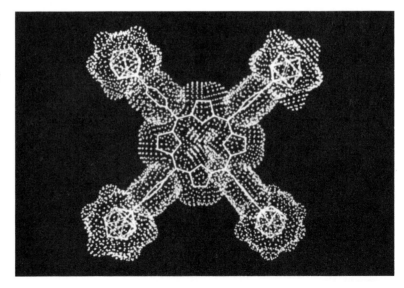

Cancer (cont.)

and development of cells involved in the immune system and blood formation. It is particularly vital to the normal development of *neutrophils*, white blood cells that protect against bacterial infection. Many cancer patients who receive *chemotherapy* (drug treatment) become vulnerable to infections because chemotherapy drastically reduces neutrophil levels.

In May 1989, two of the discoverers of G-CSF, Janice L. Gabrilove and Malcolm A. S. Moore of Memorial Sloan-Kettering Cancer Center in New York City and their colleagues reported that they had completed the first tests of genetically engineered G-CSF. Patients with advanced bladder cancer who were undergoing intensive chemotherapy treatment received G-CSF; all of them were able to complete their chemotherapy. But 29 per cent of another group of patients who had chemotherapy without receiving G-CSF were unable to complete chemotherapy because their neutrophil levels fell too low.

The study also showed that patients receiving G-CSF required fewer treatment days with antibiotics, suggesting that the growth factor reduces infection risks in patients on chemotherapy. Tests are now underway at Memorial Sloan-Kettering and elsewhere to test G-CSF in patients undergoing chemotherapy for a particular type of lung cancer and in patients with immune disorders characterized by a lack of neutrophil production.

Chemotherapy for colon cancer.
In May 1989, the FDA announced expanded use of a drug called *levamisole* in combination with the approved cancer drug 5-fluorouracil (5-FU) in some patients soon after they have undergone surgery for colon cancer. Levamisole stimulates the immune system and has anti-cancer effects.

A preliminary study first reported in 1986 by cancer treatment experts showed that a combination of levamisole and 5-FU produced a statistically significant reduction in cancer recurrence or a delay in onset of recurrence. Levamisole will be made available under special FDA regulations that enable drug manufacturers to release promising drugs to desperately ill patients before complete testing has been done. Levamisole will be distributed by NCI throughout the United States.

☐ Patricia A. Newman-Horm

In the Special Reports section, see ANSWERS TO YOUR QUESTIONS ABOUT BREAST CANCER. In WORLD BOOK, see CANCER.

Surprising information on how the brain generates spontaneous emotional expressions in babies was reported in March 1989 by psychologists Catherine T. Best and Heidi F. Queen of Wesleyan University in Middletown, Conn. They reported that, unlike adults, infants show greater emotional intensity on the right side of the face. Previous studies have found emotional expressions are more intense on the left side of the face among right-handed adults.

For their study, Best and Queen made computer copies of photographs of 10 infants between the ages of 7 and 13 months. Six of the babies were smiling; four were crying. Each half of a face was combined with its mirror image. For example, the left side of a crying face was flopped over to create a complete face.

University students then rated the intensity of the emotional expressions in each composite image. The expressions in the right-sided composites were rated more intense than the expressions in the left-sided composites.

Most psychologists believe that the adult pattern of greater emotional intensity on the left side of the face reflects the influence of the brain's right side. This part of the brain, called the right hemisphere,

Child Development

Emotional about-face

Composite photographs of mirror images of the right and left sides of babies' faces reveal greater emotional intensity on the right side, according to researchers at Wesleyan University in Middletown, Conn. In adults, expressions are more intense on the left side. The researchers suggest that in infancy, the right hemisphere of the brain, which controls the left side of the face, dampens emotional expression, resulting in more intense expressions on the right side. They theorize that as the brain matures, this function passes to the left hemisphere, which controls the right side of the face.

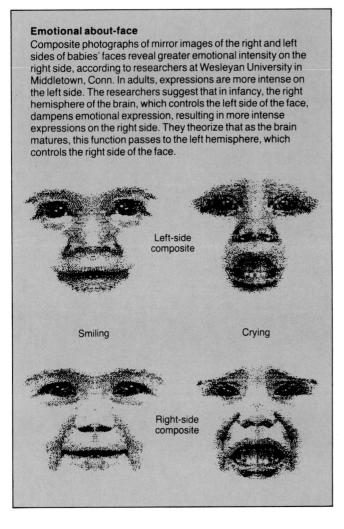

Left-side composite

Smiling

Crying

Right-side composite

Child Development (cont.)

controls many muscles on the left side of the face. Studies of brain-damaged patients who are right-handed indicate that the right hemisphere is crucially involved in experiencing emotion and recognizing facial expressions. The left brain hemisphere, which controls much of the right side of the face, may help to inhibit emotional displays, thus contributing to more intense expressions on the left side of the face.

Best and Queen's study suggests the right hemisphere matures more quickly during infancy than the left hemisphere. The main responsibility for restraining spontaneous emotions may pass to the left hemisphere as children gain more volun-tary control over emotions in the preschool years, Best said.

Children and media violence.
There is "a small but genuine association" between exposure to media violence and increased aggression among children, according to a report released in April 1989 by the American Medical Association (AMA) in Chicago. The AMA report was a review and analysis of numerous studies on children and media violence.

The report noted that not all children are affected in the same way by media violence. Researchers have not yet pinned down all the characteristics of children most likely to react aggressively in response to violent programs. Some of those characteristics, however, may be an aggressive temperament, a violent family environment, identification with aggressive media characters, and a belief that media programs are real. The report also noted that programs in which only the "bad guy" is killed and in which violence is presented as something to be cheered may arouse aggression in all viewers.

Testing intelligence. A simple test of infants' visual memory and intelligence shows promise as a tool for identifying mentally retarded children as early as 7 months of age, according to an August 1988 report by psychologist Joseph F. Fagan III of Case Western Reserve University in Cleveland. Mental retardation often is not diagnosed until a child is at least 4 years old. The test may enable child development specialists to identify such children earlier and so provide them with specialized educational programs.

Fagan's test of infant intelligence is based on previous observations that most babies look longer at new images than they do at familiar ones. Fagan contends that the ability to remember and discriminate between images is an indication of basic thinking abilities.

For the study, Fagan and his coworkers presented infants with slide projections of faces and abstract

Child Development (cont.)

patterns. Two images, one already presented and the other unfamiliar, were then shown together. The amount of time the infants looked at the familiar and unfamiliar slides was recorded.

Fagan and his team then tested the children's intelligence quotient (IQ) periodically between the ages of 2 and 7. They found that the children who had preferred to look at the unfamiliar image scored higher on the IQ tests than those who looked longer at the familiar image.

Fagan and his co-workers also gave the visual test to 128 infants at risk for mental retardation because of premature birth or neurological problems. Of 104 infants with normal test scores, 101 had normal IQ's at age 3. Of the 24 infants with low scores on the visual test, however, half had IQ's in the retarded range at age 3.

Some educators and psychologists oppose testing infants in an effort to predict later intelligence. They say that the prediction that a child will be a slow learner may lead parents and teachers to treat the child in ways that make the expectation come true. And at any age, intelligence tests do not reflect a person's ability in all areas, such as the ability to get along with others or artistic creativity. But high IQ has consistently been linked to greater scholastic and occupational achievement.

Benefits of self-control. Preschool children who are able to pass up a small reward available immediately in exchange for a larger reward in the future cope better with frustration and stress as teen-agers. That conclusion was reported in May 1989 by psychologists Walter Mischel and his colleagues of Columbia University in New York City.

In the early 1970's, Mischel and his co-workers tested 53 children aged 4. For the test, a researcher showed each child a pair of treats—two small cookies and five pretzel sticks—and then left the room. To get the five pretzels—considered the preferred treat—the youngsters had to wait for the researcher to return 15 minutes later. The children could, however, get the cookies anytime before that by pressing a buzzer.

The researchers found that when the treats were hidden from sight before the researcher left the room, the children were able to wait longer than when the treats were in plain view. In addition, the way the children thought about the treats significantly affected their self-control, the researchers said. The children asked for the cookies sooner if they were instructed to focus on "arousing" features of a treat, such as the

Infant intelligence test
Two faces—one familiar, one unfamiliar—are presented to an infant, *below left,* during an intelligence test developed at Case Western Reserve University in Cleveland. The amount of time the infant looks at each face is then recorded, *below.* Infants who looked longer at the unfamiliar image scored higher on intelligence tests in childhood than infants who preferred the familiar image.

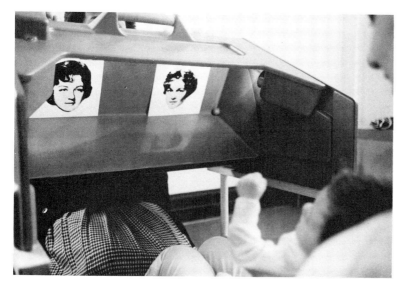

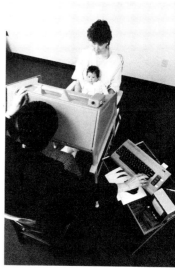

taste and crunch of a pretzel. The children were able to wait longer if they were told to imagine "abstract" qualities of a reward, such as thinking about pretzel sticks as long, brown logs.

The researchers contacted the children and their parents 10 years later. They found that the children who delayed gratification longer were, as teen-agers, considered to be more attentive, goal-oriented, and intelligent by their parents. Their parents also reported that the children were better able to resist temptation and cope with stress.

Shy outlooks. Contrary to some previous studies, shy children are not more likely to develop mental disorders as they grow older, according to research reported in November 1988 by a team headed by psychologist Avshalom Caspi of Harvard University in Cambridge, Mass. Caspi and his co-workers found, however, that enduring shyness during boyhood appears to undermine the stability of a young man's work and family life.

According to the study, men who were shy as children marry, have children, and enter stable careers later than men who were not shy. They also tend to achieve less status in their jobs and switch jobs and separate or divorce more often.

In contrast, the researchers said, shy girls appear to experience little difficulty in early adulthood. As adults, they are more likely than other women to marry, have children, and become homemakers. The researchers noted, however, that because women are now routinely entering the work force, shy females may no longer move so easily through young adulthood.

The researchers based their findings on information collected in a project begun in 1928 with 214 newborn babies. The shyness of the children was estimated from interviews with their mothers and teachers. Most of the subjects were then interviewed at ages 30 and 40.

Roots of deception. Children as young as 3 years old can mask their emotional expressions intentionally while attempting to deceive an adult, according to research reported in May 1989 and directed by psychologist Michael Lewis of the University of Medicine and Dentistry of New Jersey in Newark. The study indicates people adopt deceptive strategies in the first few years of life. It also suggests that adults find it difficult to distinguish between children who are lying and those who are telling the truth.

Lewis and his co-workers videotaped 15 boys and 18 girls, all about 3 years of age, during a laboratory test. Each child sat with his or her back to a table and was told that a researcher was putting out a toy. The children were instructed not to peek. They were also told that they could play with the toy when the researcher returned.

The researcher then left the room and returned either after the child peeked at the toy or after 5 minutes. The child was asked, "Did you peek?" The question was repeated if no response was given.

Only 4 children—3 girls and 1 boy—did not look at the toy. A total of 11 children, 9 of them boys, looked at the toy and admitted it. Another 11 children, 8 of them girls, looked at the toy but denied peeking. Seven children gave no response.

Sixty university students who viewed videotapes of the children responding to the researcher's question were unable to determine which children were truthfully denying peeking and which were lying.

Overall, the girls were just as likely as the boys to look at the toy. But the girls were much more apt to deny having done so. Lewis suggested this was because girls may experience more shame after breaking a rule, leading them to deny their offense. Lewis also theorized that girls are more interested in social approval and may lie to avoid displeasing an adult, as well as to avoid punishment.

☐ Bruce Bower

In WORLD BOOK, see CHILD.

Childbirth
See Pregnancy and Childbirth

Contraception
See Birth Control

Being fitted with an artificial crown—a process that requires several visits to the dentist—can be accomplished in less than an hour using one of several computerized reconstruction systems being tested in 1989. (An artificial crown is a replacement for the part of the tooth above the gum.) The systems, called *CAD-CAM* (computer-aided design/computer-aided manufacturing) systems, are being evaluated at several dental schools in the United States.

Restoring a tooth by adding a crown is necessary when a large portion of the tooth has been destroyed, most often by decay. Usually, so little of the tooth remains that filling the tooth is not feasible.

To make a crown, the dentist currently grinds down the outer layers of the tooth, leaving a stub to which the new permanent crown will be attached. The dentist then makes a model of the stub, called an impression. The impression is then sent to a dental laboratory, which uses it as a guide for the base of the replacement tooth. Meanwhile, the patient is fitted with a temporary crown. When the permanent crown is finished, the dentist removes the temporary crown and cements the permanent crown in place.

CAD-CAM systems allow this process to take place in less than one hour and in one office visit. Using the new system, the dentist places a tiny video camera on the top of the tooth to be reconstructed. A picture of the tooth stub—actually a three-dimensional computer image showing the contours of the tooth in great detail—is then displayed on a monitor. Using the monitor, the dentist makes any necessary modifications. The computer then directs the operation of a milling machine. This machine uses diamond disks to grind a ceramic block to create a crown fitting the design specifications. The entire process takes less than 15 minutes.

According to CAD-CAM developers, the new technology offers benefits beyond speed. The system eliminates the need for a temporary crown and for the repeated use of anesthesia, often required when the tooth is being ground down and the decay removed. The developers also believe that a computer-created crown fits more snugly to the remaining tooth. An imperfect fit may weaken a crown. In addition, a gap between the remaining tooth and the crown may become a breeding ground for bacteria, which cause future tooth decay and gum disease.

Fighting gum disease. Newly discovered chemical properties of the

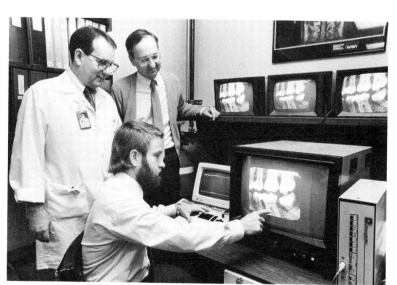

Detecting gum disease
Researchers at Washington University in St. Louis, Mo., study computerized images of dental X rays for early signs of gum disease. By using a computer system to enhance the image, researchers can detect even small amounts of the bone loss that occurs as gum disease progresses. The images may also reveal subtle changes in the bones that occur before they begin to deteriorate.

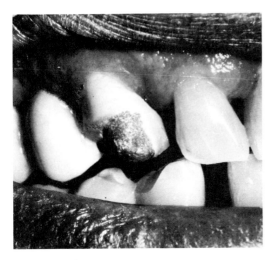

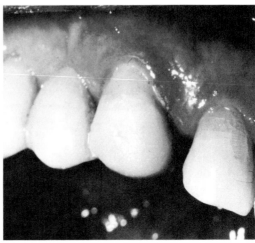

Speedy repair
The damaged porcelain covering an artificial metal bridge, *above,* can be repaired in place in less than 15 minutes using a new adhesive called Cover Up. Ordinarily, the bridge must be removed and sent to a dental laboratory, where more porcelain is fused to the metal. The adhesive, which bonds plastic to metal, allows the dentist to quickly rebuild the bridge with a plastic composite, *above right.*

Dentistry (cont.)
commonly used antibiotic tetracycline may provide a potent weapon against gum disease. This finding was reported in May 1989 by dental researcher Lorne Golub and colleagues at the State University of New York at Stony Brook.

While studying the effect of tetracycline on the bacteria that cause gum disease, the researchers found that the antibiotic also inactivated the enzyme collagenase. This enzyme, which is produced by the bacteria, destroys collagen, the major protein in the fibers of connective tissue, bone, and cartilage. Collagen fibers hold the teeth in the jawbone. The researchers discovered that tetracycline greatly slowed the destruction of collagen in the gums of patients with gum disease.

Golub and his colleagues acknowledged that the long-term use of tetracycline to treat gum disease would be unwise because the bacteria could develop a resistance to the antibiotic. To sidestep this problem, they hope to modify the chemistry of tetracycline to remove its antibacterial qualities while retaining its ability to inactivate collagenase. □ Kenneth L. Siegel

In WORLD BOOK, see DENTISTRY; TEETH.

Diabetes

A simple test that should help identify people who may develop diabetes was reported in June 1989 by researchers at the University of Pittsburgh School of Medicine in Pennsylvania. Diabetes is a disease in which the body fails to produce or efficiently use the hormone *insulin* to maintain normal levels of sugar in the blood.

The prediabetes test checks the relatives of insulin-dependent, or Type I, diabetics for their risk of getting the disease. People with Type I diabetes take daily injections of insulin to control their blood sugar.

The test is significant because early diagnosis of diabetes is critical to slowing down or preventing some of the disease's serious health consequences, such as heart disease, blindness, and kidney damage. People found to be at risk could become candidates for possible future treatments for preventing the disease. Research related to the test may also shed new light on whether diabetes is an inherited disease, the result of an environmental factor, or a combination of both.

Developed by medical researcher Massimo Trucco and his colleagues at the University of Pittsburgh, the prediabetes test uses genetic engineering techniques to detect whether a particular portion of a gene contains a particular se-

Diabetes (cont.)

quence of molecules. Trucco's research group earlier had found that the absence of that sequence of molecules at that location makes a person 107 times more likely to develop Type I diabetes.

Blood sugar and health. Evidence mounted in late 1988 that diabetics who carefully control their blood sugar level may reduce their risk of developing many of the complications of diabetes. In November, researchers at the University of Wisconsin in Madison reported that even a small improvement in blood sugar control may decrease the incidence of *retinopathy*, a condition in which blood vessels in the *retina* (the light-sensitive part of the eye) gradually break and bleed, causing blindness.

The researchers studied 1,897 people with diabetes over a four-year period. Those who reported difficulty controlling their blood sugar levels were twice as likely to develop retinopathy than those who reported good control.

But tight control over blood sugar levels is not without its risks, the scientists warned. They cautioned that such control can cause severe health problems, including *hypoglycemia* (extremely low levels of sugar in the blood).

Fat and diabetes. Researchers at the Center for Human Nutrition at the University of Texas Southwestern Medical Center in Dallas reported in September 1988 that they had evidence supporting the controversial claim that a diet high in fat may be better for people with diabetes than one low in fat. The preliminary finding contradicts the recommendation by the American Diabetes Association, the Canadian Diabetes Association, and other diabetes groups that diabetics should eat foods low in cholesterol and saturated fats and high in complex carbohydrates, such as beans and grains. Such a diet is believed to reduce the risk of heart disease, often a complication of diabetes.

The researchers focused their study on people with noninsulin-dependent, or Type II, diabetes. People with Type II diabetes produce insulin but cannot use it properly. They usually control their blood sugar through diet, though many also take oral drugs. The researchers carefully controlled the diets of 10 people with Type II diabetes, giving half a low-fat, high-carbohydrate diet and the other half a low-carbohydrate diet that was high in a type of fat called monounsaturated fat, especially olive oil. After about a month, the groups switched diets.

At the end of the study, the researchers found that the diet high in fat produced better levels of blood sugar and lower levels of cholesterol. Some scientists said the results showed the need for additional long-term studies to determine the health impact of different types of fat in the diet of diabetics.

Pancreas alternative. The artificial pancreas moved closer to reality in 1989. Such a device, surgically implanted under the skin, would mimic the function of the *pancreas* (the organ that produces insulin) by sensing levels of sugar in the body and automatically delivering a proper dose of insulin. In people with Type I diabetes, the pancreas either stops producing insulin or produces an insufficient amount of the hormone. Researchers believe an artificial pancreas could lead to

In September 1988, the National Diabetes Data Group (NDDG) in Bethesda, Md., reported that diabetes is a growing health problem among black Americans. Black women are especially vulnerable, the NDDG noted. As many as 1 in 4 black women aged 55 and older has the disease.

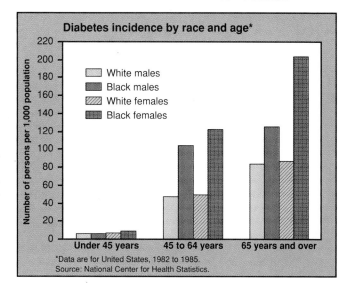

Diabetes incidence by race and age*

Number of persons per 1,000 population

☐ White males
■ Black males
▨ White females
▦ Black females

Under 45 years   45 to 64 years   65 years and over

*Data are for United States, 1982 to 1985.
Source: National Center for Health Statistics.

Figuring insulin dosages
A handheld computer that helps diabetics adjust the amount of their daily insulin dosage received approval from the U.S. Food and Drug Administration in late 1988. Diabetics enter data such as their blood sugar level and food intake into the computer, which then calculates the proper insulin dose. The computer is manufactured by the Healthware Corporation of Durham, N.C.

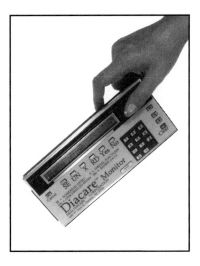

Diabetes (cont.)
major improvements in management of the disease and could eliminate the need for diabetics to assess their blood sugar levels by pricking their fingers several times a day to draw blood samples.

Scientists at the University of New Mexico in Albuquerque and at Johns Hopkins University in Baltimore announced in February that they had developed a small, needlelike electrode that can be implanted just under the skin in the abdomen and used to sense sugar concentrations in the body's tissue. The device was to undergo tests in animals and humans in late 1989.

Benefits of relaxation. People with Type II diabetes may significantly improve their ability to deal with increases in blood sugar following meals if they practice relaxation techniques. That was the conclusion of a study reported in June 1989 by researchers at Duke University Medical Center in Durham, N.C.

Medical researcher Richard S. Surwit evaluated 20 patients for their *glucose tolerance*—their body's response to an increase in blood sugar—after half of them had practiced muscle relaxation and biofeedback techniques for several weeks. (Biofeedback is a process of learning to mentally control certain bodily processes—such as heart rate—that ordinarily cannot be controlled voluntarily.) The glucose tolerance of the group that had relaxation training improved an average of 20 per cent, with the glucose tolerance of some people in the group improving as much as 30 per cent.

Surwit said that overall diabetes management might be improved by scheduling relaxation sessions after meals. The study also indicated that the central nervous system may somehow be involved in blood sugar control in diabetes.

☐ William H. Allen

In WORLD BOOK, see DIABETES; INSULIN.

Digestive System

Several researchers at the Digestive Disease Week meetings held in May 1989 in Washington, D.C., documented the accuracy of a technique called *endoscopic ultrasonography* in determining the extent of cancers of the stomach and pancreas. This method has also been useful in producing images of rectal cancers and cancers of the *esophagus* (the food passage leading from the mouth to the stomach).

In this technique, a physician inserts into the body a flexible tube called an *endoscope*. Running the length of the tube is an *optical fiber*, a hair-thin strand of glass or plastic that conducts light to the inside of the body. An eyepiece and tiny

lenses connected to the fiber enable the physician to view the inside of the body through the fiber to guide the endoscope to the correct location.

Mounted on the end of the tube that is guided into the body is a device called an *ultrasonic probe*. Wires running the length of the endoscope connect this device to an ultrasound machine, which includes a televisionlike screen.

The probe emits high-frequency sound waves, some of which bounce off internal organs and return to the probe. This device translates the returned waves into electric signals, which travel by wire to

Digestive System (cont.)

the ultrasound machine. The machine, in turn, uses the signals to create an image of the organs on its screen.

Doctors are using this technique to replace conventional ultrasonography, in which the sound waves are generated outside the body. In the conventional method, the presence of bones and intestinal gas may interfere with the view of the organ that the doctor is studying. The new technique avoids this problem. Another advantage of the endoscopic technique is that it can use higher frequencies of sound, resulting in sharper images.

New test for hepatitis. A screening test for a newly discovered hepatitis virus was announced in April 1989 and promises to slash the rate of transmission of *hepatitis* (a disease of the liver) through blood transfusions. Blood banks routinely screen donated blood for two previously identified hepatitis viruses, known as A and B. Yet as many as 7 to 10 per cent of patients who receive transfusions catch hepatitis from the blood. About 90 to 95 per cent of these cases are caused by viruses other than A and B, which scientists call non-A non-B (NANB) virus.

Scientists at the Chiron Corporation in Emeryville, Calif., announced in April 1989 that they had developed a technique to screen blood for an NANB virus they called *hepatitis C virus*, which is believed to be the cause of most cases of hepatitis transmitted by transfusions. See INFECTIOUS DISEASES.

Non-A Non-B hepatitis occurs 5 to 12 weeks after transfusion. It tends to be more mild than acute cases of hepatitis A or B. In 40 to 60 per cent of cases, however, NANB hepatitis develops into chronic hepatitis and *cirrhosis*, a type of permanent and progressive damage to the liver.

Physicians often can halt the progress of cirrhosis by removing its cause. Unfortunately, however, there is no recognized treatment for chronic hepatitis. So cirrhosis due to chronic hepatitis remains unchecked. For this reason, the ability to screen blood and blood products to prevent hepatitis C is of great importance to public health.

Treatments for gallstones.
Researchers continued to make progress during 1988 and 1989 in the study of *gallstones* (pebblelike masses of cholesterol and mineral salts that sometimes form in the gall bladder or one of its ducts). One new treatment involves a substance called *ursodeoxycholic acid*, which became available for use on gallstones in the United States in January 1989. This substance replaces

Microbes and ulcers
Campylobacter pylori bacteria (arrows) have been linked to the most common form of *gastritis* (an inflammation of the stomach) and many ulcers of the stomach and *duodenum* (the upper part of the small intestine). Doctors are experimenting with antibiotic treatments for these diseases.

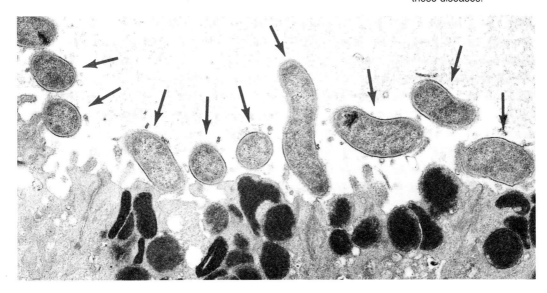

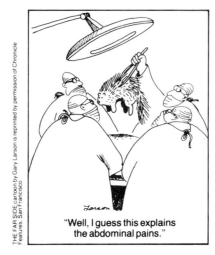

THE FAR SIDE cartoon by Gary Larson is reprinted by permission of Chronicle Features, San Francisco.

"Well, I guess this explains the abdominal pains."

Digestive System (cont.)

chenodeoxycholic acid, which has been associated with such side effects as a poisoning of the liver; diarrhea; and a tendency to raise the level of low-density lipoprotein (LDL) cholesterol in the blood, which may contribute to a narrowing of the arteries.

In a functioning gall bladder, ursodeoxycholic acid can dissolve gallstones that contain too small an amount of mineral salts to appear in X-ray images. In addition, ursodeoxycholic acid is used along with another gallstone treatment involving *extracorporeal shock-wave lithotripsy* (ESWL), in which waves of pressure break up the stones.

In ESWL treatment the waves are generated inside a machine, transmitted through water inside a bag touching the patient's skin, and focused on the area containing the gallstones. Images produced by a separate ultrasound machine help surgeons focus the waves, which enter the patient's body without damaging tissue and strike the stone. After the ESWL machine is used, the patient takes ursodeoxycholic acid or chenodeoxycholic acid to help dissolve the remaining fragments of stone.

The initial use of ESWL, reported in 1984, was to break up kidney stones. In 1986, West German researchers announced the first use of ESWL to smash gallstones. This use has not yet received the approval of the United States Food and Drug Administration (FDA), but medical centers throughout the United States are testing ESWL machines that smash gallstones to gather data needed for approval.

Because drug or ESWL therapy leaves the gall bladder intact, new gallstones can form after the treatment. While new stones may form in 50 per cent of nonsurgical patients, physicians are developing strategies to reduce this percentage. One strategy involves the use of aspirin to alter the mucus in the gall bladder in a way that may

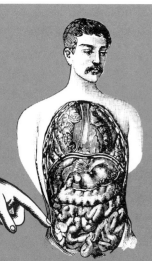

Facts in brief on the appendix

What is the appendix?
The appendix is a thin, worm-shaped pouch about 3½ inches (9 centimeters) long that is attached to the first part of the large intestine.

What is the function of the appendix?
In human beings, the appendix has no known function.

What is appendicitis?
Appendicitis is an inflammation of the appendix, resulting from a bacterial infection that causes the appendix to swell and fill with pus. Symptoms include early, intermittent pain in the navel region, later localizing to the lower right-hand corner of the abdomen; nausea; fever; and constipation or diarrhea. The lower abdomen becomes tender, and touching increases the pain.

Who gets appendicitis?
Each year, about 1 person in 500 has an attack of appendicitis. The disease is most common among males between the ages of 10 and 30, and is rare in children who are less than 2 years old.

What should I do if I suspect appendicitis?
Do not give laxatives. Consult a physician immediately. Failure to seek help promptly could result in a burst appendix, leading swiftly to a serious infection of the abdominal lining. If the doctor determines that the appendicitis is acute, he or she almost certainly will recommend an immediate appendectomy.

How is an appendectomy performed?
The patient receives general anesthesia, then the surgeon makes an incision in the lower right-hand side of the abdomen and removes the appendix. The patient usually leaves the hospital within a week.

Digestive System (cont.)

affect the formation of stones.

One complication of ESWL therapy is *pancreatitis* (inflammation of the pancreas), when relatively large fragments of stone pass through the common bile duct into the *duodenum* (the upper end of the small intestine). These stones block the duct that leads from the pancreas to the duodenum.

Physicians continued to experiment during the year with the dissolving of gallstones with a chemical called *methyl tert-butyl ether* (MTBE). In a technique reported in 1986, the surgeon inserts a thin tube into the gall bladder. The bile

in the gall bladder is then replaced with MTBE. The tube, however, must first pass through the liver.

Researchers in West Germany are experimenting with a newer technique that avoids passing a tube through the liver. The physicians guide a tube through an endoscope, the common bile duct, and the cystic duct, to the gall bladder. The doctors then release the MTBE through the tube to dissolve the stones. □ James L. Franklin

In the Special Reports section, see THE INSIDE STORY ON ULCERS. In WORLD BOOK, see DIGESTIVE SYSTEM; GALLSTONE; HEPATITIS; STOMACH.

Drug Abuse

See Alcohol and Drug Abuse

Drugs

Two new arthritis drugs were marketed in the United States in 1988 and 1989. Diclofenac, sold under the trade name Voltaren by Geigy Pharmaceuticals of Ardsley, N.Y., was introduced in the fall of 1988, and flurbiprofen, sold as Ansaid by The Upjohn Company of Kalamazoo, Mich., was marketed in early 1989. Both belong to a group of medications called *nonsteroidal anti-inflammatory drugs* (NSAID's), which also includes aspirin and ibuprofen.

The new drugs are considered as effective as other NSAID's in relieving the pain and inflammation of arthritic disorders. Individuals vary, however, in how they respond to medication, and some may experience greater benefit by using one of these new drugs than they did from previous therapy. Although new in the United States, diclofenac has been marketed in other countries for a number of years. In fact, internationally it is the drug most frequently prescribed for arthritis.

Certain precautions still apply to the use of these new NSAID's. They must not be taken by patients who experience asthma, hives, or other allergic-type reactions when they take aspirin or any other NSAID. For such patients, the new NSAID's pose the risk of a serious, and even fatal, allergic reaction. In addition, NSAID's may irritate the lining of the digestive tract, causing stomach

upsets and ulcers. Most NSAID's are less likely than aspirin to cause gastrointestinal side effects, but such reactions can occur.

The NSAID's reduce inflammation primarily by inhibiting the formation of *prostaglandins*, chemical compounds that play a variety of roles in the body, including the development of inflammation. Some prostaglandins, however, also perform a beneficial function in protecting the lining of the stomach. When these prostaglandins are depleted by the action of an NSAID, the lining becomes more susceptible to ulcers, which may become life-threatening

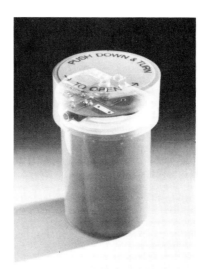

Monitoring pill-taking

A battery-operated drug container helps doctors monitor patient compliance with drug treatment. The lid of the oversized pill bottle contains electronic microcircuitry that records the time and number of container openings. This information can be transferred to a computer disk for analysis to determine if patients were taking their medication at correct intervals.

Drug Resistance: When Germs Fight Back

For many years, nearly all people who contracted gonorrhea, a sexually transmitted disease, were cured by the antibiotic penicillin. But on Sept. 1, 1989, the Centers for Disease Control in Atlanta, Ga., recommended that the drug no longer be widely used for gonorrhea treatment. Why? Some strains of the gonorrhea bacteria have, in a sense, learned to defend themselves against the antibiotic.

Penicillin is not the only "wonder drug" that is losing its power to kill disease-causing microorganisms. Scores of other drugs designed to wipe out bacteria, parasites, fungi, and viruses no longer seem as wonderful as they once did. In 1989, for example, physicians began reporting that some AIDS patients were no longer being helped by zidovudine (AZT) and other drugs used to combat viral infections.

The drugs themselves have not changed, however. It is the microbes they are designed to combat that have developed the ability to ward off attacks by drugs to which they once succumbed.

They have done so through the process of *genetic mutation*. As a group of microbes reproduce, the genetic material in the organisms occasionally undergoes a slight change, or *mutation*. Because microorganisms are extremely simple organisms with relatively few genes, small genetic changes can make a big difference in the way the organisms function. Occasionally, such genetic changes confer resistance to a specific drug.

For example, some bacteria have mutated in such a way that they produce an enzyme biologists call *penicillinase*, which inactivates penicillin. Other penicillin-resistant bacteria have undergone genetic mutations that resulted in an alteration in the way in which their cell walls are formed. Because penicillin kills bacteria by disrupting the formation of cell walls, these bacteria are not harmed by the drug.

Like penicillin, most drugs that are effective against viral, fungal, and parasitic infections also act by interfering with some process essential to the infectious organism's ability to thrive or reproduce. And, like penicillin-resistant bacteria, other drug-resistant microbes have undergone genetic changes that slightly alter the drugs' targets.

Unfortunately, drug treatment for infections actually promotes the growth of drug-resistant microbes. This is because when a drug kills off susceptible strains of a microbe, resist-ant strains no longer have to compete with them for nutrients, and they multiply.

Infections with resistant bacteria have become a serious problem in hospitals where patients with many different types of infections are being treated with many different types of drugs. There, patients being given a drug that effectively eliminates one type of microbe may, through contact with other patients, become infected with a microbe resistant to the drug.

Drug-resistant infections are also becoming a problem in other environments—such as schools and day-care centers—where people are in close contact. The problem also affects livestock, most probably due to the use of antibiotics in animal feed.

As drug resistance affects more and more microbes, scientists and physicians are searching for ways to combat it. Doctors have been able to help prevent the spread of re-

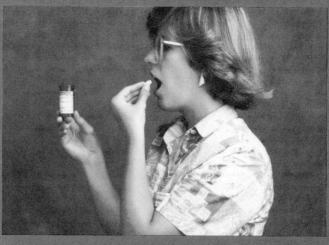

Take antibiotics only when necessary.

sistant microbes by ordering tests to determine whether the strains responsible for a patient's infection are resistant to the drugs normally used to treat it. Usually, they are then able to prescribe a drug that the microbes are still susceptible to.

Microbiologists are also trying to keep a step ahead of quickly mutating microbes by creating new drugs or modifying old ones to overcome resistance. Another way to combat the problem of drug resistance is through vaccination, which activates the immune system so that it combats infection before drug treatment becomes necessary.

Most scientists agree that the easiest and best way to control drug resistance is by using the drugs only when they are truly necessary. And just as doctors should prescribe drugs only when they are needed, patients should take drugs only as prescribed.

For example, the person who takes penicillin left over from a previous illness when he or she has a cold or the flu is engaging in a futile exercise. Colds and influenza are caused by viruses, and penicillin, like most antibiotics, is effective only against bacteria. But taking the antibiotics will give any penicillin-resistant bacteria present in the body an advantage over the nonresistant strains. The next time the person develops an infection that requires treatment with penicillin, it may be useless.

Ultimately, the only ones to benefit from improperly used drugs are the microbes.

□ Beverly Merz

Drugs (cont.)

if they cause heavy bleeding or *perforate* (eat through) the wall of the stomach. Although most patients tolerate NSAID's well, serious complications result in some patients.

Preventing stomach ulcers. A synthetic prostaglandin derivative—called misoprostol and marketed as Cytotec by G. D. Searle & Company of Skokie, Ill.—was introduced in early 1989 for the prevention of NSAID-induced stomach ulcers in patients at high risk of complications from a stomach ulcer. Although all patients being treated with an NSAID over a long period of time are at risk to develop ulcers, some are at greater risk—for example, smokers and people over age 60, those with a history of ulcer, and those being treated with a corticosteroid. By replacing the prostaglandins that have been depleted due to NSAID therapy, misoprostol helps protect the stomach lining. It is much more effective than previously marketed drugs in preventing NSAID-induced stomach ulcers and represents an important advance for many arthritis patients.

Misoprostol, however, may produce contractions of the uterus and must not be used by pregnant women. It also should not be used by women of childbearing age unless the patient is at high risk of NSAID-induced ulcers.

Heart and blood vessel disorders. In early 1989, nicardipine—sold as Cardene by Syntex Laboratories, Incorporated, of Palo Alto, Calif.—became the newest of a class of drugs known as *calcium antagonists*. Calcium antagonists increase the flow of blood through arteries by reducing the amount of calcium that enters muscle cells in the artery walls. This prevents spasms in the walls of the arteries, which can cause *angina* (chest pain) in the case of arteries that serve the heart, or complications leading to death or brain damage in the case of *cerebral* (brain) arteries. Nicardipine is prescribed for cardiovascular disorders, such as angina.

More noteworthy, perhaps, was

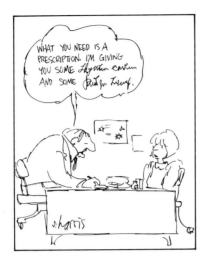

Drugs (cont.)

the marketing in 1989 of the calcium antagonist, nimodipine—sold as Nimotop by Miles Incorporated Pharmaceutical Division of West Haven, Conn. Nimodipine is unique among calcium antagonists because it has a greater effect on cerebral arteries than on other arteries.

As a result of this action, it helps combat neurological problems that occur following a *subarachnoid hemorrhage* (SAH). An SAH is bleeding into the space between the membranes that surround the brain. It is frequently caused by the bursting of a *cerebral aneurysm*, a balloonlike bulge that forms in a weakened area of a cerebral artery or vein (in the Special Reports section, see WHAT EVERYONE NEEDS TO KNOW ABOUT STROKE).

Despite improvements in surgical technique, many SAH victims die or suffer severe brain damage. Spasm of cerebral arteries often occurs following an SAH, and this accounts for many of the complications that contribute to brain damage and death. By expanding the cerebral blood vessels, nimodipine helps reduce or prevent spasm.

Because of nimodipine's effect on cerebral blood vessels, researchers have begun to investigate the drug in treating conditions such as migraine, Alzheimer's disease, and stroke-related complications. As of August 1989, however, there were insufficient data to evaluate nimodipine's potential in treating these disorders.

Allergy relief. Astemizole—marketed as Hismanal by Janssen Pharmaceutica Incorporated of Piscataway, N.J.—became available in 1989 as a new *antihistamine*, drugs used mainly for hay fever and other allergies. It is long-lasting, permitting convenient once-a-day dosing. In contrast to most other antihistamines, astemizole is unlikely to cause drowsiness. In this regard, it is similar to terfenadine, better known as Seldane, an antihistamine

Banishing baldness?
A man applies Rogaine, the only approved medication for baldness, to his scalp. In August 1988, the United States Food and Drug Administration approved Rogaine as a prescription drug. Its active ingredient is minoxidil, which has been used for treating high blood pressure. Rogaine generally requires nearly four months of treatment before hair growth can be seen and must be continued or newly grown hair will be lost.

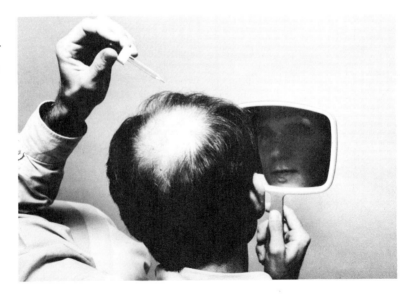

Drugs (cont.)

that has been widely prescribed since its introduction in the United States in 1985.

Astemizole provides a good example of the importance of not combining food with medications. The body's absorption of astemizole may be reduced by up to 60 per cent when it is taken with meals. Therefore, it should be taken on an empty stomach—at least two hours after or one hour before a meal.

Treating gallstones. In October 1988, Ciba Pharmaceutical Company of Summit, N.J., introduced Actigall—generic name ursodiol—a naturally occurring bile acid used for dissolving *gallstones* (pebblelike masses that form in the gall bladder or one of its ducts). Gallstones often cause pain and may require surgery, but the new drug may help patients for whom surgical removal of the stones would be risky. About 85 per cent of gallstones are composed primarily of cholesterol. Ursodial helps dissolve those stones, but does not work on those made of insoluble calcium salts.

The new drug has fewer side effects than a comparable drug, chenodiol (sold as Chenix), which causes diarrhea in many patients. The development of ursodiol represents an advance in the nonsurgical treatment of gallstones. It is not ef-

fective in all patients, however, and it is estimated that up to 50 per cent of patients whose stones are dissolved experience a recurrence of stones within five years after discontinuing therapy.

Helping hair grow. The first prescription drug for the treatment of hair loss was approved by the U.S. Food and Drug Administration on Aug. 17, 1988. The active ingredient is minoxidil, which had been used previously to treat high blood pressure. A well-recognized side effect of minoxidil prescribed for this purpose is increased hair growth. Upjohn marketed the drug (under the trade name Rogaine) in a solution applied directly to the scalp. The drug is effective in restoring hair only for those with thinning hair due to male pattern baldness, the inherited type of baldness that starts at the crown of the head.

Although the product has been ineffective in some individuals, others have experienced good results. At least four months of continuous use is generally required before new hair growth appears. The new growth of hair is not permanent and will fall out within a few months if treatment is discontinued.

□ Daniel A. Hussar

See also HEALTH POLICY; KIDNEY. In WORLD BOOK, see DRUGS.

Many children with unexplained *sensorineural hearing loss*—hearing loss caused by a defect of the inner ear or the auditory nerve—may be suffering from a condition called *perilymphatic fistula*, two research teams in the United States reported in 1989. A perilymphatic fistula is a condition in which fluid, called *perilymph*, leaks from the *cochlea* (the inner-ear structure that converts sound waves to nerve impulses) into the middle ear.

The symptoms of a perilymphatic fistula can include severe dizziness or hearing loss, or both. Those same symptoms, however, are also caused by several other ear disorders. That fact, and the absence of

any specific test for a fistula, makes the condition difficult to diagnose. In most cases, exploratory surgery is the only means of confirming that a fistula is present.

In adults, perilymphatic fistulas are usually caused by a head injury or a severe pressure change in the ear. Childhood fistulas, on the other hand, are frequently associated with anomalies of the inner ear.

A fistula can lead to total, irreversible deafness in one or both ears (in most cases, only one ear is affected). Fortunately, unlike most conditions causing sensorineural hearing loss, this disorder can be successfully treated with surgery.

Ear and Hearing

Noisy farm work

Operating tractors and other farm machinery without enclosed cabs can cause hearing loss early in life, Wisconsin researchers reported in 1989. They said farmworkers who are exposed to high levels of noise should wear ear-protection devices.

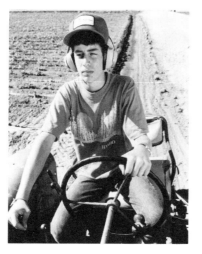

Ear and Hearing (cont.)

In February 1989, ear specialist Charles M. Myer and his colleagues at the University of Cincinnati College of Medicine in Ohio reported on a study of 26 children with sudden, fluctuating, or progressive sensorineural hearing loss. Exploratory surgery revealed that 13 of the patients—50 per cent—had perilymphatic fistulas.

The results of a much larger study were published in April by James S. Reilly, an ear specialist at the University of Alabama Medical Center in Birmingham. Reilly reported that in many cases, the abnormalities that give rise to fistulas can be de-

tected with a type of X-ray machine called a *computerized tomography* (CT) *scanner.*

Reilly and his associates studied 244 children with unexplained sensorineural hearing loss. CT scans showed probable abnormalities of the inner ear in 57 of the children. Forty-two of those patients underwent exploratory surgery, and 15 of those 42—6 per cent of the original group of 244—were found to have perilymphatic fistulas.

It thus appears that in a large group of children with sensorineural hearing loss of unknown cause, at least 6 per cent will have a perilymphatic fistula. Reilly recommended that children with sensorineural hearing loss undergo frequent hearing tests and a CT scan to look for possible deformities of the inner ear.

Farming hard on teen-agers' ears.

Teen-agers who spend much of their time operating such noisy farm machinery as tractors and combines are about twice as likely as other young people to suffer hearing loss. That finding was reported in June 1989 by investigators at the Marshfield Medical Research Foundation in Wisconsin.

The researchers tested the hearing of 872 students at 12 Wisconsin high schools. They found that 71 per cent of the students who lived on farms and operated heavy

Penicillin and amoxicillin, at $5 to $6 for a 10-day treatment, are the traditional drugs for the treatment of infections of the middle ear in children. Because some strains of bacteria have become resistant to these agents, doctors have turned to several other drugs to combat many middle-ear infections.

Alternative drugs against childhood ear infections

Drug	Effects	Price
Pediazole, a combination of two antibiotics—erythromycin and a sulfa drug	Inhibits bacteria from producing proteins and folic acid, a chemical the bacteria need in order to reproduce themselves	About $18
Cefaclor (trade name Ceclor)	Like penicillin, prevents bacteria from forming new cell walls	About $30
Septra or Bactrim, a combination of a sulfa drug and trimethoprim, a synthetic compound that enhances the action of sulfa drugs	Inhibits folic acid production by bacteria	About $12
Augmentin, a combination of amoxicillin (the most commonly prescribed form of penicillin for ear infections) and clavulanate, a compound that prevents amoxicillin's breakdown by bacteria	Prevents bacteria from forming new cell walls	About $25
Cefixime (trade name Suprax)	Prevents bacteria from forming new cell walls	About $24

Source: Children's Medical Center, Dallas.

Ear and Hearing (cont.)

equipment without protecting their ears had impaired hearing in at least one ear, compared with only 36 per cent of students who were from farming families but did not operate machinery. Earlier studies by other researchers had found hearing losses in adult farmers. Those hearing deficits, it now appears, begin in the teen years or even earlier.

Ear microphone. An extremely sensitive microphone that can be inserted into the ear to detect sounds emitted by the cochlea was introduced in early 1989 by scientists at Etymōtic Research in Elk Grove Village, Ill. The device should enable doctors to detect problems of the cochlea in patients, such as infants, who are unable to cooperate in conventional hearing tests.

The microphone picks up sounds known as *Kemp echoes.* A Kemp echo is a clicking noise made by the cochlea in response to a similar sound projected into the ear by a medical instrument. When the patient's hearing is normal, the Kemp echo has a certain pitch, but it changes when the cochlea is defective.   □ George W. Allen

In WORLD BOOK, see DEAFNESS; EAR.

A 72-year-old Pensacola, Fla., man in April 1989 became the first heart patient in the United States to receive a device that enables his doctors to defibrillate his heart over telephone lines should he have another heart attack. *Defibrillation* is a procedure that corrects *ventricular fibrillation*, the abnormal trembling of the heart that usually occurs during a heart attack. During the procedure, the patient's heart is given a jolt of electricity through special pads placed on the chest. The shock helps to restore normal heartbeat and circulation. If defibrillation is not given within a few minutes of a heart attack, brain damage or death may result.

The telephone device, called MDphone, eliminates the need for heart attack patients to wait for emergency medical personnel to arrive to perform defibrillation. The device can transmit an *electrocardiogram* (a printed record of the heart's electric currents) over telephone lines to a hospital, enabling the physician to administer an electric shock if necessary over the phone link. Since the device received approval from the United States Food and Drug Administration in 1987, three hospitals have installed the equipment,

Emergency Medicine

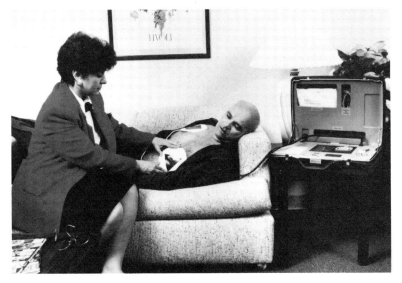

Help for heart patients
A woman places electrodes—part of a new device called MDphone—on the chest of a man suffering a heart attack. MDphone allows doctors at a nearby hospital to assess a patient's condition by telephone and, if necessary, signal the device to give electrical jolts to restore a normal heartbeat.

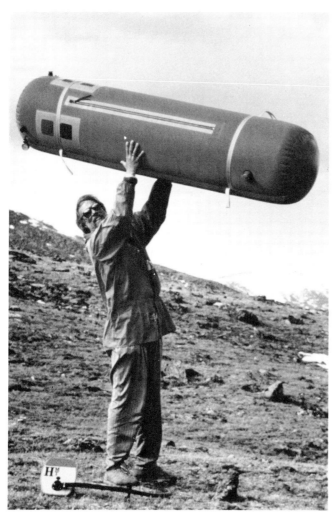

can then defibrillate the patient's heart if necessary.

Emergencies in the air. Although millions of people travel by airplane every year, little is known about the number and type of medical emergencies that occur during flights. Researchers at the University of Washington and the King County Department of Public Health, both in Seattle, published a study in March 1989 that shed light on such emergencies.

The researchers found in a year-long study of passengers arriving at the Seattle-Tacoma International Airport that the frequency of in-flight emergencies was only 1 per 39,600 inbound passengers, or 1 per 753 inbound flights. The most common complaints during flights involved motion sickness, chest pain, abdominal pain, shortness of breath, asthma attacks, and allergic reactions. Seizures and unconsciousness among people with diabetes also occurred. In many of the cases, the emergencies involved the worsening of existing illnesses.

The researchers suggested that the medical kits required on commercial jetliners should contain drugs for treating heart failure, seizures, and severe motion sickness. The medical kit currently required by the U.S. Federal Aviation Administration contains drugs for such illnesses as *angina* (chest pain that occurs when an artery is unable to carry enough blood to the heart), allergies, and diabetes. The kit is also equipped with a blood pressure cuff, stethoscope, syringes and needles, and other instruments.

The Washington researchers also recommended that flight attendants receive training similar to that given to emergency medical technicians. Although all commercial airlines provide basic first-aid training for flight attendants and other crew members, only a few teach life-support techniques.

☐ Robert D. Powers

In the People in Health Care section, see RESCUING YOUNG LIVES: INSIDE A TRAUMA CENTER. In WORLD BOOK, see HEART.

Saving climbers' lives
Igor Gamow, a scientist at the University of Colorado in Boulder, holds up a nylon bag he created to help mountain climbers suffering from *altitude sickness,* an often fatal condition caused by a lack of oxygen in the air. A climber who begins to suffer from altitude sickness climbs into the bag. It is then inflated by an air pump to simulate the oxygen-rich atmosphere found at lower altitudes.

Emergency Medicine (cont.)
which is manufactured by MEDphone Corporation of Paramus, N.J.

The MDphone consists of two separate units. One is a base unit located in a hospital; the other is a portable unit for the patient, which is contained in a briefcase. When the patient or a bystander opens the briefcase, the device automatically dials the base unit at the hospital. An alarm alerts hospital staff and a two-way speakerphone enables the physician to communicate with the person operating the portable unit. Adhesive pads wired to the portable unit are placed on the patient's chest, transmitting the electrocardiogram to the hospital. The physician

Vietnam veterans won two major legal challenges in 1989 aimed at securing compensation for illnesses and deaths they claimed were caused by exposure to the defoliant Agent Orange. During the Vietnam War (1957-1975), thousands of soldiers in Southeast Asia were exposed to Agent Orange, which contains an extremely poisonous chemical called dioxin. Veterans have contended that exposure to the defoliant caused cancer in themselves and birth defects and cancer in their offspring years after the war ceased.

Because of the settlement of an 11-year-old class-action lawsuit, approximately 30,000 veterans and 18,000 families of veterans who have died became eligible to receive awards of up to $12,800 from the manufacturers of Agent Orange. Veterans and their children who subsequently develop illnesses thought to be related to Agent Orange exposure will be allowed to apply for compensation benefits until Dec. 31, 1994.

Vietnam veterans won a second legal victory on May 8, 1989, when federal Judge Thelton Henderson rejected Veterans Administration (VA) rules for accepting medical claims based on exposure to Agent Orange, saying that the VA had failed to give veterans "the benefit of the doubt." The judge ordered the VA to reevaluate thousands of applications that had been rejected. He found that the VA had improperly required veterans to prove that there was a cause-and-effect relationship between their exposure to Agent Orange and their subsequent illnesses.

The veterans had argued successfully that the United States Congress, by enacting a 1984 federal statute, wanted to help veterans receive compensation and therefore required only that they prove that Agent Orange increased the risk of contracting certain illnesses rather than require conclusive proof of a cause-and-effect relationship. Henderson noted that, when awarding benefits to veterans for other injuries, the VA had accepted the same type of statistical evidence offered in the disputed Agent Orange claims. After the ruling, the VA announced that it would not appeal the decision and would reconsider more than 30,000 claims.

Radon update. The U.S. Public Health Service in September 1988 recommended that most U.S. homes be tested for the presence of radon, a naturally occurring radioactive gas that may seep out of some types of soil and enter indoor spaces. Chronic exposure to this odorless and colorless gas may cause up to 20,000 deaths from

Environmental Health

Radon detection
A worker analyzes the air in a Pennsylvania home for the presence of radon, a naturally occurring radioactive gas whose cancer-causing potential worried many health experts in 1988 and 1989.

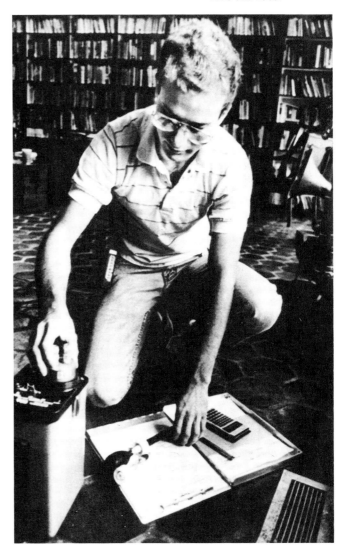

Potential health hazards at nuclear weapons plants

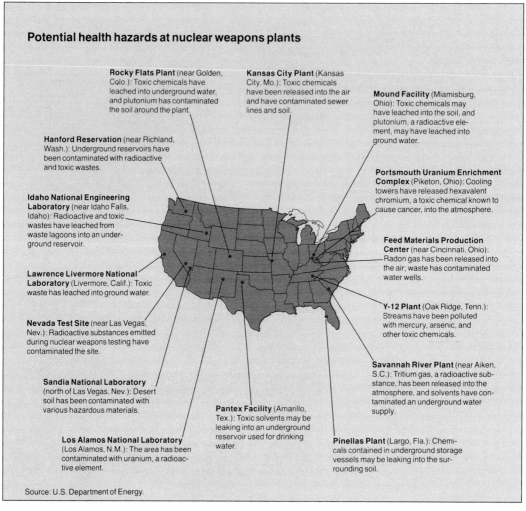

Rocky Flats Plant (near Golden, Colo.): Toxic chemicals have leached into underground water, and plutonium has contaminated the soil around the plant.

Kansas City Plant (Kansas City, Mo.): Toxic chemicals have been released into the air and have contaminated sewer lines and soil.

Mound Facility (Miamisburg, Ohio): Toxic chemicals may have leached into the soil, and plutonium, a radioactive element, may have leached into ground water.

Hanford Reservation (near Richland, Wash.): Underground reservoirs have been contaminated with radioactive and toxic wastes.

Portsmouth Uranium Enrichment Complex (Piketon, Ohio): Cooling towers have released hexavalent chromium, a toxic chemical known to cause cancer, into the atmosphere.

Idaho National Engineering Laboratory (near Idaho Falls, Idaho): Radioactive and toxic wastes have leached from waste lagoons into an underground reservoir.

Feed Materials Production Center (near Cincinnati, Ohio): Radon gas has been released into the air; waste has contaminated water wells.

Lawrence Livermore National Laboratory (Livermore, Calif.): Toxic waste has leached into ground water.

Y-12 Plant (Oak Ridge, Tenn.): Streams have been polluted with mercury, arsenic, and other toxic chemicals.

Nevada Test Site (near Las Vegas, Nev.): Radioactive substances emitted during nuclear weapons testing have contaminated the site.

Savannah River Plant (near Aiken, S.C.): Tritium gas, a radioactive substance, has been released into the atmosphere, and solvents have contaminated an underground water supply.

Sandia National Laboratory (north of Las Vegas, Nev.): Desert soil has been contaminated with various hazardous materials.

Pantex Facility (Amarillo, Tex.): Toxic solvents may be leaking into an underground reservoir used for drinking water.

Los Alamos National Laboratory (Los Alamos, N.M.): The area has been contaminated with uranium, a radioactive element.

Pinellas Plant (Largo, Fla.): Chemicals contained in underground storage vessels may be leaking into the surrounding soil.

Source: U.S. Department of Energy.

Nuclear weapons plants and laboratories at various sites in the United States have contaminated the environment, according to a preliminary report released in December 1988 by the U.S. Department of Energy. Whether the contamination poses significant hazards to health is unknown. Cleanup is expected to cost $66 billion to $110 billion.

Environmental Health (cont.)
lung cancer in the United States each year. In April 1989, the EPA urged school systems to test their classrooms for radon contamination after a survey of 3,000 classrooms in 16 states found unsafe radon levels in more than half of the rooms.

Polluted air around the globe. Air pollution has become an international health problem, according to a 1988 report issued by the United Nations World Health Organization (WHO) and Environment Program. The WHO compared the levels of five airborne contaminants—suspended particles (dust and smoke), carbon monoxide, sulfur dioxide, lead, and nitrogen dioxide—in sev-

eral of the world's largest cities. These measurements indicated that two-thirds of the world's city dwellers are exposed to air-pollution levels that exceed health standards. The problem has worsened as population, industrialization, and traffic congestion have increased.

The cities whose air was most polluted with sulfur dioxide (a poisonous by-product of the combustion of coal and oil) are Milan, Italy; Seoul, South Korea; and Rio de Janeiro, Brazil. Milan's air-pollution levels of sulfur dioxide were three times higher than the level deemed acceptable by WHO. This dramatically high level is linked to the fact that Milan is situated in a river val-

Environmental Health (cont.)
ley, which traps polluted air.

The dustiest and smokiest cities of those measured were Kuwait, Kuwait; New Delhi, India; and Beijing. In Kuwait, the levels of these particles were eight times higher than the WHO guidelines. In Beijing, the level was five times higher. By comparison, the amount of dust and smoke in Chicago and New York City was at or only slightly exceeding the WHO guideline. The report noted that the highest levels were generally found in areas plagued by windblown dust. Dust, however, is not as serious a health threat as the fine smoke particles that are the by-products of coal combustion and some industrial processes.

Carbon monoxide pollution is a serious problem in Paris: Parisians breathe more than three times the amount judged acceptable by the WHO. An extremely poisonous gas, carbon monoxide, which is produced by automobile engines, can be lethal, particularly at high altitudes or in confined spaces.

Paris also topped the list in airborne lead pollution, which is linked to the fact that gasoline sold in France contains lead. In countries where leaded gasoline is restricted, such as Japan and the United States, the levels of lead in the air did not exceed the WHO standards.

The three cleanest cities studied were Vancouver, Canada; Copenhagen, Denmark; and Melbourne, Australia. Despite their reputations for being severely polluted, New York City, Tokyo, and London were ranked in the middle of the cities studied.

The report blamed unplanned urban growth for most air pollution and cited motor vehicles, energy consumption, and industrial activity as the major causes of this form of pollution. The report also found that although industrialized nations were attempting to curb air pollution, undeveloped nations were sacrificing air quality in their drive to become more industrialized.

Asbestos banned. On July 6, 1989, the U.S. Environmental Protection Agency (EPA) imposed a gradual ban on the manufacture, use, and export of most products made of asbestos. Asbestos, any of a group of fiberlike minerals useful for their heat-resistant properties, is a known health hazard that causes about 10,000 deaths in the United States every year. The first phase of the ban is scheduled to take effect in August 1990, and the last in 1996.

□ Laura M. Lake

In the Special Reports section, see LEAD'S HIDDEN DANGERS. In WORLD BOOK, see AGENT ORANGE; AIR POLLUTION; ENVIRONMENTAL POLLUTION.

In some cases of mild *hypertension* (high blood pressure), exercise alone may be sufficient to control the condition, eliminating the need for drug therapy, according to the findings of two separate studies. The results of the studies were reported in April 1989 at a meeting of the American College of Cardiology in Anaheim, Calif.

The larger of the two studies, led by cardiologist John Kostis of the University of Medicine and Dentistry of New Jersey in Newark, involved 86 men with an average age of 57 years. The study participants had *diastolic blood pressure* readings ranging from 95 to 105. Diastolic blood pressure is the pressure in the artery when the heart relaxes between beats. "Mild hypertension" is classified as a diastolic pressure ranging from 90 to 104.

The study participants were divided randomly into two groups. One group exercised at least three times a week; went on a diet that lowered their intake of salt, fat, and alcohol; and attended weekly sessions on how to manage stress in their lives. The other group received either propranolol, a drug used to treat hypertension, or a *placebo* (an inactive substance). Those who received the placebo were later switched to propranolol; those who received propranolol were later

Exercise and Fitness

Low-Impact Exercise: Easier on the Body?

Until recently, the slogan of the fitness buff was "no pain, no gain." Many people of all ages and levels of physical fitness pushed their bodies to the limit. But in their zeal to become fit, many dedicated exercise buffs found themselves sidelined with injuries.

Certain factors increase the chance of injury, such as previous injuries or beginning to exercise after a period of inactivity. The risk of injury appears to be proportional to the increase in activity.

Experts also noted, however, that many injuries stemmed from "high-impact" activities such as jogging, in which the repetitive impact of the exercise places stress on joints, muscles, and other tissues. When aerobic dance classes became popular, for example, some participants began turning up in doctors' offices with similar injuries; a 1985 study found that participants in aerobic dance classes began to show the same kind of injuries found in marathon runners.

The toll of injuries has prompted people to look for better alternatives. Many have turned to moderate or "low-impact" exercise.

Health experts generally recommend low-impact exercises as appropriate for the unfit person as well as for the physically fit who want to avoid strenuous exercise or who want to gradually increase the amount of exercise they are doing. These activities have few jarring or bouncing movements, because one foot is usually kept on the ground at all times. As a result, they put less stress on the legs, joints, and spine than do many other types of exercise.

A variety of activities can be classified as low-impact exercise. Fitness walking—brisk walking at speeds of 3½ to 5 miles (5.6 to 8 kilometers) per hour—is a low-impact exercise. So are cross-country skiing, swimming, and cycling. These activities involve gliding or pumping movements that are easy on the joints and muscles.

An increasingly popular activity is low-impact aerobics. Instead of the jumping and running that occur in high-impact aerobics, low-impact aerobics involve low kicks, high steps, side-to-side lunges, and large upper-body movements.

Does low-impact exercise actually reduce the rate of injury? According to epidemiologist Steve Blair of the Institute for Aerobics Research in Dallas, there are few statistics on injuries, and so it's not clear whether low-impact exercise actually is less likely to cause injuries than high-impact activities. But many health experts believe it's reasonable to assume that low-impact sports are a sensible alternative, especially for sedentary people.

Low-impact exercise can provide most of the same health benefits—such as strengthening the cardiovascular system by regularly increasing one's heart rate—that come from high-impact activities. In fitness walking and low-impact aerobics, strong upper body movements can push up the heart rate.

Like all physical activities, low-impact exercises can cause muscle soreness and injuries unless they are done properly. The nature of such injuries is not yet clear. But no matter what form of activity you choose, health experts stress the importance of consulting a physician before starting any exercise program.

□ James Skinner

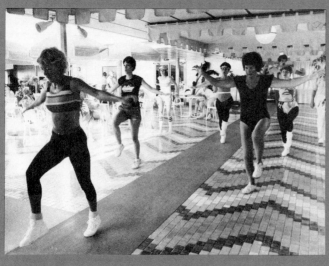

A low-impact exercise class stresses low kicks and arm swings.

Exercise and Fitness (cont.)

switched to the placebo. This group received no counseling regarding exercise, diet, or stress.

At the end of the six-month study, the researchers found that the group that exercised and received no drugs had an average blood pressure reduction of almost 13, compared with 8 for those who received propranolol and 4.5 for those who received a placebo for the last three months of the study.

The second study, conducted by rehabilitation specialist Kerry Stewart of Johns Hopkins University in Baltimore, compared men who exercised and took drugs for hypertension with those who only exercised. This study found that the combination of drug therapy and exercise did not control blood pressure any better than exercise alone.

The Johns Hopkins study involved 52 men between the ages of 25 and 59 who had diastolic pressures ranging from 90 to 105. The study participants were divided randomly into three groups. One group received a placebo, the second received propranolol, and the third received diltiazem, another drug used to treat hypertension. All three groups took part in a 10-week exercise program.

At the end of the study, the 19 patients who took the placebo had an average *systolic pressure* (the pressure in the arteries when the heart contracts) of 131 and an average diastolic pressure of 89. (Blood pressure readings are expressed by giving the systolic pressure over the diastolic pressure, so the average blood pressure of the placebo group was 131 over 89, or 131/89.) This compared with 138/88 for the 17 on diltiazem and 132/88 for the 16 who received propranolol.

Stewart concluded that in some cases of mild hypertension, exercise alone may be sufficient to control blood pressure. In other cases, exercise may enable some people with mild hypertension to lower the dosage of their medication.

Exercise reduces fats. Exercise alone can reduce levels of fat in the blood and may thus help prevent heart disease, according to the results of a study reported in May 1989 by researchers at the Rockefeller University in New York City and Adelphi University in Garden City, N.Y. The study suggested that those who have trouble losing weight still benefit from exercise.

The study demonstrated that men who exercised but who maintained constant body weight still had reduced levels of *triglycerides* (fat molecules) and *lipoproteins* (substances that are part fat and part protein) in their blood. Six men be-

Americans have been shifting away from such high-intensity activities as running and aerobics, according to an annual survey by the National Sporting Goods Association. Participation in those sports peaked in 1984 and subsequently leveled off or declined. The only sports to show an increase in participation are walking, bicycling, and golf.

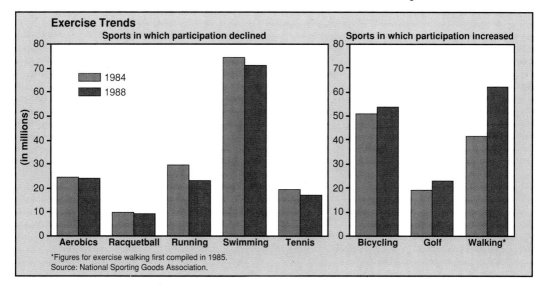

Exercise Trends

Sports in which participation declined — 1984, 1988 (in millions): Aerobics, Racquetball, Running, Swimming, Tennis

Sports in which participation increased: Bicycling, Golf, Walking*

*Figures for exercise walking first compiled in 1985.
Source: National Sporting Goods Association.

Sports appropriate for teen-agers with medical problems

Type of sport

Contact	Limited contact	Noncontact and strenuous	Noncontact and nonstrenuous
Football	Baseball	Aerobics	Archery
Ice hockey	Basketball	Running	Golf
Martial arts	Bicycling	Swimming	
Soccer	Gymnastics	Tennis	
Wrestling	Horseback riding	Track	
	Skating	Weightlifting	
	Skiing		
	Softball		
	Volleyball		

Recommendations for participating in sports

Medical condition	Contact	Limited contact	Noncontact and strenuous	Noncontact and nonstrenuous
Hypertension				
mild	Yes	Yes	Yes	Yes
moderate	*	*	*	*
severe	*	*	*	*
Inguinal hernia	Yes	Yes	Yes	Yes
Missing kidney	No	Yes	Yes	Yes
Neurologic				
History of trauma to head or spine, frequent concussions	*	*	Yes	Yes
Convulsive disorder—				
Well controlled	Yes	Yes	Yes	Yes
Poorly controlled	No	No	Yes†	Yes††
Missing ovary	Yes	Yes	Yes	Yes
Asthma	Yes	Yes	Yes	Yes
Sickle cell trait	Yes	Yes	Yes	Yes
Enlarged spleen	No	No	No	Yes
Missing or undescended testicle	Yes**	Yes**	Yes	Yes

*Requires individual assessment   †No swimming or weightlifting   **Requires protective cup   ††No archery

Source: The American Academy of Pediatrics Committee on Sports Medicine.

Every adolescent should undergo a complete physical examination before participating in sports, because certain activities should be ruled out for people with various health problems.

Exercise and Fitness (cont.)
tween the ages of 22 and 33 with normal levels of fat in their blood were put on a seven-week exercise program. The program consisted of running on a treadmill for an average of 15 miles (24 kilometers) a week. The calorie intake of the study participants was increased so that they maintained their original body weight during the study.

Blood samples were taken after meals. One group of lipoproteins, *very low-density lipoproteins* (*VLDL's*), were measured, because people with high levels of VLDL's in their blood are at risk for heart disease. The researchers found that although the men in the exercise program ate more to maintain their

original body weight, they were able to lower the amount of fat in their bloodstream. VLDL levels were 32 per cent lower than prior to the exercise program.

Weight loss key. Weight loss appears to be effective in raising levels of high-density lipoproteins (HDL's)—the so-called good cholesterol that helps lower the risk of heart disease, according to a study reported in November 1988 by researchers at Stanford University in Stanford, Calif.

The study involved 155 overweight men. They were divided into three groups—a group that went on a diet to lose weight, a

Exercise and Fitness (cont.)
group that exercised to lose weight, and a third group that followed their usual habits of eating and exercising. At the end of the yearlong study, the diet group had lost an average of about 16 pounds (7 kilograms) per person, the exercise group had lost an average of about 9 pounds (4 kilograms) per person, and the control group that neither dieted nor exercised maintained a constant weight average. Both the dieters and the exercisers raised their HDL levels by about 7 per cent, while HDL levels remained unchanged for the control group.

The study focused on HDL's be-cause people with high levels of HDL have a lower risk of heart disease. The HDL's help remove cholesterol from cells so that it can be taken out of the blood by the liver.

The researchers concluded that losing weight—either by dieting or exercising—raises HDL levels. Exercise in itself, however, may not boost HDL levels unless it contributes to weight loss.

☐ Rod Such

In the Special Reports section, see Steroid Abuse: Turning Winners into Losers. In World Book, see Physical fitness.

Several studies reported in 1988 and 1989 indicated that users of contact lenses, especially those who wear or care for their lenses improperly, have a greater risk of eye damage and vision impairment than previously thought.

Hard news for soft-lens users. In September 1988, the preliminary results of the largest study to date of contact lens use were reported by the United States Food and Drug Administration (FDA). The results were from a survey of 22,584 people who wore various types of contact lenses, including hard and soft contact lenses that must be removed and cleaned daily, and extended-wear soft contact lenses that were designed to be removed and cleaned as infrequently as once every 30 days.

The aim of the study, conducted by researchers from Harvard Medical School in Boston, was to determine which type of lens was responsible for *corneal ulcers*—patches of dead tissue on the cornea, the eye's transparent outer covering, that can result from infection with microorganisms. Such organisms can be transmitted to the eye by contaminated contact

Eye and Vision

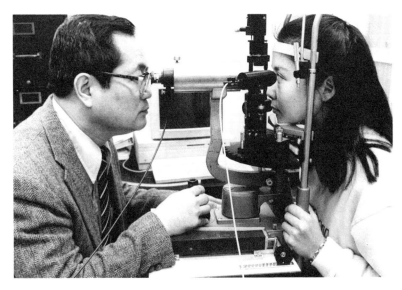

Early cataract detection
Chemist Nai-Teng Yu of the Georgia Institute of Technology in Atlanta uses a low-intensity laser he helped develop to determine if an eye patient is prone to *cataracts* (clouding of the lens). Cataracts often develop to an advanced stage before being detected. Because the sensitive laser can detect the proteins that eventually form cataracts, the experimental technique may help physicians in early detection.

Eye and Vision (cont.)

lenses. Corneal ulcers can lead to severe loss of vision.

The researchers found the lowest rate—1 case in 2,000 people annually—among users of daily-wear lenses, both hard and soft. There was 1 case of corneal ulcers a year in every 500 people who used extended-wear lenses. People with extended-wear contact lenses who had undergone surgery to remove the lens of the eye had the highest rate of corneal ulcers—1 case for every 200 people each year. (The lens is a transparent structure of the eye that helps focus light.)

The annual rate of other serious reactions, such as scratching the cornea when inserting the lens, followed a similar pattern, the researchers found. It was 1 in 300 among users of daily-wear lenses, 1 in 100 among users of extended-wear lenses, and 1 in 50 among users of extended-wear lenses who had lens-removal surgery.

Extended-wear retraction. In May 1989, the FDA requested manufacturers of extended-wear soft contact lenses to change package labels to reflect a reduction in maximum wearing time from 30 days to 7 days. The FDA also required manufacturers to strengthen warnings that wearing the lenses could lead to *ulcerative keratitis*—an inflammation that produces corneal ulcers.

Ulcerative keratitis is the result of infection by microorganisms. Because soft contact lenses absorb large amounts of water, they can become reservoirs of such infectious organisms if they are not properly disinfected.

The FDA request was based on data from the same survey used in the corneal ulcer study. According to the results of the study, an estimated 21 people in every 10,000 with extended-wear contact lenses develop ulcerative keratitis each year, while only 4 of every 10,000 with daily-wear lenses do so. Thus, the researchers computed the overall risk of ulcerative keratitis to be 4 to 5 times greater for people with extended-wear lenses.

The researchers determined, however, that the risk of ulcerative keratitis could be reduced by properly cleaning and rinsing the lenses and the lens case. On the basis of that determination, the FDA decided not to prohibit the sale of extended-wear soft lenses but to reduce the recommended wearing time and continue to monitor contact lens users for the occurrence of ulcerative keratitis.

Homemade solutions. Because many infections related to the use of contact lenses result from inadequate lens sterilization, the FDA in

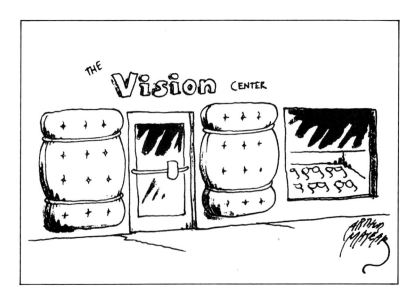

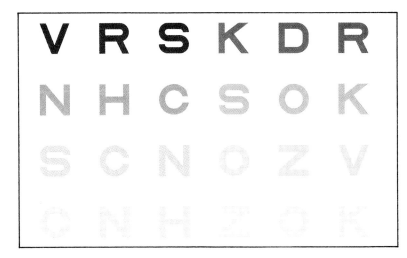

New eye chart
A new eye chart designed to measure the eye's sensitivity to contrasts was introduced in 1988. Known as the Pelli-Robson chart, it consists of letters the same in size but with declining contrast. This type of test promises to detect some visual disorders, such as glaucoma and diabetic retinopathy, at an early stage. Such disorders often are not detected by the use of standard eye charts, which have rows of letters that decline in size.

Eye and Vision (cont.)

February 1989 sent letters to about 50,000 eye-care specialists asking them to warn patients against using homemade salt solutions to rinse or soak contact lenses. The homemade solutions are generally made by dissolving salt tablets in distilled unsterilized water.

The FDA warned that the water in such homemade solutions may be contaminated with bacteria and *acanthamoeba*, a single-celled organism. Acanthamoeba infection is still relatively rare in the United States but its incidence has been increasing within the last five years. It is difficult to eradicate once it has invaded the eye, often producing extensive corneal scarring and resulting in blindness.

Colored contact lenses. People who wear certain tinted contact lenses to alter their eye color may look better but they often see worse, according to a study reported in December 1988. After some patients fitted with a particular type of colored lens complained of hazy peripheral vision, researchers at Tulane University of Louisiana and Louisiana State University Medical Center, both in New Orleans, tested the effects of wearing that type of lens on 10 women with normal vision. To eliminate vision defects as a source of the complaints, the researchers chose women with normal vision. The lens that was tested is colored by applying tiny opaque blue, green, or aqua dots on the surface. The lens also has a transparent central section, which is designed to fit over the *pupil*, the circular opening of the eye through which light passes to the lens.

The researchers administered the Goldmann Visual Field test, a standard assessment of the scope of vision, to the 10 women. They found that the *visual fields* of 9 of the women decreased from 21 per cent to 47 per cent when the women were wearing the lenses. (Visual field is the area in front of the eye in which an object can be seen without moving the eye.) The 10th woman had no change in visual field with the lenses.

The researchers concluded that in some cases, the clear zone of the lens was too small to accommodate the wearer's pupil, and that in others it was not centered over the pupil. They advised contact lens specialists to fit that type of tinted lens so that the clear zone is directly over the pupil.

Sun exposure and cataracts. In December 1988, researchers from Johns Hopkins University in Baltimore reported evidence for a strong link between exposure to sunlight and the formation of *cataracts*—opaque regions on the lens of the eye that can impair vision.

Eye and Vision (cont.)

Earlier studies had indicated that people who live in regions where sunlight is more intense tend to develop cataracts at a faster rate than people who live in cloudier regions. Some studies had indicated that cataract development is closely related to exposure to a component of sunlight known as *ultraviolet-B radiation*. In contrast to ultraviolet-A radiation, which passes through the lens of the eye, most ultraviolet-B radiation is absorbed by the eye. The Johns Hopkins team wanted to determine to what extent exposure to ultraviolet-B radiation increases the chances of developing the three most common types of cataracts. These are nuclear cataracts, in the back two-thirds of the lens; subcapsular, at the base of the lens; and cortical, located on the front third of the lens.

To do so, they studied 838 men over age 30 who had worked on boats on nearby Chesapeake Bay. Each man was asked to estimate the number of hours he had spent in the sun since age 15 and to answer detailed questions about his use of sunglasses and protective hats, which screen out ultraviolet-B radiation. The researchers used the data to calculate each man's cumulative ultraviolet-B exposure. They excluded from the study 2 men who had been born with cataracts and

12 men who had lens damage resulting from a blow or wounds. The examinations revealed that 111 men had cortical cataracts, 229 had nuclear cataracts, and 14 had subcapsular cataracts.

When the researchers compared the development of the three types of cataracts with the amount of exposure to ultraviolet light, they found no association between ultraviolet-B exposure and the development of nuclear and subcapsular cataracts. They did find, however, a greater than threefold increase in the number of cortical cataracts among men who had the highest exposure to ultraviolet-B radiation. Moreover, the average annual exposure to ultraviolet-B was 21 per cent higher in men who had some type of cataract than in men with normal lenses.

The Johns Hopkins team concluded that, although other factors such as the normal aging process contribute to the development of cortical cataracts, exposure to ultraviolet-B also plays a role. They recommended several measures to minimize ultraviolet-B exposure, among them avoiding the sun from 10 a.m. to 2 p.m., when ultraviolet-B radiation is the strongest; using glasses with ultraviolet-B absorbing lenses; and wearing a hat with a brim.   □ Beverly Merz

In WORLD BOOK, see EYE.

Financing Medical Care

The push for health coverage of uninsured people became more intense in the United States in 1988 and 1989. In 1989, Senator Edward M. Kennedy (D., Mass.) reintroduced legislation to require employers to provide medical coverage to most workers, along with creation of a new program to cover the uninsured unemployed. The Senate Labor and Human Resources Committee approved the Kennedy bill.

Other proposals for universal health coverage were introduced by various groups, including national commissions and physicians' groups. With public opinion polls showing a majority of Americans favoring workplace-based insur-

ance, legislation mandating employee coverage appeared to be the most politically attractive solution, though small employers promised an all-out fight against it.

Some states did not wait for the federal government to act. Massachusetts' plan for universal coverage was bogged down by funding shortfalls and political opposition, but Hawaii passed and funded universal coverage for its residents. Bills proposing some form of broad or universal coverage were introduced in most state legislatures.

A growing sense of urgency on the issue was spurred by release in November 1988 of the federal gov-

Financing Medical Care (cont.)
ernment's National Medical Expenditures Survey, which found a 38 per cent rise in the number of uninsured since 1977, to 37 million. Also, a poll published in March 1989 found that 61 per cent of Americans preferred a Canadian-style, government-funded health care system over their own.

"Catastrophic costs" coverage.
On Jan. 1, 1989, the first phase of Medicare "catastrophic" coverage began in the United States, following passage of major federal legislation in 1988. The legislation, designed to protect 33 million elderly and disabled Medicare participants, was intended to address the problem of huge medical bills for extensive care that can leave many senior citizens without savings.

The new law gives Medicare participants unlimited hospital benefits for the year after the patient makes an initial payment. This annual deductible, which was $560 in 1989, will rise each year with inflation. Starting in 1990, the new law will phase in assistance in paying for prescription drugs. It places a $1,370 ceiling on out-of-pocket payment for doctor services.

These services are funded by increased payments by the beneficiaries. For most Medicare clients, the cost is expected to be modest, perhaps an additional $125 per year by 1993. But for about 1.6 million beneficiaries—those with enough income to pay income tax—a surcharge of up to $800 a year is being assessed beginning in 1989, rising to $1,050 in 1993.

Many beneficiaries launched a vigorous protest against the increased payments. Support for their protests came from a Congressional Budget Office study that claimed more money would be collected than was needed. Administrators of the Medicare program countered by claiming that the prescription drug program would be underfunded without the higher payments. Senator Lloyd M. Bentsen, Jr. (D., Tex.) sought to reduce the maximum payment, but President Bush threatened to veto any legislation containing such a provision.

New payment plan. Another controversy erupted over Medicare's desire to trim payments to physicians. One idea for a new payment system known as the *relative value scale* (RVS) was proposed separately by medical economist William Hsiao of Harvard University in Cambridge, Mass., and by the Physician Payment Review Commission (PPRC), a panel formed to study Medicare physician payment.

The two RVS proposals attempt to revalue various medical services.

Surcharge* for Medicare's catastrophic care plan
(per single beneficiary)

Annual income	Annual surcharge	
	1989	1993
$ 5,000-15,000	$ 0.0	$ 0.0
15,000-20,000	78.12	116.52
20,000-25,000	197.88	250.56
25,000-30,000	306.96	401.28
30,000-35,000	370.68	702.00
35,000-40,000	678.36	1,021.68
40,000-45,000	800.00†	1,050.00†

*In addition to a basic premium
†Maximum surcharge

Source: Joint Committee on Taxation.

A new law intended to protect 33 million elderly and disabled Medicare participants from "catastrophic costs" for long-term care went into effect on Jan. 1, 1989. The additional services provided by the plan will be funded by increased payments by the beneficiaries, in the form of a surcharge. The amount of the surcharge, which is linked to the income of the beneficiary, will cost up to $800 in 1989, rising to $1,050 in 1993.

Food

See Nutrition and Food

Financing Medical Care (cont.)

Traditionally, Medicare payments have been based on guidelines that favored *procedures* (such as surgery) over *cognitive care* (such as counseling patients); thus, payments to procedure-oriented physicians have been many times higher than those to other physicians. The RVS plans seek to integrate physicians' time, mental effort and judgment, technical skill, physical effort, and psychological stress into a new scale that revalues various treatments. The results will likely increase the pay of cognitive specialists and reduce surgeons' pay.

The American College of Surgeons opposed the RVS approach and sought a special surgical pay scale. Internal medicine groups supported the RVS. The American Medical Association, a broad-scale organization of doctors, finally voiced support for a modified RVS. In June 1989, the Ways and Means Committee of the U.S. House of Representatives voted to approve use of the scheme beginning in October 1991, and congressional passage seemed a possibility in 1989.

The committee, however, also tied use of an RVS to a plan that would set a maximum for total Medicare payments to physicians, beginning in 1989. If that total were exceeded, the next year's payments to physicians would be cut.

Accounting change. In February 1989, the Financial Accounting Standards Board, a group of professional accountants that dictates accounting rules for businesses, made a decision that many businesses had feared. It announced its intention to require businesses to list unfunded health benefits for retirees as liabilities, rather than as assets. With estimates of such unfunded benefits ranging as high as $400-billion, the announcement set off a storm of protest from beleaguered employers. Many companies offer medical benefits for retirees until they qualify for Medicare or for as long as they live. In many cases, the companies do not have the total reserves necessary to fund these benefits. Under the new procedures, businesses will either have to fund the benefits or list them as unfunded liabilities on their balance sheets.

The new requirements outlined the underlying problem of health care financing: the shrinking number of U.S. residents and firms that can afford health care or health insurance coverage without some form of help.

□ Emily Ann Friedman

In WORLD BOOK, see MEDICAID; MEDICARE.

Genetics

Scientists at the National Institutes of Health (NIH) in Bethesda, Md., opened a new chapter in medical genetics in May 1989 with the insertion of a foreign (nonhuman) gene into human cancer patients. The experiment, designed to enable cancer-killing cells to be tracked in the patients' bodies, was conducted after months of investigation into the safety and ethics of the technique. The gene-insertion procedure is not a form of *gene therapy*, which would involve replacing defective genes in cells with functional ones, but it is a step toward that goal.

The researchers, under the direction of molecular biologists Steven A. Rosenberg, R. Michael Blase,

and W. French Anderson, first extracted cancer-fighting cells called *tumor infiltrating lymphocytes* (TIL's) from patients with advanced cases of cancer. The TIL's were then grown in laboratory cultures rich in *interleukin-2* (IL-2), an immune-system substance that stimulates certain white blood cells and increases their disease-fighting ability.

Before administering the TIL's to the patients, the scientists inserted into the cells copies of a gene, taken from a bacterium, that made the cells resistant to the antibiotic neomycin. A harmless virus carried the gene into the cells.

Genetics (cont.)

The transferred gene will help the investigators track the TIL cells as they move through the bodies of the patients. The TIL cells that are removed from the subjects will be exposed to neomycin; if the cells survive, the scientists will know they contain the foreign gene. In this way, the scientists will be able to tell where the TIL's that were treated with IL-2 end up in the body. The objective is to learn why this therapy works with some cancer patients but not with others.

The use of viruses to carry genes into human cells is likely to become a standard technique in medicine. In most cases, this probably will be done as part of gene therapy. The successful transfer of the bacterial gene into TIL's was an important step toward that goal.

Cystic fibrosis gene found. The discovery of the gene responsible for cystic fibrosis was reported in August 1989 by researchers at the University of Michigan in Ann Arbor and the Hospital for Sick Children in Toronto, Canada. Cystic fibrosis is one of the most common and deadly of all genetic diseases.

About 30,000 children and young people in the United States have cystic fibrosis. Some 12 million Americans carry the cystic fibrosis gene, which is a faulty version of a gene that is vital to the normal functioning of the lungs and pancreas. Only people who inherit two copies of the faulty gene—one from each parent—develop the disorder.

The disease causes a build-up of thick mucus in the lungs and pancreas and is invariably fatal. Patients, who rarely live past their 20's, usually die of lung infections.

Geneticists said cystic fibrosis may now be a candidate for gene therapy. They said it might prove possible, using a virus carrier, to insert normal copies of the gene into the lung and pancreas tissue of cystic fibrosis patients, thereby overcoming the harmful effects of the faulty gene.

The genetics of schizophrenia.
Among other disorders that may

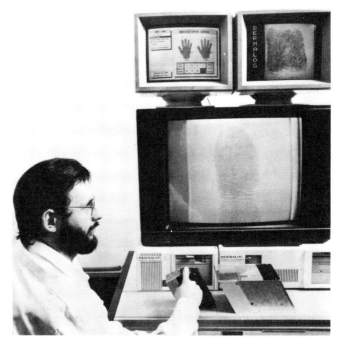

one day be treated by gene therapy is schizophrenia, a serious form of mental illness that apparently has a genetic basis. In November 1988, researchers in Great Britain and the United States reported conflicting data that indicate how complex the genetics of schizophrenia may be.

Although schizophrenia takes a number of forms, it typically is characterized by delusions, hallucinations, and general disorientation. The disorder is known to run in families, and biologists have long suspected one or more abnormal genes are involved.

The British research team, led by psychiatrist Robin Sherrington at the University of London, studied the *deoxyribonucleic acid* (DNA)—the molecule genes are made of—from 104 members of seven families from Iceland and England. The families all had a history of schizophrenia. The researchers found that many of the family members had an identical segment of DNA on chromosome 5. Chromosomes are threadlike structures in the cell nucleus that carry the genes.

In the United States, a research

Fingerprint forecasts
Gunther Müll, founder of the Institute for Dermatoglypics in Hamburg, West Germany, examines an enlargement of a fingerprint, which will be analyzed by computer for certain telltale characteristics that indicate whether a couple has an increased risk of having a baby with one of 10 genetic disorders, including Down's syndrome.

Close-up of DNA
The first detailed image of unaltered deoxyribonucleic acid (DNA), the molecule of heredity, was released in January 1989 by scientists at Lawrence Berkeley Laboratory and Lawrence Livermore National Laboratory, both in California. The picture was made with an instrument called the scanning tunneling microscope, which can distinguish individual atoms.

Genetics (cont.)

group at the Yale University School of Medicine in New Haven, Conn., reported a contrary finding in a study of 157 members of a large Swedish family with a history of schizophrenia. The scientists, under the direction of geneticist Kenneth Kidd, found no evidence that the family members had a DNA segment in common on chromosome 5.

The contradictory findings of the two research groups indicate that schizophrenia is caused by different genes in different families. If so, that would not be surprising; earlier in the 1980's, molecular biologists discovered that several, varying genes

are involved in manic depression, another common form of mental illness. Biologists also believe that there may be nongenetic forms of schizophrenia.

Work continues on the families studied by Sherrington and Kidd. The disorder is so complex, however, that it likely will take years to determine how genetic and environmental factors interact to cause it.

The human genome project. The genes involved in schizophrenia are buried in a staggering amount of genetic material, including as many as 100,000 genes and many more DNA segments of unknown function. Taken together, this genetic information is called the *human genome*. In late 1988, the American scientific establishment began an ambitious project to identify all human genes and determine the complete *sequence*—the order of some 3 billion DNA subunits called *bases*—of the genome. The huge endeavor, which may take 15 years, is expected to shed new light on genetic disorders, the regulation of growth and development, and the evolutionary history of the human species.

The early phases of the genome project will concentrate on devising new technologies to speed up the sequencing process and on developing a detailed map—that is, pinpointing the precise locations on the chromosomes of all genes—of the human genome. Up to now, only about 1,500 human genes have been mapped to specific chromosomes or regions of chromosomes; the sequence of bases of about 600 other genes has been determined.

Many of the genes that have been mapped are associated with genetic disorders, including Huntington's disease, cystic fibrosis, and muscular dystrophy. Because of the massive amount of genetic material in the genome and the large number of bases separating the genes that have been mapped, there are many large gaps in current maps.

The safety of prenatal diagnosis. In March 1989, the medical genet-

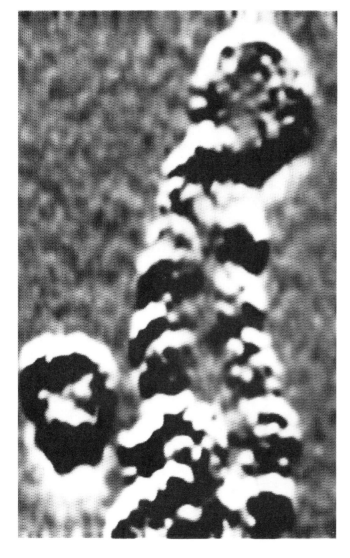

Genetics (cont.)

ics community reported the results of a long-awaited collaborative study on the safety of *chorionic villus sampling* (CVS), a technique for diagnosing genetic disorders in the fetus during the first *trimester* (three months) of pregnancy. The study concluded that the procedure is generally effective and safe, though it does slightly increase the risk of miscarriage.

The sampling is accomplished by inserting a catheter through the vagina and the *cervix* (the narrow passage at the lower end of the uterus). A small piece of tissue is then taken from the *chorionic villi*, projections of a membrane called the *chorion*, which surrounds the fetus. This tissue, which is genetically identical to the fetus, can be analyzed in the laboratory for a variety of chromosomal abnormalities.

Since its introduction in the United States in the early 1980's, CVS has grown in popularity because it can be done as early as 7 to 9 weeks after conception and results can be obtained in 1 week or less. Amniocentesis, the older and more established prenatal diagnostic technique, is done after the 16th week of pregnancy, and results are not available for 2 to 4 weeks. With CVS, therefore, the pregnant woman can make reproductive decisions—such as obtaining a therapeutic abortion, if desired—much earlier in the pregnancy.

Many physicians, however, have expressed concern that CVS is riskier for both the mother and the fetus than amniocentesis. To investigate the possible hazards of CVS—as well as its effectiveness—seven medical centers in the United States in the mid-1980's began a joint study of the procedure. The study compared 2,278 women who underwent first-trimester CVS with 671 women who had amniocentesis at 16 weeks into their pregnancy.

The researchers were able to make genetic evaluations of the fetus in 97.8 per cent of the CVS group and 99.4 per cent of the amniocentesis group. The accuracy of the diagnoses was very high in both groups. With regard to risk, the CVS group had an 0.8 per cent higher chance of miscarriage than the amniocentesis group.

The authors of the study concluded that chorionic villus sampling is "a safe and effective technique for the early prenatal diagnosis of [genetic] abnormalities, but that it probably entails a slightly higher risk of procedure failure and of fetal loss than does amniocentesis."

☐ Joseph D. McInerney

In WORLD BOOK, see CELL; GENETICS.

A combination of two female hormones whose production falls during *menopause* (the time of life when menstruation ends) may safely help older women reduce blood cholesterol levels and, thus, their risk of developing coronary artery disease. That conclusion was reported in January 1989 by researchers at the University of Western Ontario in London, Canada. The study provides additional support for the common practice of prescribing hormone supplements for postmenopausal women.

Women who have not yet gone through menopause—which usually occurs sometime between the ages of 45 and 50—are less likely to suffer from heart disease than are men. In addition, the level of cholesterol, a fatlike substance, in their blood is usually low. High blood levels of certain types of cholesterol may contribute to the development of heart disease.

At menopause, both blood cholesterol levels and the rate of heart disease rise. Many studies have linked these increases with the drop in the production of the female hormone estrogen that occurs during menopause. Estrogen supplements, however, can increase the risk of developing other health problems, chiefly cancer of the uterus. Taking progesterone, another female hor-

Glands and Hormones

Glands and Hormones (cont.)

mone, in combination with estrogen seems to reduce the health risks that may result from the use of estrogen alone.

For their study, the Canadian researchers treated 18 postmenopausal women with estrogen and progesterone for three years. They reported that the hormone treatment lowered blood cholesterol levels in the women. In addition, they reported drops in the women's blood levels of triglycerides and lipoproteins, substances that play a role in *atherosclerosis*, a build-up of fatty deposits and other substances in the walls of arteries.

Stimulating growth. Contrary to common medical belief, administering a male hormone to spur the development of teen-age boys with *constitutional delayed growth* will not prevent them from reaching their final adult height. That conclusion was reported in December 1988 by researchers at the State University of New York Health Sciences Center in Syracuse.

Children with constitutional delayed growth appear normal but for unknown reasons develop at a much slower-than-normal rate. Most children with this condition eventually attain their normal adult height by their early 20's. But their slow growth rate—and delayed sexual development—often cause serious psychological problems.

Some doctors have treated boys with this condition with male hormones. But other doctors have criticized the practice as not only unnecessary but harmful as well, because they believe that the treatment might prematurely halt bone growth.

The researchers treated 15 undersized boys in their early teens with testosterone, a male hormone, once a month for an average of 14 months. As expected, the researchers found that the hormone stimulated the boys' physical and sexual development. After the treatment ended, however, the boys continued to grow. All the boys reached their final adult height, as calculated from growth tables.

Kidney stones. The tendency of some people to develop kidney stones may be an inherited condition related to the defective action of an enzyme produced by red blood cells. (Kidney stones are hard, pebblelike masses, commonly composed of a calcium compound, that form in the kidneys.) That conclusion was reported in October 1988 by researchers from the University of Milan in Italy.

In general, the reason kidney stones form is unknown. But the most common abnormality associ-

Hormones and test scores

Women's performance on tests of reasoning ability and manual dexterity is linked to monthly fluctuations in female sex hormones, according to a controversial study reported in November 1988 by psychologists at Western Ontario University in London, Canada. The researchers reported that women do better on tests involving verbal skills and precise hand movements when estrogen levels are high.

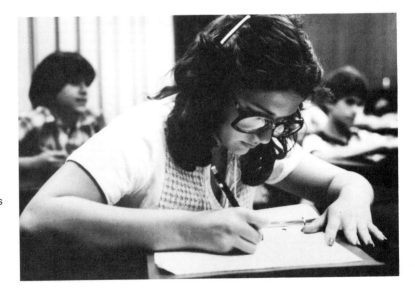

Glands and Hormones (cont.)

ated with kidney stones is a higher-than-normal level of calcium in the urine, a condition called *idiopathic hypercalciuria*. For their study, the Italian researchers examined the blood of 38 patients with idiopathic hypercalciuria. They found higher-than-normal levels of an enzyme produced by red blood cells that controls the amount of calcium excreted by the kidneys into the urine. They concluded that the higher levels of this enzyme resulted in higher levels of calcium in the urine. This, in turn, increased the likelihood of developing kidney stones.

The researchers also tested enzyme levels in families with no history of idiopathic hypercalciuria. They found that parents and their children tended to have similar levels of the enzyme under study. They also found the levels of calcium in the urine corresponded to the levels of the enzyme in the body. The researchers concluded that an inherited tendency to produce increased levels of the enzyme may play a role in the development of kidney stones. □ William Jubiz

In WORLD BOOK, see GLAND; HORMONE.

Health Care Facilities

United States health care organizations faced a variety of challenges in 1988 and 1989. Hospitals and health maintenance organizations (HMO's) were under particular stress.

Hospitals. Pressure on hospitals came in several forms. In 1988, the American Hospital Association (AHA) reported, hospitals made no profit, or excess revenue (income that exceeds expenses), in providing care to patients, down from the meager 1987 figure of 0.1 per cent profit from patient care. Profits from other sources of revenue, however, such as from rent and investment income, averaged 4.8 per cent, up slightly from the 1987 figure of 4.7 per cent.

Outpatient visits to hospitals continued to soar in 1988. The number of visits rose 5.9 per cent over 1987 levels to more than 92 million emergency room visits and 50 million clinic visits.

Rural institutions continued to founder in 1988. The Prospective Payment Assessment Commission, which monitors Medicare payment policy, reported in 1989 that rural hospital admissions have declined by 5 per cent each year since 1981. Low occupancy rates, declining reimbursement from government and private insurers, and difficulties in retaining medical staff all reportedly contributed to the decline.

Of 81 community hospitals reported by the AHA to have closed in 1988, 43 were rural hospitals. That raised to 206 the number of rural facilities closed since 1980.

Steps were being taken to address the crisis, however. Congress and the Administration of President George Bush both sought to raise Medicare payments for rural hospitals. Equally significant was intervention by state legislatures to help rural hospitals change their operations and mission in order to survive. For example, Montana allowed rural hospitals to become "medical assistance facilities." The designation would enable them to provide a few basic services, such as outpatient care and emergency stabilization, without meeting the strict and often costly requirements demanded of a large urban hospital. A state-funded program in California was pursuing a similar plan, and legislation to allow such experiments in other states was pending in Congress.

Medical waste. Although hospitals were not found directly responsible, they were put in the spotlight in 1988 when used syringes, needles, vials of blood, and other medical wastes washed up on United States beaches. After the situation caused public outcry, Congress passed a

Medical waste
Used syringes and hypo-
dermic needles, along with
other medical waste prod-
ucts, washed up on United
States beaches during the
summer of 1988, prompt-
ing investigations into how
hospitals and other health
care facilities dispose of
waste products that could
threaten public health.

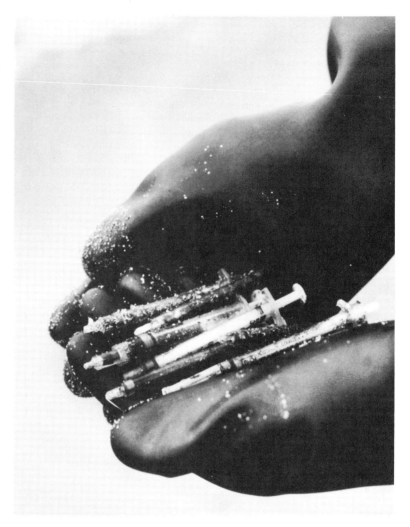

Health Care Facilities (cont.)
law in October requiring the Environmental Protection Agency (EPA)
to track the disposal of medical
wastes. The EPA launched a 10-
state pilot project in 1989.

Quality of care. The quality of hospital care continued to be a source
of concern in 1988 and 1989. The
Joint Commission on Accreditation
of Healthcare Organizations
(JCAHO), which accredits most hospitals, announced that as of July 1,
1989, hospitals failing to meet its
standards would be given "conditional accreditation" status and
would lose their accreditation if they
failed to improve. The JCAHO
planned to reveal which hospitals

received conditional accreditation to
the Health Care Financing Administration (HCFA), which administers
the Medicaid and Medicare programs. The HCFA reimburses hospitals with Medicare and Medicaid
payments only if they have been
accredited by the JCAHO.
   In the past, the JCAHO informed
the federal government only about
which hospitals failed or passed
inspection for accreditation. The
JCAHO will also allow less time for
corrective action by hospitals with
conditional status than had been
permitted in the past.

Nursing homes were criticized for
the quality of the care they provide

Health Care Facilities (cont.)

in a December 1988 report by the Department of Health and Human Services. The report indicated that in 1987, 44.8 per cent of the nursing homes surveyed failed to handle food in a safe and sanitary manner, 25.3 per cent failed to properly administer drugs, and 21.4 per cent had problems with cleanliness and sanitation.

The 75-volume, state-by-state survey rated about 15,000 nursing homes according to various standards of care. The report was contested by nursing homes, but its findings were supported by some organizations that lobby on behalf of senior citizens. The report was also criticized for being too mild by other organizations concerned with nursing home care.

HMO's. InterStudy, a research group that tracks HMO trends, reported that as of Jan. 1, 1989, 31.94 million Americans (13 per cent of the U.S. population) were enrolled in HMO's. This figure represents an increase of 5.4 per cent over January 1988, one of the smallest gains in HMO growth since 1977.

Some HMO's showed signs of instability. Maxicare, one of the nation's largest for-profit HMO's, declared bankruptcy in 1989. At the

100 years of health care
Two celebrated health care institutions were 100 years old in 1989. They were Johns Hopkins Hospital in Baltimore and the Mayo Clinic in Rochester, Minn. Since it opened in 1889, Johns Hopkins Hospital, *below,* has treated more than 20 million patients. The Mayo Clinic—one of the world's largest medical centers—began as a clinic for surgical patients in 1889, founded by William Worral Mayo and his two sons, *right,* Charles H. Mayo (left) and William J. Mayo. The clinic became known as the Mayo Clinic in 1903.

Health Care Facilities (cont.)

same time, the HCFA's attempt to enroll more Medicare beneficiaries in HMO's in an effort to save money for the Medicare program showed little progress. The total number of Medicare enrollees in HMO's remained stable at approximately 1-million. Furthermore, a record 44 HMO's dropped out of the Medicare program in 1988, citing insufficient reimbursement levels.

AIDS inpact on hospitals. Most patients with acquired immune deficiency syndrome (AIDS) are being treated in just 5 per cent of the nation's hospitals, threatening those facilities with financial disaster, according to a study reported in August 1989. The study of 322 hospitals was conducted by the National Public Health and Hospital Institute, a private research group in Washington, D.C. Because large numbers of AIDS patients are uninsured or are covered by Medicaid, which pays only part of the treatment cost, hospitals have lost an average of more than $3,500 per AIDS patient, the study found.

□ Emily Ann Friedman

See also FINANCING MEDICAL CARE. In WORLD BOOK, see HOSPITAL.

Health Policy

A yearlong ban on the use of human fetal tissue in federally funded medical research remained in effect in the United States in mid-1989, though an advisory committee to the National Institutes of Health (NIH) recommended a lifting of the ban. The controversy over the ban, which went into effect in March 1988 under the Administration of President Ronald Reagan, now must be resolved under the Administration of President George Bush.

Human fetal tissue may have a wide range of beneficial medical applications. Such tissue has been transplanted into the brains of patients suffering from Parkinson's disease with the aim of controlling the tremors that are characteristic of that disease. Fetal pancreatic cells have also been studied for possible application to treat such disorders of the brain and nervous system as spinal cord injuries, Alzheimer's disease, epilepsy and stroke, as well as immunological disorders.

The source of the fetal tissue, however, is from induced abortions, and this fact has aroused controversy. In March 1988, the Department of Health and Human Services (HHS) halted all federally sponsored research on fetal tissue until a special advisory panel could address the ethical questions raised by the research.

The 21-member panel consisted of medical, scientific, legal, ethical, and religious experts and was chaired by Arlin M. Adams, a retired federal appeals court judge. In December 1988, an NIH advisory committee voted to accept the panel's report, which said that such research was "acceptable public policy."

Adams concurred with the panel's majority, noting that "the panel has carefully weighed concerns over abortion against concerns for medical research that could improve the lot of thousands of Americans." Four members of the panel dissented, citing their belief that abortion is immoral and that the use of tissue from an abortion would thus be an immoral practice.

The panel recommended that strict guidelines be developed to prevent abuses in fetal tissue research. Among the safeguards proposed were a prohibition on the sale of tissue from aborted fetuses, and procedures to ensure that a woman would not know if her aborted fetus was to be used for medical research. The latter safeguard was intended to prevent any woman from being encouraged to have an abortion.

The panel's report was accepted by the NIH, which forwarded it to HHS Assistant Secretary Robert Windom, who had first announced the ban. The ban was to stay in ef-

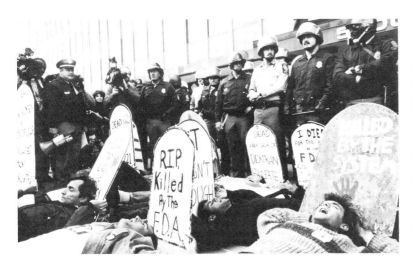

AIDS and public policy
Protesters demonstrating in Washington, D.C., in July 1988 demand that the federal government speed the approval process for drugs to treat AIDS, *left*. Others, marching in New York City in November 1988, voice their support of a controversial program to distribute free sterile hypodermic needles to drug addicts, aimed at slowing the spread of AIDS among addicts and their sexual partners, *below*.

Health Policy (cont.)
fect, however, until the panel's report was studied by Congress and the Bush Administration.

Free needles for addicts. Programs providing intravenous (IV) drug addicts with clean hypodermic needles as part of an effort to slow the spread of AIDS (acquired immune deficiency syndrome) via contaminated needles, would have the support of HHS. The declaration of support was made in a March 1989 interview by HHS Secretary Louis W. Sullivan. He stressed that such programs should be developed at the local level but that HHS would be supportive if communities implemented such programs.

New York City began a small-scale needle exchange program in November 1988. The pilot study, which was to involve 400 IV drug users awaiting drug rehabilitation, was the first government program in the United States to distribute needles to addicts.

Speeding drug approval. In an effort to hasten the U.S. approval of new antibiotics to treat infectious diseases, a group of health experts began, in February 1989, the process of updating research guidelines for pharmaceutical firms. The drug approval process for antibiotics currently can take as long as 10 to 12 years, according to Thomas R. Beam, Jr., who was on leave as an

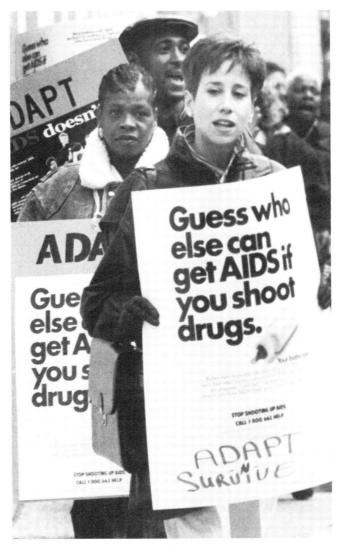

associate professor of medicine and microbiology at the State University of New York at Buffalo to direct the effort. He said that officials hope new guidelines will cut two or three years from the process of approving drugs to treat such infections as pneumonia, meningitis, and urinary tract infections.

The Food and Drug Administration (FDA) has not updated its guidelines for testing antibiotic drugs since the 1970's. The new guidelines will show companies testing prospective drugs what studies should be done, and how to ensure that the studies will meet FDA requirements. A similar effort, involving the formation of a panel of experts to find ways to hasten the approval of drugs to treat AIDS and cancer, began in 1988.

Race and access to medical care.
Blacks in general have less access than whites to physician care, according to a report in the Jan. 13, 1989, issue of the *Journal of the American Medical Association* by a team of researchers from Harvard School of Public Health in Boston, the University of Pennsylvania in Philadelphia, and the University of California, Los Angeles. The researchers based their findings on an analysis of data collected in a 1986 telephone survey (directed by

members of the research team) of 10,130 people living in the continental United States.

For economic reasons, blacks see doctors less often than do whites, the researchers found. One in every 11 blacks reported being unable to afford seeing a doctor, compared with 1 in 20 whites.

The survey also found that blacks are less likely than whites to have any type of health insurance and that they are "considerably less likely" to have private health insurance. Moreover, a greater percentage of blacks (40.5 per cent) than whites (30.0 per cent) were found to live in states with the least generous Medicaid programs.

The disparity in access to care is made worse by the fact that blacks tend to be in poorer health than whites. Blacks have a death rate that is 1.5 times higher than whites of the same age, and the infant mortality rate for blacks is twice that of whites, according to HHS. The researchers concluded that "despite progress during the past two decades, the nation still has a long way to go in achieving equitable health care for all its citizens."

☐ Rod Such

In the Special Reports section, see MEDICAL ETHICS AND THE AIDS EPIDEMIC. In WORLD BOOK, see HEALTH CARE.

Hearing

See Ear and Hearing

Heart and Blood Vessels

Researchers reported in 1988 and 1989 on several new devices that remove *plaque*—deposits of cholesterol (a fatlike compound), calcium, and other substances—from the walls of diseased arteries. A build-up of plaque on arterial walls (a condition known as *atherosclerosis*) narrows the opening through which blood flows and can be extremely dangerous. If a blood clot forms at a narrowed part of an artery that supplies blood to the heart, a heart attack can occur. The new plaque-removing devices are mounted on a *catheter* (thin tube), which a physician inserts into the artery and moves to the plaque build-up.

In October 1988, physicians from

Sequoia Hospital in Redwood City, Calif., presented results of experiments with the Simpson Atherocath to doctors attending the Annual Texas Heart Institute Symposium in Houston. The Simpson Atherocath has a slot on one side of the catheter's metal tip and a balloon on the other side.

After moving the catheter to the site of the plaque, the surgeon inflates the balloon, pushing the slot against the plaque. As a result, some of the plaque enters the slot. The doctor then advances a rotating blade down the catheter. The blade shears off the plaque and pushes it into the hollow tip of the catheter.

Heart and Blood Vessels (cont.)

The California physicians reported that they had successfully removed plaque from 92 per cent of a group of 200 patients whose *peripheral arteries* (arteries outside of the heart) were narrowed due to atherosclerosis. These were the first such patients on whom they tested the device.

Cardiologist John B. Simpson, who developed the Atherocath, reported that the device reduced the average diameter of the plaque build-up from 76 per cent of the diameter of the artery to 24 per cent of the diameter, without once puncturing or cutting the vessel. There were, however, some complications, including a complete blockage of the artery, *distal embolization* (the formation of debris into a mass outside the catheter), and blood clotting at the site of the operation. During the first three years after surgery, plaque regrew to at least half its original diameter in 16 per cent of the places from which it had been removed.

At the November 1988 Annual Scientific Session of the American Heart Association (AHA) in Anaheim, Calif., Simpson reported on the use of a modification of the Atherocath in the coronary vessels that supply blood to the heart. Simpson said that he had successfully removed plaque from such vessels in 133 patients.

Complications occurred, however, in 22 patients, and plaque built up to at least half its original diameter in 9 of 40 patients whose progress was followed for six months after surgery. Thus, initial results in the coronary vessels were not as good as in peripheral arteries.

Laser devices. Researchers tested two types of laser catheters on arteries clogged by atherosclerosis. One uses a laser beam to heat a metal tip on the end of the catheter. The tip is then inserted into the blocked area, where it burns away plaque.

Cardiologist Richard Leachman and colleagues at the Texas Heart Institute in Houston in October 1988 reported a 98 per cent success rate

with 50 narrowed peripheral arteries and a 72 per cent success rate with 117 completely blocked arteries. The major complication was puncturing of the artery, which occurred in 20 patients. Clotting and distal embolization also were reported.

The second device uses the laser beam to vaporize blockages in arteries. With this device, there is a high risk of puncturing the artery. Currently, this technique can be applied only to long, straight segments of arteries—the kind found in the upper leg.

Plaque drill. Cardiologist Jose A. Perez of the University of Texas

Laser opens arteries
A new type of laser probe opens blocked arteries by removing from their walls deposits of *plaque* (a substance containing cholesterol, calcium, and other substances). The probe, which is threaded into the artery, first emits a laser beam to penetrate the plaque. Then laser light heats the tip of the probe, vaporizing the deposit.

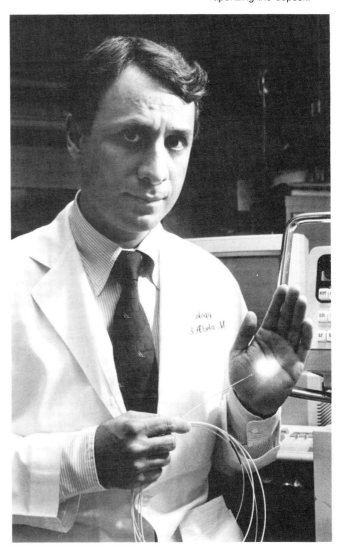

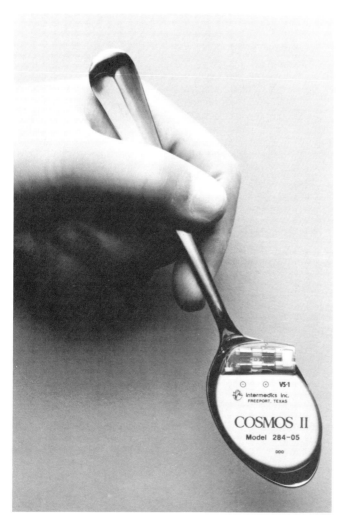

Diamond cuts plaque. Another experimental device for removing plaque resembles a dentist's burr and is tiny enough to fit inside and channel through completely blocked arteries. Robert Ginsberg, a cardiologist at Stanford University Medical Center in Stanford, Calif., reported in November 1988 that he had tested the burr on 18 patients with blocked coronary arteries and 35 patients with obstructions of leg blood vessels, with a 100 per cent success rate.

The surgeon positions the burr, which is made of stainless steel coated with diamond, by means of a wire about twice the thickness of a human hair that is threaded into the artery. During the operation, the burr spins at a rate of 180,000 rpm; blood flowing through the artery washes away the microscopic particles of plaque that are removed. Possible complications include a build-up of particles farther down in the blood vessel that could block its smaller branches.

Low cholesterol a risk? Four studies reported at the annual meeting of the AHA in Washington, D.C., in November 1988 suggest that low levels of high-density lipoprotein (HDL), the so-called "good" cholesterol, may be a major risk factor for premature disease of the coronary arteries. There are two main types of cholesterol-carrying molecules—HDL and low-density lipoprotein (LDL). The LDL molecule tends to deposit cholesterol in cells, including cells in the walls of the arteries.

Doctors know that an excessive amount of LDL cholesterol in the blood implies a high risk of heart attack, stroke, and other complications involving the blood vessels. An individual can reduce his or her level of LDL cholesterol by lowering the cholesterol and fat content of the diet.

Unlike LDL, the HDL molecule tends to prevent cholesterol from depositing on arterial walls. Thus, it is desirable to have a high level of HDL. Exercise and weight loss can increase levels of HDL. In addition, gemfibrozil, a new drug for treating

Spoon-sized heart help
The tiny Cosmos II pacemaker, produced by Intermedics, Incorporated, of Angleton, Tex., uses a single computer chip to maintain a normal heart rate. An earlier version used five chips. Cosmos II collects up to six months of information on its own performance, as do other devices, but also gathers six months of data on the patient's response.

Heart and Blood Vessels (cont.)
Health Science Center at San Antonio conducted tests during 1988 and 1989 of a catheter-mounted, drill-like tool called the *transluminal extraction catheter*. This tool has a cone-shaped end containing blades that rotate at a rate of 750 revolutions per minute (rpm) as they chop up plaque. The shavings are then vacuumed from the bloodstream through the catheter.

Perez developed the device in 1987 while at Duke University Medical Center in Durham, N.C. At Duke, he used the catheter in 36 operations on leg arteries, with a success rate of 97 per cent. By the summer of 1989, the catheter had been used in peripheral arteries only.

Heart and Blood Vessels (cont.)
high total cholesterol, increases HDL levels.

Studies such as those reported at the AHA meeting have caused concern that patients whose total cholesterol and LDL cholesterol are within normal limits but who have low HDL will be falsely reassured that they are in a low-risk group. Furthermore, some individuals with high total cholesterol—including a high HDL level—may be wrongly considered as having a high coronary artery disease risk factor. Thus, many cardiologists urge that physicians routinely measure HDL levels along with total cholesterol.

Measurements of HDL are not included in the current recommendations of the National Cholesterol Education Program (NCEP) of the National Heart, Lung, and Blood Institute. Some scientists have suggested, however, that the NCEP should recommend the measurement of HDL in a patient with only one risk factor for coronary heart disease. A low HDL measurement would then be a second risk factor.

Opponents of this change point out that cardiologists do not yet know what to do about low HDL. There is no evidence that treating patients who have low HDL levels improves their chance of avoiding coronary heart disease.

Abdominal fat is risky. Researchers at the Physical Activities Science Laboratory and the Lipid Research Centers at Laval University in Quebec, Canada, reported in the March-April 1989 issue of the journal *Arteriosclerosis* that there is an association between the amount of deep abdominal fat in obese women and low HDL cholesterol levels accompanied by high LDL cholesterol levels. The scientists measured fat around the abdominal organs and in the midthigh region by means of computerized X-ray pictures. Excess fat at the midthigh region did not show any significant relationship with lipoprotein levels.

The use of ultrasound to produce unobstructed images of the heart continued to be improved through-

out 1988 and 1989. A new technique using an ultrasonic probe was evaluated during the year. This technique differs from the standard method of imaging the heart ultrasonically in that the *probe*, the instrument that emits and receives high-frequency waves, is inserted into the body.

In the standard method, the ultrasonic device rests on the patient's chest. Waves emitted by the device pass through the skin. Some of the waves travel into the chest, where they bounce off the heart and return to the probe.

As the waves return, the probe translates them into electrical sig-

Heart restarter
An implantable restarter for the heart improves survival rates for at least two years, report researchers at the University of California at San Francisco. A wallet-sized device is implanted in the abdomen and connected to wire-mesh patches that are sewn to the heart. When the device detects a certain type of abnormal rhythm, it delivers an electric shock to the heart to restore the normal rhythm.

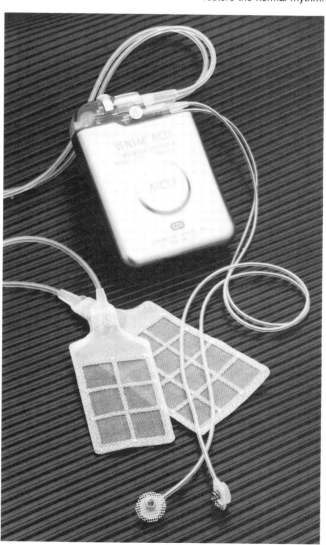

About 30 per cent of people 4 to 19 years old in the United States have cholesterol levels higher than 180 milligrams per 100 milliliters of blood, according to ongoing research begun in 1984 on about 6,000 children. The American Academy of Pediatrics, reflecting concern about such high levels, in October 1988 declared that children with levels of 176 and higher should change their diets.

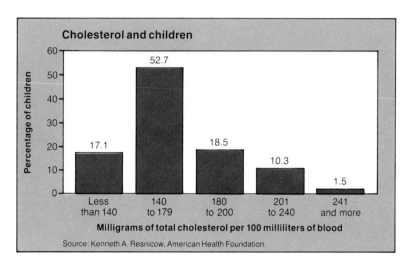

Cholesterol and children

Percentage of children

Milligrams of total cholesterol per 100 milliliters of blood				
Less than 140	140 to 179	180 to 200	201 to 240	241 and more
17.1	52.7	18.5	10.3	1.5

Source: Kenneth A. Resnicow, American Health Foundation.

Hospitals
See Health Care Facilities

Heart and Blood Vessels (cont.)
nals, which in turn create a televisionlike image of the heart. Unfortunately, many waves also bounce off ribs and the lungs, producing images that prevent the cardiologist from getting a clear view of the heart.

The new technique uses a *transesophageal* probe mounted on the end of a flexible tube 8.5 millimeters (0.33 inch) in diameter and 100 centimeters (39.4 inches) long, and placed in the *esophagus* (the food passage leading from the mouth to the stomach). Because this passage runs directly behind the heart, the resulting pictures are not only free of obstructions but also extremely sharp.

For an examination with the probe, the patient first has a local anesthetic sprayed into the throat and receives a sedative to promote relaxation. Once these measures are taken, most individuals can easily swallow the tube until the probe lies directly behind the heart. The examination usually causes little discomfort and has a low risk of complications. ☐ Michael H. Crawford

In WORLD BOOK, see ARTERIOSCLEROSIS; CHOLESTEROL; HEART; HEART ATTACK; ULTRASOUND.

Infectious Diseases

AIDS (acquired immune deficiency syndrome) continued to be a major public health problem in the United States in 1988 and 1989. The U.S. Centers for Disease Control (CDC) in Atlanta, Ga., reported that the number of U.S. AIDS cases since the disease was first identified reached 102,671 by July 30, 1989; 59,391 AIDS deaths were reported for the same period. (See AIDS.)

"Doorway" for cold viruses. Two teams of researchers reported in the March 10, 1989, issue of the journal *Cell* that they had identified the *cell receptors* used by certain viruses that cause the common cold. A cell receptor is a molecule on the surface of the cell that viruses use as a "doorway" to enter the cell. A particular part of the virus fits into the receptor much as a key fits into a lock. The virus multiplies inside the cell by forcing the cell's own "machinery" to produce more viruses.

The identification of this particular receptor, called *intercellular adhesion molecule 1* (ICAM-1), may lead to the development of a drug to combat the common cold. This drug—perhaps a nasal spray—would contain a large number of artificial receptors shaped so much like ICAM-1 that the viruses could not distinguish between the artificial receptors and the real one. The viruses would attach to both the natural and artificial receptors, but the spray would contain so many artificial receptors that most of the viruses would not reach natural receptors. So cold symptoms would be much less severe than normal.

The ICAM-1 receptor is the attachment site for about 90 per cent of the more than 100 cold-causing viruses known as *rhinoviruses*. These viruses are responsible for up to half of all common colds.

The two scientific teams that identified ICAM-1 as a rhinovirus receptor had been pursuing separate lines of research, based on two facts. The scientists knew, first, that the molecule plays a role in mobilizing certain cells that are part of the immune system and, second, that about 90 per cent of all rhinoviruses share a common receptor.

A team led by molecular biologists Jeffrey M. Greve, Michael Kamarck, and Alan McClelland of the Miles Research Center of Miles Incorporated in West Haven, Conn., was investigating the receptor used by about 90 per cent of the rhinoviruses and determined that it was identical to ICAM-1.

Researchers headed by molecular biologist Timothy Springer of Harvard Medical School in Boston had been studying ICAM-1's role in the immune system when they discovered that ICAM-1 was identical to the rhinovirus receptor.

Test for hepatitis virus. Researchers at Chiron Corporation in Emeryville, Calif., announced in April 1989 that they had developed a test to detect a newly discovered hepatitis virus called hepatitis C. Medical experts expect this development to make donated blood much safer and to lead to a vaccine for hepatitis caused by the C virus.

About 150,000 cases of hepatitis result from blood transfusions in the United States each year. Viruses known as hepatitis A and hepatitis B cause some 5 to 10 per cent of these cases. But about 75 per cent of the cases are due to the C virus. Screening donated blood for the hepatitis C virus as well as for A and B is likely to cut the number of cases of hepatitis sharply.

Measles outbreak. An outbreak of measles that began in the United States in 1984 skyrocketed in 1989. The outbreak did not spread uniformly, but rather was heavily concentrated in certain areas—and the concentrations varied widely from year to year. In 1986, for example, New York City reported 945 cases, but by 1988 the number of cases had plummeted to 52. Ohio reported only 5 cases in 1987 but 109 in 1988.

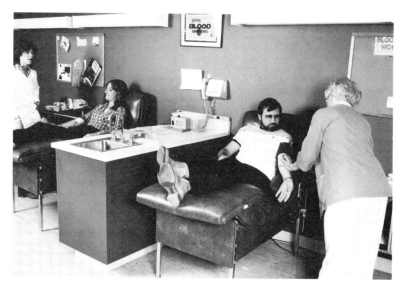

Test for safer blood
Donated blood may soon become safer, thanks to a test to screen blood for the newly discovered *hepatitis C* virus. About 4 per cent of recipients of blood transfusions catch hepatitis C, which causes inflammation of the liver, from donated blood. The test, developed by Chiron Corporation of Emeryville, Calif., may be approved for use in the United States by 1990.

Measles continues to resist elimination from the United States. A vaccine introduced in 1963 slashed the number of cases. A second vaccine appearing in 1967 was an improvement but was unstable, failing to protect many recipients. A stable vaccine was introduced in 1980, however, so today's problem is that not enough people are getting vaccinated. This problem became more severe in the first eight months of 1989, with more than 9,000 new cases reported.

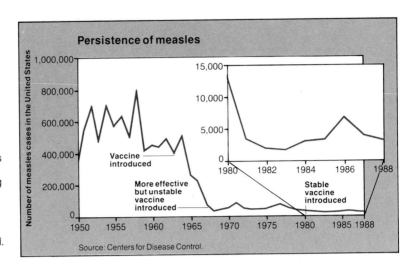

Persistence of measles

Number of measles cases in the United States

Vaccine introduced

More effective but unstable vaccine introduced

Stable vaccine introduced

Source: Centers for Disease Control.

Infectious Diseases (cont.)

In early 1989, there were large numbers of cases in Houston, Los Angeles County, and Kansas City, Mo. By mid-August 1989, more than 1,200 cases had been reported in the Chicago area—including 6 deaths.

Three groups of individuals were likely to contract measles during the current outbreak. Children who were vaccinated before they were 15 months old were vulnerable because measles *antibodies* (molecules produced by the body to fight disease) are often passed from mother to child before birth. This can prevent the vaccine from making a very young child completely immune to the disease. Preschoolers who had never been vaccinated made up a second group that federal health officials estimate might include more than half the nation's preschoolers.

The third group consisted of a small percentage of those people who were born after 1956 but before 1980 and had been vaccinated. The first vaccine for measles, prepared from dead viruses and introduced in 1963, was somewhat unsatisfactory. An improved vaccine prepared from live viruses was developed in 1967, but it became ineffective when not refrigerated properly. In 1980, a stable live-virus vaccine finally became available.

Most people born before 1957

were not at risk because they had developed immunity due to natural infection with the measles virus. Prior to the 1960's, most children caught the measles, so their bodies produced antibodies that provided lifelong immunity from later attacks.

Number of cases still small. The current outbreak involves nowhere near the number of cases common in the United States before the introduction of the first vaccine for measles in 1963. In 1952, for example, there were about 700,000 cases in the United States. By 1967, thanks to the vaccine, the number had dropped to 63,000. By 1978, there were only 27,000 cases per year, and the CDC launched a program to eliminate the disease in the United States by 1982. The program failed, but by 1983 the number of cases was only 1,500.

Each year since then, however, at least 2,500 cases have been reported to the CDC. From Jan. 1 through Aug. 26, 1989, the CDC received reports of 9,650 additional cases. □ Jay Myers

See also Drugs (Close-Up). In the Special Reports section, see The Great White Plague: A History of TB; The Puzzle of Legionnaires' Disease; When a Kiss Can Make You Sick. In the Health Studies section, see Vaccines and Your Health. In World Book, see Cold, Common; Hepatitis; Measles; Virus.

Injury
See Emergency
Medicine, Safety

A genetically engineered hormone approved on June 1, 1989, for use in the United States promises to end *anemia* (a shortage of red blood cells) in virtually all patients who undergo dialysis. In *dialysis*, artificial means are used to filter the blood. Dialysis patients are said to have end-stage *renal* (kidney) disease; the kidneys' ability to perform such vital functions as filtering waste materials from the blood and producing erythropoietin (EPO), the hormone that stimulates the bone marrow to produce red blood cells, is greatly hampered. The genetically engineered hormone, called epoietin alfa, is a form of EPO.

In mid-1989, about 100,000 patients in the United States were receiving dialysis treatments regularly. Because their kidneys produce too little EPO, more than 75 per cent of these patients are anemic. Anemia accounts for many of the symptoms of kidney failure, such as being easily tired and a decreased capacity for exercise. About 5 to 10 per cent of all dialysis patients have such severe anemia that they require periodic transfusions of additional red blood cells to raise their red blood cell counts to tolerable—but still anemic—levels.

But genetically engineered EPO can be produced in large quantities by cells grown in the laboratory. In tests on dialysis patients, the genetically engineered EPO increased red blood cell counts of almost all dialysis patients into the normal range and virtually wiped out the need for transfusions. With a higher blood count as a result of the treatment, dialysis patients have an improved tolerance for physical activity.

Side effects due to epoietin alfa included high blood pressure, seizures, and an increased risk of blood clotting, but these were infrequent. Researchers expect that the average yearly cost of this medication will be about $5,000 to $10,000 per patient.

Painkillers and kidney disease.
A report published in the May 11, 1989, issue of *The New England Journal of Medicine* provided strong evidence of a link between the regular use of certain over-the-counter *analgesics* (painkillers) and the development of chronic kidney disease. The report cited two medications—analgesic mixtures that contain acetaminophen, the active ingredient in such products as Tylenol and Anacin 3, and phenacetin. Phenacetin had been removed from the market in the late 1970's because previous studies had suggested this linkage. Acetaminophen is one of the main substances produced when the body breaks down phenacetin.

The May 1989 study compared

Kidney

Kidney drug approved
Frank E. Young, commissioner of the U.S. Food and Drug Administration, approves the use of a genetically engineered form of a hormone known as erythropoietin (EPO) to treat anemia in certain kidney patients.

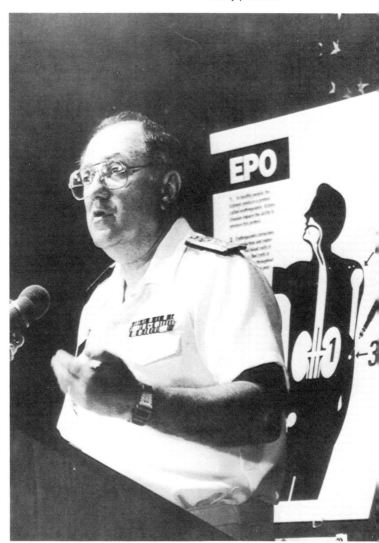

Kidney (cont.)

the history of analgesic use by a group of renal disease patients whose illness was first diagnosed in North Carolina medical centers with that of people contacted at random living near the centers. The researchers, led by epidemiologist Dale P. Sandler of the National Institute of Environmental Health Sciences in Research Triangle Park, N.C., gathered their data in telephone interviews in which they asked individuals to recall their past use of analgesics.

Sandler and her colleagues found a statistically significant association between the presence of kidney disease and the daily use of acetaminophen, phenacetin mixtures, or both. They found no such association, however, with daily use of aspirin or with weekly or occasional use of acetaminophen.

The study determined only an association, not a cause-and-effect relationship, between use of the analgesics and renal disease. It is estimated that individuals must take at least 1 kilogram (2.2 pounds) of analgesics—more than three thousand 325-milligram tablets—for renal disease to develop.

☐ Jeffrey R. Thompson

In WORLD BOOK, see KIDNEY.

Mental and Behavioral Disorders

Evidence of a physical cause for schizophrenia, a severe mental disorder, was reported in November 1988 by a team headed by psychiatrist Robin Sherrington of the University of London in England. The researchers reported that some people may have a particular gene that predisposes them to the disorder. Other researchers cautioned, however, that schizophrenia is too complex a disorder to result from a single gene.

Schizophrenia is actually a group of mental disorders characterized by severe disorganization of thinking, emotions, and behavior. Symptoms often include hallucinations, delusions, apathy, and an inability to take care of one's basic needs.

Sherrington and his colleagues found what they believe is a genetic marker for schizophrenia on chromosome 5 in seven Icelandic and English families. Each family had an unusually large number of schizophrenic members. Each human cell has 23 pairs of chromosomes carrying as many as 100,000 genes, which are composed of deoxyribonucleic acid (DNA). A *genetic marker* for a particular gene is a piece of DNA that occupies a location on a chromosome near the location of that gene.

Also in November, however, psychiatrist James L. Kennedy of Yale University in New Haven, Conn., and his co-workers reported finding no evidence linking abnormalities in that section of chromosome 5 with schizophrenia. Kennedy and his colleagues studied several generations of a Swedish family with numerous cases of schizophrenia. In May 1989, independent research teams at the University of Edinburgh in Scotland and the University of Utah in Salt Lake City also reported no link between the chromosome 5-area and schizophrenia.

The most likely explanation for the difference between Sherrington's report and the other studies, according to the Yale scientists, is that several genes are involved in schizophrenia. Even in the Icelandic and English families, for instance, not everyone with the genetic marker on chromosome 5 developed the disorder. It is likely that environmental influences determine whether a genetically susceptible person develops schizophrenia, the researchers said.

Schizophrenia medication. Many of the hundreds of thousands of people with schizophrenia who are not hospitalized can get by on about one-fifth the standard dose of fluphenazine, a commonly prescribed antipsychotic drug, according to a September 1988 report. The finding is important, said study director Gerard E. Hogarty of the Uni-

Mental Disorders (cont.)

versity of Pittsburgh (Pa.) School of Medicine, because low doses of the drug are less likely than high doses to cause *tardive dyskinesia*. This movement disorder causes involuntary jerking of the limbs and severe facial twitches. An estimated 20 per cent of people treated with antipsychotic drugs develop tardive dyskinesia to some degree.

Hogarty and his colleagues monitored 70 patients with schizophrenia for two years after their discharge from a psychiatric hospital. Those injected with one-fifth the standard dose of fluphenazine did as well overall as patients on the full dose.

Creativity and mood. People who experience relatively mild mood swings and the healthy relatives of people with *manic-depressive disorder* tend to be more creative than the general population. That finding was reported in August 1988 by psychologist Dennis K. Kinney and his colleagues of McLean Hospital in Belmont, Mass. Manic-depressive disorder, also known as *bipolar disorder*, is characterized by recurrent mood swings—alternating between episodes of frenzied euphoria and bleak despondency.

Kinney and his colleagues studied 17 people with manic-depressive disorder, 11 of their parents and siblings—none of whom had

been diagnosed as having the disorder—and 16 people with mild mood swings. The researchers also studied 33 other volunteers who had no family history of manic-depressive disorder.

The researchers rated each subject's creativity on a variety of work and free-time activities, including painting, writing poetry, and starting a business. They found that individuals with mild mood swings are most creative at work, and that individuals related to people with manic-depressive disorder show the highest creativity in their spare-time pursuits. The reason for this pattern is unclear.

Mental disorders among children. According to two large surveys, both released in December 1988, a surprisingly large percentage of children in the United States and Puerto Rico—about 20 per cent—suffer from psychiatric problems severe enough to interfere with their lives. The reports also indicated that many of these children do not receive mental health care.

In one study, psychologist Elizabeth J. Costello of Duke University Medical Center in Durham, N.C., and her colleagues examined 789 children aged 7 to 11 years who visited their pediatrician over a one-year period. Based on interviews with the children and their parents,

Brain defect and autism Researchers have found evidence of a physical difference in the brains of people with *autism,* a severe mental disorder characterized by avoidance of human contact. Using magnetic resonance imaging, neurologist Eric Courchesne of the San Diego Children's Hospital found in 1988 that certain portions of the brain (shaded area) of an autistic person, *below,* are often much smaller than those structures in a normal brain, *below left.*

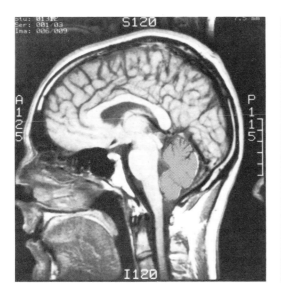

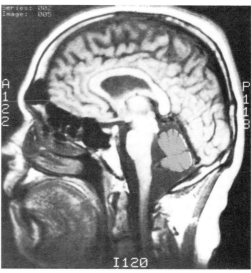

Face value of emotions

Facial expressions are not only the visible sign of particular emotions but actually may produce the emotions that they represent, according to studies reported in July 1989. Researchers found that creating a frown, *below,* produces a modest unpleasant feeling, while arranging the face into a smile, *below right,* produces a modest pleasant feeling. Facial movements may change the temperature of blood in the brain, affecting those areas that regulate emotion, researchers theorized.

Mental Disorders (cont.)

who lived in and around Pittsburgh, the researchers estimated that 22 per cent of the youngsters had one or more mental disorders.

The mental disorders most commonly diagnosed in the children included *phobia,* intense fear of a particular object or situation; *oppositional disorder,* which consists of persistent confrontations with parents and teachers, as well as temper tantrums; and *overanxious disorder,* marked by excessive worrying about the future and how one is viewed by others. Despite the widespread incidence of mental disorders, however, fewer than 4 per cent of the children were referred to a mental health professional by their pediatricians.

The second study involved a survey of 777 Puerto Rican children aged 4 to 16 by psychiatrist Hector R. Bird of Columbia University in New York City and his co-workers. They concluded that nearly 16 per cent of the children studied suffered from moderate to severe mental disorders.

The findings of the two studies may signal a major public health problem. Costello and Bird noted, however, that no one knows what happens to children with untreated psychiatric disorders as they grow older. Such disorders may have serious consequences or they may

pass with no long-lasting effects, the researchers said.

Consequences of child abuse.

Child abuse often haunts the backgrounds of individuals with borderline personality disorder, according to a study published in April 1989. Psychiatrist Judith L. Herman of Harvard Medical School in Boston and her colleagues reported that child abuse alone does not cause this disorder but plays an influential role in many cases.

Characteristics of this disorder involve intense and unstable relationships, self-destructive and impulsive behavior—such as drug abuse—suicide attempts aimed at manipulating other people, and rage alternating with a childish dependency on others.

Herman and her co-workers interviewed 21 patients with borderline personality disorder and 11 people who were not regarded as having the disorder but nevertheless had several characteristics of the condition. They also interviewed 23 people with such related psychiatric diagnoses as antisocial personality disorder, which is characterized by, for example, persistent violence and lawbreaking.

Seventeen of the 21 people with borderline personality disorder reported experiencing childhood trauma, including physical abuse,

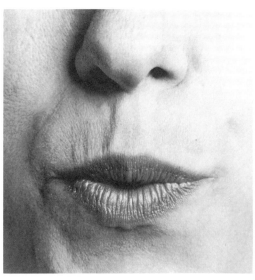

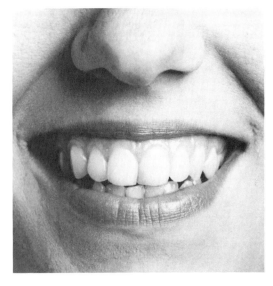

Art sick

Great art is supposed to affect us deeply. But in the last 10 years, more than 100 tourists to Florence, Italy, have been so overcome by that city's bountiful and glorious art that they have been admitted to a local hospital suffering from hallucinations, delirium, disorientation, rapid heart beat, or stomach pains.

Psychiatrist Graziella Magherini, who has documented these cases of what she has named the Stendhal Syndrome in a new book, estimates that hundreds of milder cases have likely gone unreported.

The Stendhal Syndrome is named for Marie Henri Beyle, a 19th-century French novelist who wrote under the name Stendhal. On a visit to Michelangelo's tomb in 1817, Beyle was so overcome his heart beat wildly and he thought he would fall down while walking. He finally calmed himself by reading some favorite poetry.

According to Magherini, the typical victim of the syndrome is unmarried, between the ages of 26 and 40. Most are infrequent travelers sightseeing alone or in a small group at a whirlwind pace. Most victims are from northern Europe and the United States. And more than half have already seen a psychologist or psychiatrist.

Magherini explained that when combined with the fatigue, loneliness, and confusion often involved in travel, sudden exposure to art can trigger intense reactions in certain sensitive people. The victims "took refuge in sickness because they found it impossible to tolerate a passionate relationship with an aesthetic object," Magherini said.

For example, Martha, after lengthy contemplation of Fra Angelico frescoes, returned to her hotel room and stood, dazed and mute, in a corner. Kamil, a young Czech painter, felt feverish and collapsed after seeing a painting by Masaccio.

According to Magherini, the victims recover after a few days of rest. The cure, she said, "is a heavy dose of the familiar and the mundane."

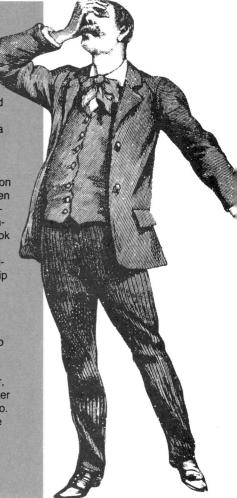

Mental Disorders (cont.)
sexual abuse, or witnessing serious domestic violence. About 60 per cent of the remaining subjects reported childhood trauma, but their abusive experiences were less frequent and less severe than those experienced by those with the disorder, the researchers said.

Violent vulnerabilities. Violent teen-agers often have a long history of violence and come from violent families, according to a long-term study of juvenile delinquents reported in May 1989. Psychiatrist Dorothy Otnow Lewis of New York University in New York City and her colleagues evaluated 95 young men aged 15 while they were at a correctional school and then again seven years later. The group consisted of 77 "very violent" subjects arrested for rape, murder, and other physically aggressive acts and 18 "less violent" subjects arrested for crimes such as shoplifting.

Violence does not always breed violence, according to Lewis. Nearly the same proportion of the "very violent" teen-agers and the "less violent" teen-agers were arrested for physically aggressive crimes as adults. But the researchers found a number of factors shared by the young men with the highest rate of aggressive criminal offenses. These included recurring psychotic symptoms; neurological problems; low

Nervous System
See Brain and Nervous
System

Nursing Homes
See Health Care
Facilities

Mental Disorders (cont.)
reading and intelligence test scores;
and an upbringing in a violent, abusive household.

Elderly abuse. Contrary to common
belief, most victims of elderly abuse
and neglect are relatively well-func-
tioning people who are mistreated
by a dependent spouse. That
finding was reported in April 1989
by psychologists Karl Pillemer and
David Finkelhor of the University of
New Hampshire in Durham. Previously, it was assumed that such
abuse was usually inflicted by family
members, often the adult children of
the victims, pushed over the edge

by the stress of caring for a frail,
dependent old person.

The report was based on the first
large-scale random sample of elderly abuse. The researchers found
that although some elderly abuse is
inflicted by emotionally disturbed or
violent family members, the typical
abuser is a spouse who depends
on the victim for money, transportation, housing, and household re-
pairs.   □ Bruce Bower

In the Special Reports section,
see No Need to Panic. In World
Book, see Child abuse; Mental illness; Schizophrenia.

Nutrition and Food

A diet rich in fruits may reduce a
person's risk of developing *oral
cancer* (cancer of the mouth and
throat). That finding was reported in
October 1988 by researcher Joseph
K. McLaughlin and his colleagues at
the National Cancer Institute (NCI)
in Bethesda, Md. The study involved
interviewing 871 people who had
oral cancer and 979 people who
were free of the disease to determine how much fruit they included
in their daily diet during their life-
times.

Those people who ate fruit regularly had half the risk of developing
cancer as those who ate fruits infre-

quently. Fruit also appeared to protect against oral cancer even
among those people in the study
who smoked or drank alcohol
heavily—habits that increase the
risk for oral cancer.

Although other scientific studies
have indicated that vitamin C and
beta-carotene (a nutrient that the
body converts into vitamin A) may
reduce the risk of this disease,
McLaughlin found that these nutrients had little or no protective effect
in the study. He suggested that
chewing raw fruits may simply clean
the mouth of potential cancer-
causing substances or that fruits

School lunches
School lunches are too
high in fat, sugar, and salt,
charged an August 1988
report by the Public Voice
for Food and Health, a
Washington, D.C.-based
consumer group. The U.S.
Department of Agriculture
rejected the group's call
for setting specific limits
on these substances in
school lunches, citing a
lack of studies indicating
what amounts are appro-
priate for growing children.

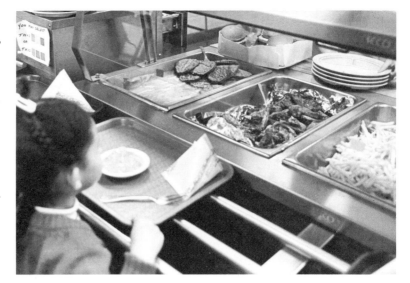

may contain some chemical compounds that help inhibit cancer.

Move over, oat bran. Researchers at the United States Department of Agriculture in Albany, Calif., reported in March 1989 that rice bran may reduce levels of *cholesterol* (a fatlike substance) in the blood at least as well as oat bran. Bran is the fiber-rich outer coat of cereal grain kernels that is usually removed when grain is milled.

In the study, the scientists fed one group of hamsters a diet in which rice bran was the only source of fiber, while another group of hamsters were fed a diet containing *cellulose*, a type of fiber that does not affect cholesterol levels. They found that the hamsters that were fed the rice bran had as much as a 32 per cent reduction in blood cholesterol levels, compared with hamsters on the other diet. High blood cholesterol has been linked with heart disease.

Rice bran—like oat bran—is rich in *soluble fiber*, a type of dietary fiber that dissolves in water. Studies have found that a diet high in soluble fiber seems to reduce the risk of heart attack by lowering the level of blood cholesterol.

Vitamin E and health. Scientists gathered at a conference sponsored by the New York Academy of Sciences in New York City in the fall of 1988 to discuss the latest findings on the health benefits of vitamin E. At the meeting, researchers from the University of Western Ontario in London, Canada, reported that vitamin E may help decrease a person's risk of developing *cataracts*. Cataracts, the clouding of the eye's natural lens, is one of the leading causes of blindness in the United States.

In the study, 350 adults were asked about vitamin E intake. Half of the adults had cataracts; the rest showed no signs of the disorder. According to the researchers, those people who took vitamin E supplements reduced their risk of developing cataracts by at least 50 per cent, compared with those who did

Drawing by D. Reilly, © 1989 The New Yorker Magazine, Inc.

Wellness Update: Thirty-year-old man starting on the twenty-five-thousand-pound oat-bran muffin he must consume over forty years in order to reduce significantly his risk of death from high cholesterol

not take the supplement. The scientists suggested vitamin E may somehow inhibit chemical changes in the lens that lead to cataracts.

Vitamin E and smoking. Researchers from the Rowett Research Institute in Aberdeen, Scotland, reported at the New York City conference that vitamin E may help counteract the effects of *free radicals* (molecules that are highly reactive chemically) found in cigarette smoke. Free radicals can react violently with other molecules in cells and have been linked to cancer and heart disease, illnesses for which smokers are at high risk.

In the study, 20 male smokers

The Milk of Human Illness

Milk has been called the "perfect" food—high in protein, calcium, and vitamins. But for some 30 million people in the United States, milk can bring little gain and much pain, in the form of abdominal cramps, gas, and diarrhea.

In fact, up to three-fourths of the world's adults have little or no ability to digest *lactose*, the sugar in milk. This condition, called *lactose intolerance*, is normal for most people of African, Asian, American Indian, and Latin-American descent, and also for many Europeans—especially those with roots in Eastern Europe or the Mediterranean.

Infants worldwide are able to digest milk because their intestines produce the enzyme *lactase*, which breaks lactose into parts that can be absorbed by the body. After infancy, lactase production gradually declines. In some people, it nearly stops altogether.

When people consume more milk than their supply of lactase can handle, bacteria in the digestive tract feed on the undigested lactose, producing gas and acids—and discomfort. The severity of the symptoms varies widely among individuals, depending on how much lactase they produce and how much lactose they consume in a given period of time. Symptoms may first appear as early as age 2 or as late as adulthood.

Lactase production may also drop temporarily or permanently from such causes as illness (including bowel disease or malnutrition), surgery in the digestive tract, radiation therapy, or use of antibiotics or other medications. Lactose intolerance, however, is not the same as milk allergy, a sensitivity to milk protein most common in young children.

Until the 1960's, lactose intolerance was considered rare because researchers had based their studies mostly on white Americans. These people usually descended from northern and western Europeans—virtually the only peoples in the world that retain much of their ability to digest lactose.

In turn, many doctors today are unaccustomed to looking for lactose intolerance and may fail to recognize it. Also, because many people drink less milk as they get older, adults who have lost some of their tolerance might show symptoms only rarely and may not see a connection to milk.

If you have frequent gas, cramps, or diarrhea, you might ask your doctor to test you for lactose intolerance. One test involves checking your breath for a high hydrogen content, which indicates poor lactose absorption. But the easiest test is just to eliminate all milk products from your diet for a few days and see if the symptoms clear up—and if they recur after you drink milk.

The inability to digest much milk is not a problem in most parts of the world, since most cuisines use little or no milk. But in America, milk is considered essential to a good diet and is used routinely in cooking and food manufacturing. Cooking food does not alter the lactose content.

Fortunately, most lactose-intolerant people can handle some lactose. The simplest way to avoid symptoms is to learn your own limits and adjust your diet accordingly.

All milk products—including all fluid milks, dry milk, cream, butter, cheese, sour cream, yogurt, and ice cream—contain lactose. Eggs, though often classed as a dairy product, have no lactose.

Milk products are common ingredients in breads, dressings, mixes, processed foods, and diet formulas. Check food labels not only for milk, but also for *whey* (the watery part of milk that separates in souring or cheesemaking). Some manufacturers label their foods in accordance with Jewish dietary laws, which restrict the use of milk; foods marked *pareve* or *parve* are milk-free.

Lactose is an inactive ingredient in some medicines. Your pharmacist can tell you whether a drug contains lac-

Lactose content of some dairy foods*	
Milks (1 cup or 244 g):	
Whole	11.4 g
Lowfat (2%)	11.7 g
Skim	11.9 g
Cheeses (1 ounce or 28 g):	
Brie	0.1 g
Cheddar	0.4 g
American	0.5 g
Blue	0.7 g
Mozzarella (part skim)	0.8 g
Processed spread	2.5 g
Other dairy products:	
Butter (1 stick or 113 g)	0.1 g
Light cream (1 cup or 240 g)	8.8 g
Lowfat cottage cheese (1 cup or 226 g)	8.2 g
*In grams (g)	
Source: U.S. Department of Agriculture.	

tose. Lactose may also be absorbed into the digestive tract from inhaled medicines used for asthma and other respiratory diseases.

Some milk products are easier to tolerate than others. Cup for cup, cream contains less lactose than milk because a larger proportion of cream is fat. Thus, butter—which is made from cream—may have less lactose than margarine, which often contains nonfat milk. Only a few brands of margarine are milk-free.

Cheese has less lactose than the milk it came from because the bacterial activity that creates cheese breaks down some of the lactose. The longer the cheese ripens, the more lactose is broken down. Thus, most aged cheeses (such as cheddar) have less lactose than most young cheeses (such as ricotta). Aged cheeses with a high fat content, such as brie, have the least lactose of all.

Active-culture yogurt may be easily tolerated because it contains live bacteria that may continue to break down lactose in the digestive tract. In addition, some studies suggest that eating yogurt daily may increase a person's tolerance of lactose. Most frozen yogurt, however, has no live cultures and thus no such advantages.

Special lactose-reduced milk products are sold under the brand name Lactaid. The same company also produces lactase enzyme in liquid form, which you can use to treat milk at home, and lactase tablets, which can be taken with milk products to aid lactose digestion.   ☐ Robin Guldman

and 20 male nonsmokers were given either 1,000 milligrams of vitamin E or a *placebo* (inactive substance) every day for two weeks. When the researchers examined the subjects' blood cells, they discovered that the cells of those smokers who did not take the vitamin E supplement appeared more vulnerable to damage by free radicals than the cells of either the smokers taking the vitamin or the nonsmokers.

Vitamin E and immunity. Researchers from Colorado State University in Fort Collins and Tufts University School of Medicine in Boston suggested that vitamin E may help the immune system of elderly people fight off bacterial or viral infections. In their study, the researchers gave 34 healthy people over 60 years old a vitamin E supplement or a placebo each day.

The researchers then studied the responsiveness of each volunteer's immune system. To do this, they injected small amounts of a foreign substance under the skin to see the activity of the volunteer's *lymphocytes*—white blood cells that are part of the immune system. (Some lymphocytes fight infections by producing *antibodies*, proteins that attack infectious organisms or foreign substances; other lymphocytes attack such organisms or substances directly.)

The researchers also added foreign substances to blood samples taken from the volunteers to simulate what might happen if a lymphocyte came in contact with a disease-causing organism. In both tests, the lymphocytes of the volunteers who received vitamin E had a better response than the lymphocytes of the volunteers who received the placebo.

Onions fight cancer? Onions may help protect against stomach cancer, according to an NCI study published in January 1989. The study, conducted in China, found that a diet rich in onions, garlic, leeks, chives, and scallions may reduce the risk of stomach cancer by as much as 40 per cent.

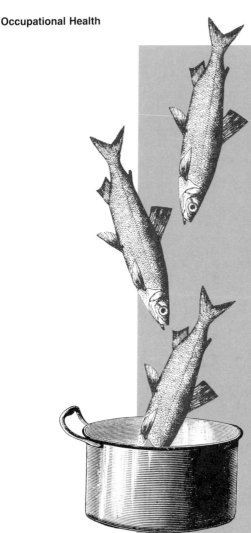

A fish tale

The next time you are about to bite into that tempting bit of sushi, consider what happened to a man in New York City. His story, as reported in the April 27, 1989, issue of *The New England Journal of Medicine*, may make you think twice about eating raw fish.

According to the *Journal*, the man went to the hospital with severe abdominal pain and was diagnosed as having appendicitis. Hours later, doctors operated with the expectation of finding and removing an inflamed appendix.

Imagine the operating team's surprise when they discovered that their patient's appendix was normal. Imagine their even greater surprise when they noticed a 1.6-inch (4.1-centimeter) reddish-brown worm moving onto the surgical drapes that surrounded the incision.

After surgery, questions about the patient's recent dining habits revealed the apparent source of the worm: raw fish served by a friend. Although the man recovered, his experience is a graphic warning of the potential hazard of eating raw fish. Salmon, cod, and other fish are often infected with worms. Fish that is properly cooked or frozen is generally safe, but people who eat fish raw may get more than they bargain for.

If a person ingests a worm, it may be killed during digestion. In some cases, like that of the New York man, the worm may stay in the digestive tract, producing symptoms similar to that of an ulcer or appendicitis.

Usually, such a wormy encounter won't cause death—but it can be very unpleasant. Sushi eaters beware!

Occupational Health
See Safety

Nutrition and Food (cont.)

The NCI study compared the diets of people who had stomach cancer with people who did not have the disease. The researchers found that the people who were free of cancer ate significantly larger quantities of these vegetables than those who had stomach cancer. The researchers also determined that the risk of stomach cancer declined the longer a person followed a diet high in onions and garlic. The people in the study who did not have cancer had been eating these vegetables regularly since childhood.

Healthier milk? In April 1989, food engineers at Cornell University in Ithaca, N.Y., reported that they had refined a technique called *supercritical fluid extraction* to produce milk that is 90 per cent cholesterol-free. In this process, milk fat is first separated from the rest of the milk. Then, under high pressure, carbon dioxide is forced through the milk fat. This separates the cholesterol-rich fat from the low-cholesterol fat. The low-cholesterol part is then put back into the milk. Although the technique can reduce the milk's cholesterol content, its overall fat content is not lowered. □ Jeanine Barone

In the Special Reports section, see MAKE MINE VEGETARIAN? In WORLD BOOK, see CHOLESTEROL; NUTRITION.

Most women who have given birth by *Caesarean section* should try to deliver vaginally in subsequent pregnancies, according to new guidelines issued in October 1988 by the American College of Obstetrics and Gynecology (ACOG). A Caesarean section is an operation to remove a baby from the uterus by cutting through the mother's abdominal and uterine walls.

In recommending subsequent vaginal delivery in the absence of medical complications as the preferred procedure, the guidelines officially reverse the long-standing practice of routinely performing a Caesarean section on women who have undergone the procedure once. Previously, the ACOG had urged doctors to consider subsequent vaginal delivery as an option.

About 25 per cent of the 3.8 million babies born in the United States each year are delivered by Caesarean section. About 33 per cent of these births are repeat Caesareans.

Although the Caesarean section is one of the safest surgical procedures, it nevertheless carries significant risks for both the mother and child. Women who undergo Caesarean section often develop infections. They are also two to four times as likely to die in childbirth as women who deliver vaginally. Babies born by Caesarean section have a greater chance of developing respiratory problems because the fluid in their lungs is not forced out by the contractions of the birth canal.

According to the ACOG, even women who have had two or more Caesarean sections should be encouraged to give birth vaginally if there are no medical complications. The ACOG estimates that from 50 to 80 per cent of women who have had a Caesarean section can successfully deliver vaginally in subsequent births.

Caesarean rate. The number of Caesarean sections performed in the United States reached a new high in 1987, but the rate of increase was the lowest since the mid-1970's, according to a study released in January 1989 by

the Public Citizen Health Research Group, a consumer advocacy group based in Washington, D.C. The group found that the percentage of Caesarean sections rose slightly in 1987, to 24.4 per cent of all births, from 24.1 per cent in 1986.

Despite the slowdown, the 1987 figure— representing about 934,000 Caesarean sections— was the highest ever reported. About 50 per cent of these procedures were unnecessary, the study concluded. The consumer group reported that these unnecessary procedures caused about 250,000 serious infections, forced patients to spend 1.1

Labor monitor
A device for detecting early signs of premature labor will register pressure changes in the uterus indicating contractions. A recorder worn over the shoulder transmits the information by telephone to the doctor. Early warning allows the doctor to stop the contractions with drugs.

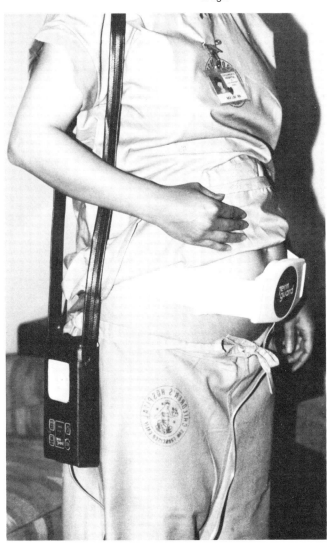

High-tech fertilization
Technicians freeze eggs and sperm for storage at a laboratory specializing in *in vitro fertilization* (IVF), a procedure in which sperm and egg are united outside a woman's body. More than 5,000 babies conceived by IVF have been born in the United States since the late 1970's. But the procedure remains expensive and even top-rated IVF clinics have success rates of only 17 per cent or less.

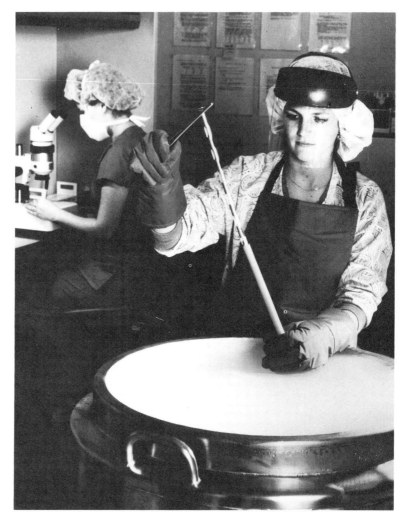

Pregnancy and Childbirth (cont.)
million extra days in the hospital, and cost more than $1 billion.

Screening for Down's syndrome.
A new prenatal screening method involving blood tests, described in a study reported in October 1988, may be an important advance in screening large numbers of pregnant women to determine if their fetuses have Down's syndrome. About 5,000 babies are born in the United States each year with Down's syndrome, the leading genetic cause of mental retardation.

The two tests currently used to identify fetuses with the disorder—amniocentesis and chorionic villus sampling—require the insertion of a needle or *catheter* (tube) into the uterus and carry a small risk of miscarriage. The tests are thus usually recommended only for women over age 35 and others considered at risk for bearing a child with Down's syndrome.

Although for any individual woman the odds of having a child with Down's syndrome increase with age—especially after age 35—about 80 per cent of children with the disorder are born to women under age 35. These younger women are typically not screened.

The new screening method, developed by researchers in the United States and Great Britain, involves measuring the levels of three

Pregnancy and Childbirth (cont.)
proteins produced by the fetus and found in the mother's blood. At about 16 weeks, the researchers found, fetuses with Down's syndrome produce abnormally high levels of two of the proteins and abnormally small amounts of the third.

To calculate the risk that the fetus has the syndrome, the blood test results and the mother's age are analyzed by computer according to a mathematical model developed by the researchers. If the risk is high, women may choose to have an amniocentesis to confirm the results. If the risk is low, however, women—especially older women, who are more likely to miscarry—may choose not to endanger the fetus by undergoing the invasive test.

Circumcision benefits? Circumcision has "potential medical benefits and advantages," the American Academy of Pediatrics reported for the first time in October 1988. According to the academy, the procedure may protect against infections of the urinary tract and kidneys.

The statement departs from the academy's previous position on circumcision, expressed in a 1971 statement, that "there are no valid medical reasons" for routinely circumcising newborns. The 1988 report stopped short of recommending the procedure, however.

Circumcision, the most common surgical procedure performed on males in the United States, involves removing the foreskin of the penis. Since 1971, the number of circumcisions performed in the United States has fallen, partly because of the academy's previous position on the procedure. In 1979, for example, 79 per cent of newborn boys were circumcised, compared with 95 per cent in the 1960's. By 1987, the percentage had fallen to 59.5 per cent, or about 1 million per year.

The academy's new position is based on research by pediatrician Thomas E. Wiswell of the Brooke Army Medical Center at Fort Sam Houston, Texas. In several studies involving more than 400,000 infants, Wiswell found that uncircumcised boys were 10 times more likely to develop infections of the urinary tract during their first year than were circumcised boys.

The academy noted, however, that the procedure also carries "disadvantages and risks." In addition, the academy reported that independent experts who reviewed Wiswell's studies suggested that the way in which he collected his data might have unintentionally biased the results. Therefore, the academy said, it considered the findings "tentative." ☐ Barbara Mayes

See also ALCOHOL AND DRUG ABUSE. In WORLD BOOK, see CHILDBIRTH.

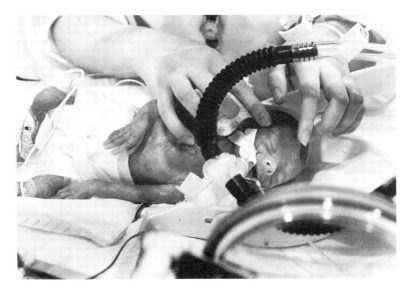

Milk with a boost
A premature infant receives a fortified version of breast milk developed at the Children's Nutrition Research Center in Houston. The new recipe combines the immune properties normally found in mother's milk that protect against infection, with the concentrated nutrients found in the cow's-milk formula usually fed to premature babies. A key ingredient in the new formula is minerals vital for healthy lungs and bones.

Respiratory System

Health kick
Aerobic dance can improve the stamina of asthma sufferers by strengthening muscles critical to breathing, according to a November 1988 report on a program in the United States called Aerobics for Asthmatics.

International trends in deaths due to asthma were reported in the November 1988 issue of the journal *Chest*. A group of New Zealand physicians investigated these trends in response to an increase in asthma-related deaths in New Zealand during the late 1970's.

The investigation covered the years from 1970 to 1985 and included data from 15 countries. New Zealand's death rate due to asthma had skyrocketed from 1.3 per 100,000 people in 1974 to 4.2 per 100,000 in 1979. Over the next six years, however, the rate had declined, with 1.85 deaths per 100,000

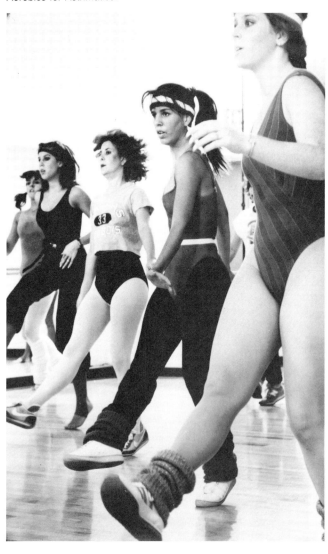

reported in 1985. Asthma death rates among the 14 other countries varied greatly, with most of the countries reporting a gradual increase during the study period. In the Special Reports section, see LIVING WITH ASTHMA.

Cigarette smoking continued to play a major role in the development of life-shortening diseases. The Centers for Disease Control (CDC) in Atlanta, Ga., said in its Nov. 18, 1988, *Morbidity and Mortality Weekly Report* that in 1985 cigarette smoking caused more than 314,000 deaths in the United States. Two-thirds of the victims were men.

The CDC calculated that these smoking-related deaths resulted in the loss of about 3.6 million years of life, or about 11½ years per victim. The statistics indicated that smoking remained the most common cause of premature death in the United States.

Three articles in the Jan. 6, 1989, issue of *The Journal of the American Medical Association* discussed trends in cigarette smoking in the United States. The articles, from the Office on Smoking and Health in the CDC's Center for Chronic Disease Prevention and Health Promotion, said that smoking was decreasing in all race and gender groups.

The decline was slower among women than men. In addition, more young women than young men were starting to smoke. This difference in start-smoking rates is responsible for a previously noted narrowing of the "gender gap" in smoking. In 1986, 33 per cent of U.S. men smoked, compared with 28 per cent of U.S. women—but the women are catching up.

Smoking in the year 2000. The CDC authors predicted that, in the year 2000, 22 per cent of United States adults, or about 40 million Americans, will be smokers. The major contributor to differences in percentages of smokers between various groups will be differences in education. The CDC researchers

Respiratory System (cont.)

estimate that 30 per cent of people with a high school education or less will smoke, compared with 10 per cent of adults with more than a high school education.

Diagnostic technique reviewed.

Lung-disease specialists in Rochester, N.Y., reported in the April 1989 issue of *Chest* on their evaluation of a well-established technique for diagnosing the cause of chronic cough. The technique, developed in 1981 by Richard S. Irwin and his associates at the University of Massachusetts in Worcester, is known as the *anatomic, diagnostic proto-*

col. Using this technique, several groups of physicians had reported that they could consistently determine the cause of the cough and decide upon an effective treatment. Of the patients who followed the prescribed therapy, Irwin reported, 97 per cent were cured of their cough.

In the recent evaluation, Robert H. Poe and colleagues at Highland and St. Mary's hospitals and the University of Rochester School of Medicine and Dentistry studied the use of the diagnostic method on 139 consecutive patients referred to lung specialists at the two hospitals. The Rochester investigators diag-

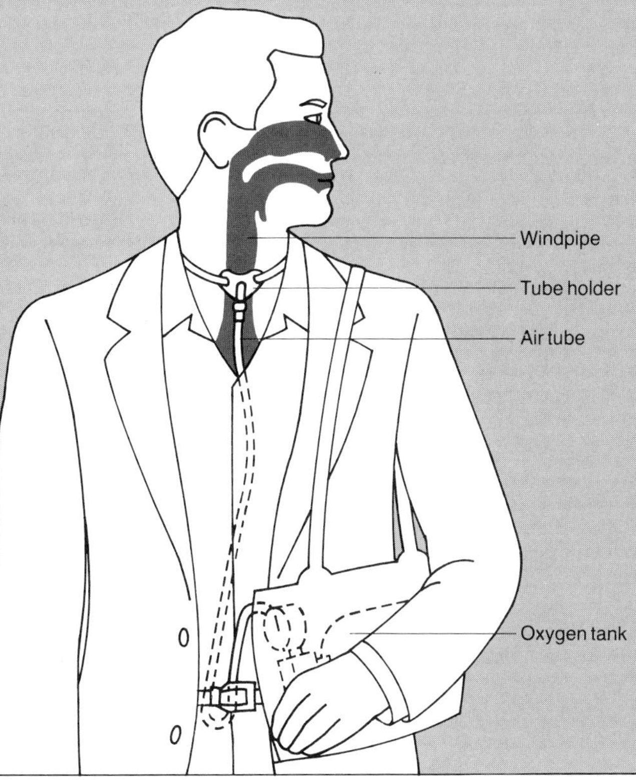

Easier breathing for patients on oxygen therapy
The Micro-Trach air tube delivers bottled oxygen through a tiny hole pierced in the throat, enabling patients to breathe more easily than they do through tubes that deliver oxygen via the nostrils. The developer of this new device is Henry J. Heimlich, a chest surgeon at Xavier University in Cincinnati, Ohio, and originator of the *Heimlich maneuver,* a first-aid technique for people who are choking.

Windpipe
Tube holder
Air tube
Oxygen tank

Respiratory System (cont.)

nosed the specific cause of the cough only 88 per cent of the time, even after running extensive diagnostic tests. Their success rate after long-term treatment was 87 per cent. Patients who did not respond well included individuals who did not follow the prescribed therapy, people who continued to smoke, and those with chronic bronchitis.

Detecting lung cancer. Doctors may be able to detect lung cancer by testing a patient's *blood serum* (the clear, fluid part of the blood). This diagnostic advance was reported in the December 1988 issue of the *American Review of Respiratory Diseases* by physicians Brian S. Schepart and Mitchell L. Margolis of the Medical College of Pennsylvania in Philadelphia and the Philadelphia Veterans Administration Medical Center.

Schepart and Margolis tested the serum with laboratory-produced proteins called *monoclonal antibodies*. Natural antibodies are produced by the body's immune system to help destroy germs and cancer cells. They recognize and attach to these "foreign invaders" by means of identifying molecules on the invaders called antigens. In the tests, the monoclonal antibodies made by Schepart and Margolis attached to one type of antigen produced by lung cancer cells.

The researchers performed the test on serum from 61 patients under the care of lung specialists at the Veterans Administration Medical Center. Monoclonal antibodies attached to antigens in the serum of 12 of 18 patients diagnosed as having lung cancer.

Eight patients had *false positive* results. (A false positive result incorrectly indicates that the substance being tested for—in this case, lung cancer cells—is present.) Two of the false positives were in patients who had cancerous tumors elsewhere in their bodies. One patient who was thought to have a false positive reaction because his chest X ray was normal turned out to have a small cancerous lung tumor.

Because lung cancers that have not yet entered advanced stages produce antigens that can be detected in the blood, this test promises to have a tremendous impact on the ability to discover cancers at an early stage, to monitor patients' response to therapy, and to detect recurrences of cancer. It is still too early to use this test in routine physical examinations.

□ Robert A. Balk

In the Special Reports section, see THE GREAT WHITE PLAGUE: A HISTORY of TB. In WORLD BOOK, see LUNG; SMOKING.

Safety

A major study of school bus safety issued on May 8, 1989, recommended against requiring the installation of seat belts in the 390,000 school buses in the United States. The study, conducted by the National Academy of Sciences (NAS) at the request of Congress, found that other measures would be more effective and less costly in protecting the 25 million children who ride school buses each day. Among the measures, the study suggested raising the height of school bus seat backs from the standard 20 inches (51 centimeters) to 24 inches (61 centimeters) to provide extra protection in the event of a crash.

Requiring seat belts on all school buses would cost $40 million per year and prevent 1 death and several dozen serious injuries, the study said. In contrast, raising seat-back heights would cost only $6 million per year and prevent 3 deaths and about 95 serious injuries.

The study found that 10 children are killed each year while in a moving bus. About 40 children, however, are killed while trying to board or leave a bus. Many of these victims are struck by their own school bus. To prevent such accidents, the study recommended better training of school bus drivers and better safety instruction for students.

Safety (cont.)

The NAS study also strongly recommended that school districts operating buses built before 1977 replace them with newer models as rapidly as possible. Pre-1977 buses lack a variety of safety features, the study noted.

Buckling up works. Automobile safety belts received a strong endorsement from the first study to use medical data to evaluate their effectiveness. The study, reported in December 1988, was conducted by researchers at the University of Illinois in Chicago and other institutions.

The researchers found that among 1,364 accident victims, seat belts reduced the severity of injury by 60 per cent, hospital admissions by 65 per cent, and hospital costs by 66 per cent. Previous evidence about the importance of wearing seat belts was based on police records.

Keeping kids safe. United States Surgeon General C. Everett Koop in February 1989 urged a nationwide effort to prevent childhood accidents, the leading cause of death among children. Koop said that preventable injuries kill more children than all childhood diseases com-

A cat with a cause
Casual T. Cat warns parents about the dangers of childhood accidents in a 30-second public service television announcement released by the American Academy of Pediatrics in May 1989.

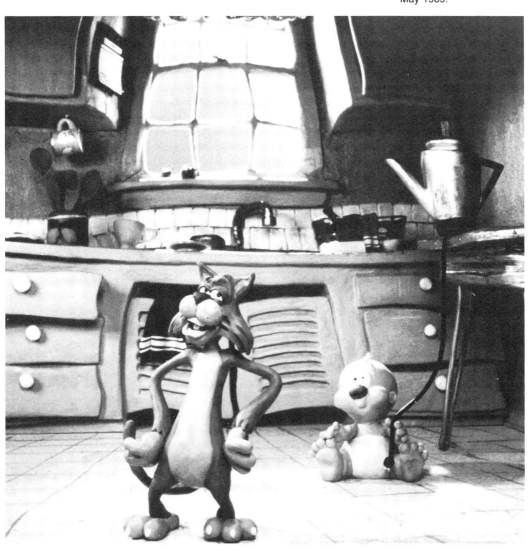

Food Fears

The public's confidence in the safety of apples and other fresh fruit and vegetables grown in the United States was seriously shaken in February 1989. That month, the U.S. Environmental Protection Agency (EPA) and the Natural Resources Defense Council (NRDC), a Washington, D.C.-based consumer group, made separate announcements about the potential hazards of pesticide residues on some of these foods.

On February 1, the EPA said it planned to speed up the process to ban a suspected cancer-causing chemical called *daminozide*. The chemical, sold under the trade name Alar, is sprayed on red apples and other fruits grown in the United States to give them a fresh and uniformly ripe appearance. Although the EPA initially said that only 5 per cent of the U.S. apple crop is treated with Alar, the agency later reported that the figure actually may be closer to 15 per cent.

According to the EPA, 5 out of every 100,000 people exposed to Alar during their lifetime run the risk of developing cancer. The NRDC said the threat is higher for children, who eat more apples and processed apple products, such as applesauce, than for adults. Although preliminary tests indicated that Alar poses a cancer risk, the EPA said the risk level was not great enough to ban the chemical until tests show conclusively that Alar is an imminent health hazard.

The EPA's action drew strong criticism from consumer advocates and environmental-ists who said the agency should withdraw the chemical immediately from the market. Concern over Alar was so great that some parents and school administrators stopped serving apples and apple products to children at home and in school cafeterias. In June, Alar's manufacturer, Uniroyal Chemical Company Incorporated of Middlebury, Conn., responded to the outcry by voluntarily halting U.S. sales of the chemical.

The EPA's Alar announcement was followed on February 20 by the release of a two-year NRDC study on children's dietary exposure to pesticides. The study, which focused on the chemical residues found on 27 foods most frequently eaten by children, said that at least 5 out of every 20,000 people may develop cancer as a result of exposure to pesticides before age 6. The study said that more than 6,000 preschool children today may develop cancer because of pesticide residues.

The EPA quickly responded to the NRDC's findings, stating that the study exaggerated the potential hazard to children by as much as 10 times, and that it used out-of-date government pesticide data. The EPA said that pesticide residues pose little health hazard because the amounts of pesticide residue permitted on foods are well below what is considered dangerous. The agency added that it already takes into account the higher exposure children may have to pesticides when setting residue limits.

Although pesticides can be dangerous if used improperly, many scientists agree with the EPA that pesticides are present in foods in such small amounts that they do not pose a serious health threat—even

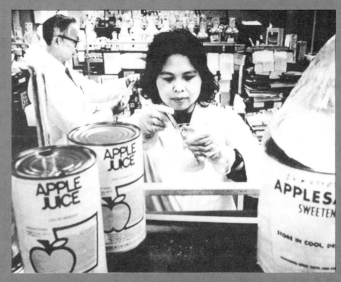

A chemist tests apple products for the chemical Alar in 1989.

to children. In fact, some say that people run a much greater risk of developing cancer and other serious diseases from smoking, drinking alcohol, and eating a diet that is high in animal fats.

The nationwide concern about food safety renewed debate about how pesticides are regulated and monitored. The EPA sets allowable pesticide residue levels in food, and licenses the use of more than 45,000 pesticides and other chemicals. It falls to the U.S. Food and Drug Administration (FDA) and to the 50 states to enforce these regulations.

Some critics suggest that the federal government should strengthen its regulatory standards on pesticides. The NRDC called for the FDA to routinely monitor more pesticides and said that the EPA should move more quickly to ban potentially dangerous chemicals.

There are some steps consumers can take to reduce their exposure to pesticide residues. Experts recommend buying only domestically grown produce or fruits and vegetables that are grown *organically* (without the use of pesticides or other chemicals). They also suggest rinsing all produce thoroughly with water and peeling or removing skins or outer leaves before eating. Cooking produce also eliminates some residues.

The debate over pesticides is far from over. But health experts generally agree that the confusion should not stop Americans from eating fresh fruits and vegetables, which contribute to good health.

☐ Mary Krier

Safety (cont.)
bined. About 8,000 children under age 14 die each year in accidents, and about 50,000 are permanently disabled.

The leading causes of accidental death among children are automobile and bicycle accidents, drowning, fires, and burns. Koop, who served as honorary chairman of the National Safe Kids Campaign, said adults must ensure a safe home environment for children. National Safe Kids is an organization of civic and health groups that are trying to reduce childhood accidents through public education.

Fruit scare. Fresh fruit imported from Chile disappeared temporarily from grocery stores in March 1989 after federal health inspectors discovered traces of cyanide in two seedless red grapes imported from the South American country. Although the amount of cyanide was too small to harm a child, the U.S. Food and Drug Administration (FDA) advised consumers to discard all fruit from Chile and on March 13 imposed a quarantine on imports of Chilean fruit.

Chile supplies virtually all of the grapes sold in the United States during the winter, as well as nectarines, plums, and other fruit. Government officials in Chile blamed terrorists for the sabotage. The FDA lifted the quarantine on March 17 after inspections of Chilean fruit showed no further contamination.

Helmets for bicyclists. Researchers at the University of Washington School of Medicine in Seattle, and other institutions, reported on May 25, 1989, that bicycle safety helmets could substantially reduce the risk of head injury among America's 85 million bicyclists. The study found that wearing helmets reduces risk of serious head injury by 85 per cent. Head injuries are the main cause of death in about 80 per cent of the 1,300 biking fatalities that occur annually.

Air safety. Lapses in security and accidents involving aging aircraft caused a surge in public concern

Safety

Fruit scare

A grocery store posts a sign to reassure shoppers that its fruit is not from Chile after federal health inspectors found traces of cyanide in two seedless grapes imported from the South American country on March 13, 1989.

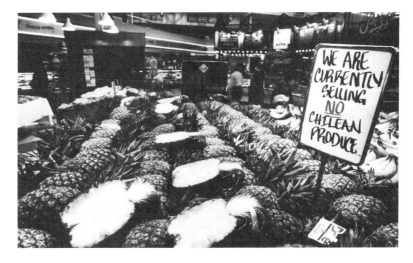

It's in the bag

A technician adjusts the position of a mannequin during a test of passenger-side airbags for automobiles. Airbags on the driver side became a standard safety feature of many 1990 model cars introduced by U.S. automakers in September 1989.

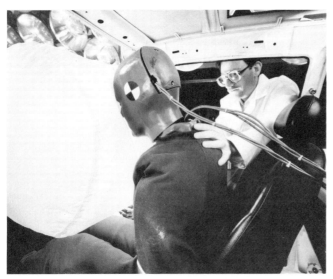

Safety (cont.)

about the safety of air transportation during 1988 and 1989. On Dec. 21, 1988, a Pan American World Airways jetliner flying from London to New York City exploded and crashed into the village of Lockerbie in southwestern Scotland, killing 270 people. Investigators blamed the crash on a terrorist bomb made from a plastic explosive that could not be seen on airport X-ray screening devices.

The bombing led to stricter security rules at airports around the world. On April 3, 1989, the U.S. Federal Aviation Administration (FAA) said it would install up to 100 new bomb screening devices that can detect plastic explosives at dozens of airports in the United States and other countries. The FAA also decided to require airlines to buy more effective conventional X-ray detectors.

But the agency said it would not issue public warnings of terrorist threats against airlines. Relatives of victims of the Lockerbie crash had requested that such warnings be given. They argued that passengers should have the right to decide whether to ignore a bomb threat or choose a different airline. The FAA, however, said that public warnings make it more difficult to investigate terrorist threats.

Aging aircraft. The FAA on May 18, 1989, ordered airlines to make major modifications in older Boeing 727, 737, and 747 aircraft. The new practices were adopted as a result of a spectacular accident on April 28, 1988, in which an Aloha Airlines Boeing 737 jet lost part of the top of its *fuselage* (body) while flying over Hawaii. On May 23, 1989, the NTSB blamed Aloha Airlines for the accident. The board criticized Aloha's inspection and maintenance program for failing to detect cracks caused by metal fatigue in the 19-year-old jet.

This incident had been followed by several others. In one, which occurred on Feb. 24, 1989, nine pas-

Safety (cont.)

sengers died when they were sucked through a hole that opened in the fuselage of an 18-year-old United Airlines Boeing 747 jet flying over the Pacific Ocean. Investigators blamed the accident on failure of a cargo bay door. Also, a 15-year-old United Airlines jet with a disabled hydraulic system—crucial equipment needed for maneuvering the plane—crashed in Sioux City, Iowa, on July 19. At least 112 people died.

The new FAA order requires stricter procedures for ensuring the safety of older aircraft. Previously, airlines were expected to periodically inspect jetliners for cracks, corrosion, and other problems and to replace any components found defective. The new approach sets an age limit on aircraft parts considered critical for safety.

Cutting collisions. A long debate between the airline industry and the U.S. government over the need for collision warning devices ended on Jan. 5, 1989, when the FAA ordered all commercial aircraft to install the devices by December 1991.

The FAA's action resulted from a 1986 midair collision over Cerritos, Calif., that killed 82 people and from numerous near-misses between jetliners and small planes. A collision device determines whether two planes are too close and then tells the jetliner's pilot to climb, descend, or maintain the same altitude to avoid a collision.

Job injuries rise. The U.S. Bureau of Labor Statistics on Nov. 15, 1988, reported the first increase in job-related injuries and illnesses since 1984. The bureau said that more than 6 million cases had occurred in 1987, including 351,000 more injuries and 53,000 more illnesses than in 1986. Americans in 1987 lost 48.8 million days of work because of job-related injuries, compared with 45.4 million in 1986.

Officials said that part of the increase was due to government action encouraging companies to report accidents and illnesses. The number of workers killed in occupational accidents decreased—from 3,610 in 1986 to 3,400 in 1987.

Toxin limits. On Jan. 13, 1989, the U.S. Occupational Safety and Health Administration (OSHA) issued regulations intended to protect about 21 million people exposed to toxic and hazardous substances in the workplace. The agency placed new limits on exposure to 164 substances and strengthened existing regulations on 212 others. The substances range from such well-known hazards as carbon monoxide and gasoline fumes to poisonous gases such as hydrogen cyanide. They include a number of potential hu-

Safer stairs

Wearing a padded suit to protect herself, a Georgia Institute of Technology researcher walks down a special staircase that will collapse when she blocks an electric eyebeam. A camera will record exactly how she falls. Researchers took such spills in 1988 and 1989 to gather information on how people hurt themselves on stairs. The data will be used to make stairs safer.

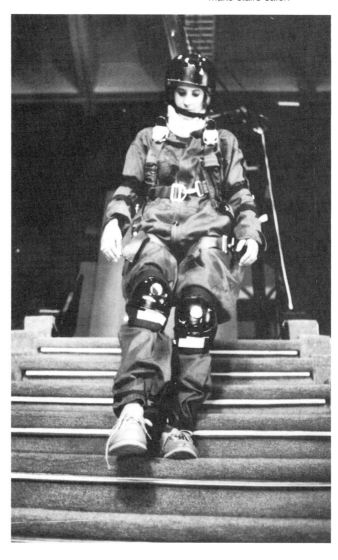

Safety (cont.)

man *carcinogens* (cancer-causing substances) and *mutagens* (agents that cause mutations).

The action was called the most far-reaching ever taken by OSHA, which in its 17-year history had issued regulations on only 24 substances. OSHA, which is part of the Department of Labor, estimated that the regulations would save 700 lives per year.

Drug tests stay. In what the federal government termed "a major contribution to railroad safety," the Supreme Court of the United States on March 21, 1989, ruled that engi-

neers and other railroad employees can be required to undergo tests for drug and alcohol use following accidents. The decision came in a suit brought by railroad unions, which objected to regulations issued in 1985 by the Federal Railroad Administration. The regulations required railroad crewmen involved in major accidents to provide blood and urine samples for drug testing.

☐ Michael Woods

In the People in Health Care section, see RESCUING YOUNG LIVES: INSIDE A TRAUMA CENTER. In WORLD BOOK, see SAFETY.

Sexually Transmitted Diseases

Pregnant women with a history of recurrent genital herpes infections rarely pass on the disease to their infants, according to research reported in 1988. Genital herpes infections during pregnancy are associated with complications and deaths in infants, but unless the pregnant woman is infected with herpes for the first time, she has a very low risk of passing on the infection to her infant.

There are several reasons why. For one, the *cervix*, the part of the uterus through which a baby passes at birth, is not frequently involved with recurrent infections, whereas it is commonly involved during first, or primary, infections. Second, the virus that causes genital herpes, herpes simplex type 2, is present in smaller amounts and for a shorter period of time during recurrent infections than during a primary infection. Finally, the presence of the mother's *antibodies* (disease-fighting proteins) against the virus probably protects against an infection of the infant.

These studies argue against routinely testing pregnant women for genital herpes in order to reduce the risk of herpes among infants. Instead, careful evaluation of a newborn baby is more effective in identifying early symptoms.

Herpes without symptoms. Reports from both the Centers for Disease Control (CDC) in Atlanta, Ga., and the University of Pittsburgh in Pennsylvania in 1988 and 1989 showed that the vast majority of individuals infected with herpes simplex virus type 2 say they had no symptoms. Based on a nationally representative sample of the population, researchers estimated that nearly 30 million Americans were infected with genital herpes viruses and that most were unaware of their infection.

Other evidence, however, suggested that truly *asymptomatic* (without symptoms) herpes is not as widespread as the study results indicated. Many infected patients apparently fail to recognize small ulcers as symptoms of genital herpes. In one study, for example, after infected women who reported no symptoms were taught how to recognize symptoms, about half of the women correctly identified ulcers or other signs of the infection during the next five months, according to researchers at the University of California at San Francisco and the University of Washington in Seattle.

The researchers noted that certain risk factors are associated with truly asymptomatic herpes, including a large number of sexual partners during a person's life, a history of sexually transmitted diseases, and past or present sexual partners

Sexually Transmitted Diseases (cont.)
with genital herpes. More than two-
thirds of those women who had evidence of asymptomatic herpes,
however, had no known risk factors.

Human papillomavirus (HPV) is a
sexually transmitted infection that
causes genital warts. Studies in
1988 and 1989 linked particular
strains of HPV with cervical cancer.
As a result, researchers have been
looking at newly developed tests
both to detect the presence of an
HPV infection and to identify the
particular strain of the virus responsible for the infection.

The virus often causes no symptoms. When symptoms do occur in
persons infected with HPV, they are
variable. In women, genital warts
may be visible on the *vulva* (the external part of the female genital organs) or hidden from view within the
vagina. When found on the cervix,
the warts are frequently microscopic
and can be best diagnosed with an
instrument known as a *colposcope*.
When men get genital warts, they
usually occur on the outer skin of
the penis.

Unfortunately, while warts can be
removed chemically, surgically, or
with lasers, they frequently recur.
The reported cure rate averages
only 20 per cent. Women with a history of HPV or genital warts should
receive annual Pap smears to reduce the risks of suffering serious
consequences from undiagnosed
cervical cancer.

New chlamydia approaches.
Chlamydia is the most common sexually transmitted disease in the
United States caused by bacteria.
But efforts to control chlamydia
have been hampered by the relative
difficulties of arriving at a diagnosis
and treatment.

In 1989, investigators reported
successful use of a doctor's office
test for chlamydia that may assist in
identifying and ultimately controlling
this bacteria. The new test was evaluated in 47 physicans' offices and
was more than 90 per cent accurate, compared with the same type
of test that is performed in a standard laboratory.

Generally, sexually active people
are considered at risk for chlamydia
if they are under 25, are pregnant,
have multiple sexual partners or
partners with genital symptoms, or
have had a new partner within the
last several months. Because of the
widespread nature of chlamydia,
people with certain symptoms—
including a noticeable cervical or
urethral discharge or bleeding
caused by swabbing the cervix—
should be tested.

□ Willard Cates, Jr.

In WORLD BOOK, see VENEREAL
DISEASE.

The facts about human papilloma virus

What it is: a highly contagious sexually transmitted virus. Some types of
the virus have been linked to cervical
cancer.

Symptoms: The only visible symptom
is genital warts, often appearing as tiny
whitish lumps, larger reddish-brown
lumps, or, more typically, cauliflower-
like growths. The warts usually appear
in and around the vagina and anus, on
the penis, or on the cervix. The virus
also causes growths that are invisible
to the naked eye. The types of the virus
that cause the invisible growths are
most strongly linked to cancer.

Treatment: Cryotherapy (freezing
unwanted tissue) with liquid nitrogen is
the preferred treatment for visible
warts. The underlying viral infection
cannot be cured. Women with cervical
warts should have regular Pap tests to
detect evidence of precancerous or
cancerous growths.

People infected with HPV in the United
States: **10 million to 20 million**

New cases of genital warts per year:
                 500,000 to 1 million

Number of U.S. women diagnosed with
cervical cancer per year: **16,000**

U.S. deaths from cervical cancer per
year: **7,000**

Source: Centers for Disease Control; American Cancer Society.

Skin

A drug that increases the normal rate of wound healing was successfully tested in human beings for the first time by researchers at the University of Louisville in Kentucky; Emory University in Atlanta, Ga.; and Vanderbilt University in Nashville. The research team, headed by biochemist Gregory L. Brown of the University of Louisville, reported their results in the July 13, 1989, issue of *The New England Journal of Medicine*.

The drug is a genetically engineered version of *epidermal growth factor*, a protein produced by the body to stimulate the growth of skin cells. Epidermal growth factor was first discovered in 1960, but tests to see if it could be used as a drug to speed healing were not possible until genetic engineering techniques made it possible to produce significant amounts of the protein.

Brown and his colleagues tested the drug in 12 adults who had areas of healthy skin removed from the thigh to cover wounds caused by severe burns or other injuries. In each patient, two identically sized patches of skin were taken from the thigh and transplanted to the injured areas. Every 12 hours, the researchers applied a cream containing a small quantity of epidermal growth factor to one of the areas on the thigh and applied a cream without the factor to the other area. Every day, the scientists took photographs of the areas and compared the rates of healing.

The skin grew at rates that varied from patient to patient, but in every one, the site treated with the growth factor healed more rapidly than the untreated site. On average, the skin healed 1½ days faster if treated with the growth factor. The researchers, who studied their patients for up to one year after treatment, found no side effects from the new drug.

The amount of growth factor used for the study was small, so there is a possibility that wounds treated with a larger dose of the drug may heal even more quickly. Even a small decrease in healing time is beneficial, however, because it translates into a decrease in the amount of time patients suffer pain. By late July 1989, further tests of the safety and effectiveness of this experimental drug—as well as other related growth factors—had begun.

Cutaneous T-cell lymphoma. A promising treatment for a type of cancer affecting the skin and other organs was described in August 1988 by dermatologist Richard L. Edelson of the Yale University School of Medicine in New Haven, Conn. Edelson, along with dermatologists at several universities in the United States and Europe, reported preliminary results in 1987. Their treatment helps patients with *cutaneous T-cell lymphoma*. This uncommon cancer affects T cells—a type of white blood cell—and is characterized by widespread skin lesions containing large numbers of these malignant T cells.

The treatment involves giving a patient a drug called *8-methoxypsoralen*, which occurs naturally in some fruits and vegetables. Cells that have taken in the drug can be damaged when they are exposed to light.

After the patient has swallowed the drug, some white blood cells are removed from the patient's bloodstream and irradiated with light of the ultraviolet A wavelength. This damages the cells containing 8-methoxypsoralen, which are then returned to the patients' bloodstream. The damaged cells "vaccinate" the patient by stimulating the immune system to destroy other abnormal white blood cells, including the cancerous T cells.

Edelson and his colleagues treated 37 patients who had not benefited from other treatments and were expected to survive less than three years. The skin lesions of 9 patients completely disappeared, and those of 18 other patients improved. Cancer in two of the patients was in complete remission—that is, the symptoms of the disease had disappeared—at least 29

Skin (cont.)

months after the treatment was stopped.

Such results are extraordinary with a disease for which there has been little other treatment. The therapy was approved by the FDA in 1988, and studies are now underway to determine the applicability of the technique to other cancers and other diseases.

Treatment for psoriasis. Cyclosporine, a drug widely used to prevent rejection of organ transplants, may be effective in the treatment of psoriasis, according to a report by dermatologists in the *British Journal of Dermatology* published in late 1988. Psoriasis is a chronic skin disease characterized by itchy, scaly red patches on the elbows, scalp, and other parts of the body. Cyclosporine is of special benefit to psoriasis patients who also have a form of arthritis associated with the disorder. The drug has been shown to cause dramatic improvement in both conditions.

To determine whether cyclosporine will have a permanent role in the treatment of psoriasis, however, the risks associated with its long-term use at low doses must be established. At the high doses typically given to transplant recipients, the drug can cause kidney damage and high blood pressure and increase the risk of cancer.

Port-wine stain birthmarks in young children can now be removed without scarring using a special type of laser, according to dermatologist Oon Tian Tan and colleagues at the Boston University Medical Center. Port-wine stain birthmarks, pink to purplish-red patches that usually occur on the face and neck, are caused by malformed blood vessels in the skin. The new procedure is a modification of the laser treatment used for adults with the birthmarks, which caused an unacceptable amount of scarring in children.

The Boston University dermatologists reported in February 1989 that the *tunable dye laser*, which can selectively destroy tissue of a partic-

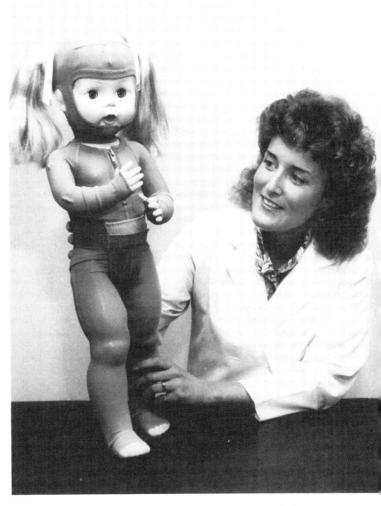

Suit for burn victims
A doll dressed in a special pressure suit that reduces scarring after severe burns is displayed by a representative of the company that makes the suit. The doll is used to help young students adjust to the changed appearance of a classmate recovering from burn injuries.

ular color, completely cleared the skin of 35 children with disfiguring port-wine stain birthmarks and caused scarring only if the treated area was accidentally injured after the procedure. The laser is tuned to emit a pulse of blue-green light that is absorbed by hemoglobin, a red substance in blood. As the hemoglobin absorbs the light, it becomes hot, destroying the malformed blood vessels but leaving other tissue unharmed.

☐ Tania J. Phillips and Jeffrey S. Dover

In the Special Reports section, see Treating the Severely Burned. In World Book, see Skin.

Smoking

Up in smoke

On March 1, 1989, R. J. Reynolds Tobacco Company pulled the plug on Premier, a smokeless cigarette. Premier was not a hit with smokers, who said it had an unpleasant taste and odor.

Smoking continues to be "the single most important preventable cause of death in our society," said United States Surgeon General C. Everett Koop on Jan. 11, 1989, the 25th anniversary of the U.S. government's first report on the health consequences of smoking. Koop marked the occasion by releasing the latest government report on smoking. That report noted that smoking takes more lives annually than had been thought. According to previous estimates, smoking killed about 300,000 Americans a year. But in 1985, the latest year for which figures are available, smoking was responsible for about 390,000 deaths, Koop said.

Since the first surgeon general's report was issued in 1964, there has been a considerable drop in the number of people who smoke. In 1965, 40 per cent of adults smoked. By 1987, that figure had dropped to 29 per cent.

Even so, as many as 55 million Americans still smoke, despite scientific evidence that the habit causes lung cancer and other illnesses. According to the 1989 report, smoking is most prevalent among blacks, blue-collar workers, and less-educated Americans.

Smokeless cigarette. In March 1989, the R. J. Reynolds Tobacco Company announced that its plans to market a "clean" cigarette had gone up in smoke. The company had introduced the cigarette—called Premier—in late 1988, billing it as a "virtually smokeless" cigarette that warmed rather than burned its tobacco and would not produce any ash or odor.

R. J. Reynolds spent more than $300 million to develop, manufacture, and advertise the product. But in marketing tests in Tucson, Ariz., and St. Louis, Mo., Premier failed miserably with smokers, who complained the cigarette gave off a plastic taste and a foul smell.

Critics of Premier also said that the cylinder inside the cigarette containing tobacco extracts and other flavoring could be packed with substances other than tobacco, such as crack, a highly addictive form of cocaine. Surgeon General Koop and several health organizations had insisted that Premier be classified as a drug-delivery system and be subjected to strict regulations by the U.S. Food and Drug Administration.

Cervical cancer link. Researchers at the University of Utah School of Medicine in Salt Lake City reported in March 1989 that women who smoke or who are exposed to *passive smoke*—the cigarette smoke

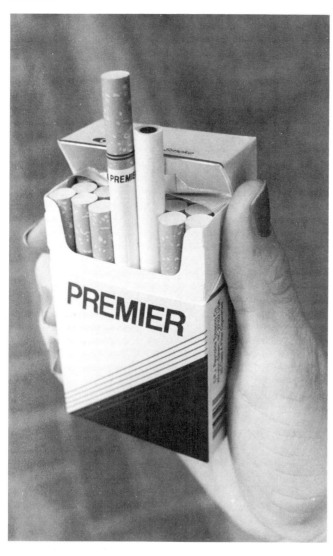

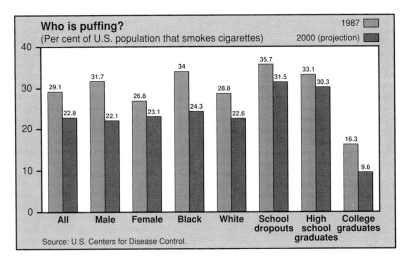

Who is puffing?
(Per cent of U.S. population that smokes cigarettes)

1987 □
2000 (projection) ■

	All	Male	Female	Black	White	School dropouts	High school graduates	College graduates
1987	29.1	31.7	26.8	34	28.8	35.7	33.1	16.3
2000	22.8	22.1	23.1	24.3	22.6	31.5	30.3	9.6

Source: U.S. Centers for Disease Control.

Fewer people in the United States will be lighting up cigarettes by the year 2000, according to a January 1989 report from the U.S. Centers for Disease Control in Atlanta, Ga. The greatest decrease in smoking will be among males and blacks, the report said.

Smoking (cont.)

that lingers in the air after it is exhaled by others—run a greater risk of developing cancer of the *cervix* (the narrow end of the uterus) than women who do not come in contact with smoke. Previous studies had demonstrated the connection between smoking and cervical cancer, but the Utah study broke new ground by examining the connection to passive smoke.

To best assess the effects of passive smoke, the researchers studied women who were members of a religious group that does not permit smoking. They found that women exposed to passive smoke for three or more hours a day were three times more likely to develop cervical cancer than those who did not encounter the smoke.

No safe cigarettes. Smokers who switch to so-called *low-yield* or *light* cigarettes are doing nothing to lessen their risk of heart attack, according to a study reported in June 1989 by researcher Julie R. Palmer at the Boston University School of Medicine. Low-yield cigarettes, which are popular among women, are advertised as being lower in tar and nicotine than other types of cigarettes.

In a study of more than 3,000 women, Palmer and her colleagues found that those who smoke low-yield cigarettes run the same risk of heart attack as those who smoke

regular brands. That risk is four times greater than for nonsmokers.

Hurting the heart. In January 1989, a group of Boston researchers found that heart disease patients who smoke are three times more likely to suffer chest pains and inadequate blood flow to the heart than nonsmokers. The researchers said the study gave the most direct evidence yet of the link between smoking and heart disease.

The researchers attached heart monitors to 24 smokers and to 41 nonsmokers; both groups were monitored 24 hours a day. The researchers found that smokers expe-

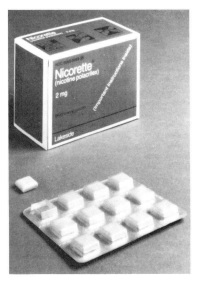

To chew or not to chew
A study released in March 1989 by researchers at the University of Vermont in Burlington raised doubt about the effectiveness of Nicorette, a nicotine gum that is prescribed by doctors to help people stop smoking.

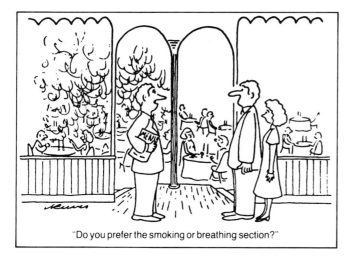

"Do you prefer the smoking or breathing section?"

WHR's—more fat around their waist than their hips—run a greater risk of developing these diseases.

The researchers were unable to explain the changes they saw in the weight and WHR of volunteers who stopped and then restarted smoking. They found that when volunteers gave up smoking, their weight increased more than their WHR. When volunteers restarted smoking, however, their weight decreased while their WHR increased.

It's never too late. A six-year study reported in November 1988 by researchers at the University of Washington in Seattle and the Mayo Clinic in Rochester, Minn., challenged the common notion that elderly people who quit smoking gain no significant health benefits over those who continue to smoke. The study compared 807 people aged 54 and older who quit smoking the previous year with 1,086 elderly people who continued the habit.

The death rate of those who kept smoking was 70 per cent higher than for those who stopped, the scientists reported. Among those over age 65 who stopped smoking, the death rate from heart attack dropped nearly 50 per cent.

□ William H. Allen
In WORLD BOOK, see SMOKING; TOBACCO.

Smoking (cont.)
rienced more—and longer—episodes of decreased blood supply to the heart than nonsmokers.

Where the fat is. Smoking can lead to a harmful redistribution of body fat that may make smokers more prone to heart disease and diabetes, according to a study reported in February 1989 by researchers at the National Institute on Aging in Bethesda, Md. The study, which involved 1,122 men, found that smokers had much larger waist-to-hip circumference ratios (WHR's) than nonsmokers. Studies have shown that people with high

Stroke

Two studies reported in 1989 indicate that ticlopidine, a recently developed drug, prevents strokes more effectively than aspirin. Like aspirin, ticlopidine inhibits blood clotting. Blood clots in the brain are a major cause of stroke.

In one study, reported in June, researchers in the United States and Canada set out in 1986 to determine whether ticlopidine can protect people who have had a minor stroke from having a more serious stroke or a heart attack. Ticlopidine was given to 525 of 1,053 patients who had suffered a recent minor stroke, and 528 received a *placebo*, a pill with no active ingredients.

During the three years of the

study, 15.3 per cent of the placebo group, but only 10.8 per cent of the ticlopidine group, had a stroke or heart attack or died of related causes each year. Those figures translated into a 30 per cent lower risk of stroke, heart attack, or death for those taking ticlopidine.

The other study, reported in February, began in 1981 and involved 3,069 patients at 55 U.S. medical centers. All the patients had either suffered a small stroke from which they had fully recovered or had experienced some of the warning signs of stroke, such as a temporary numbness or loss of vision.

Stroke (cont.)

The patients were randomly assigned to receive either ticlopidine or aspirin. The group taking ticlopidine had 21 per cent fewer strokes and 13 per cent fewer stroke deaths than did the group taking aspirin. The U.S. government has not yet approved the drug for sale.

Estrogen and stroke. The female hormone estrogen can protect women who have undergone *menopause* (cessation of menstruation, usually between the ages of 45 and 50) from stroke. That finding was reported in August 1988 by researchers at the University of Southern California in Los Angeles.

Beginning in 1981, the investigators mailed a health questionnaire to residents of a retirement community near Los Angeles. Questionnaire recipients were asked to give their medical history and to tell whether they took estrogen after menopause.

Over a six-year period, 8,807 women returned usable questionnaires. Of those women, 4,962 said they took estrogen. During the course of the study, 1,019 of the women died, 63 of them from strokes. Only 20 of those stroke deaths occurred among the women who had used estrogen.

Balloons for the brain. A new technique to prevent *intracranial vaso-spasms*, a common and deadly complication of strokes, was reported in November by a group of researchers at the University of California at San Francisco. Intracranial vasospasms are constrictions of blood vessels in the brain that often occur after strokes caused by brain *hemorrhage* (bleeding due to a ruptured blood vessel).

The San Francisco team used a technique called *subluminal angioplasty*, in which a hair-thin *catheter* (tube) is inserted into one of the large blood vessels in the groin and threaded up into the brain.

Once the catheter has reached a narrowed vessel, the physician inflates a tiny balloon attached to the catheter tip. The balloon expands the vessel walls as it is inflated. When the vessel has been restored to its normal diameter, the balloon is deflated and the catheter withdrawn.

Nine of the 13 patients who underwent the procedure improved markedly. The researchers concluded that it might be valuable in treating many of the 20,000 people in the United States each year who have vasospasms following a brain hemorrhage.   □ Beverly Merz

In the Special Reports section, see WHAT EVERYONE NEEDS TO KNOW ABOUT STROKE. In WORLD BOOK, see STROKE.

Teeth
See Dentistry

Urology

Advances continued in 1988 and 1989 in *urology*—the branch of medicine dealing with the kidneys, ureter, bladder, and male sex organs. One area featuring important advances involved new methods of treating *benign* (noncancerous) enlargement of the prostate gland.

In some cases, an enlarged prostate compresses the *urethra* (the tube carrying urine from the bladder through the penis), causing such problems as an increased frequency of urination. The compression may even completely block the urethra, calling for immediate medical attention.

The conventional treatment for benign enlargement of the prostate is a surgical procedure called *transurethral prostatectomy* (TURP), in which the portion of the prostate gland that is compressing the urethra is cut away. In cases of severe blockage, the physician usually removes the entire prostate.

Heating technique. Urologists Stuart D. Boyd of the University of Southern California in Los Angeles and Mark Zerbib of Hospital Cochin in Paris described studies using a new method that uses heat to shrink the prostate at the American Urological Association (AUA) national meeting held in May 1989 in Dallas. The technique involves threading a

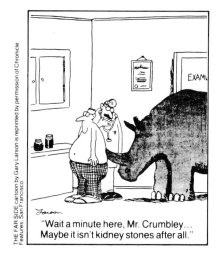

THE FAR SIDE cartoon by Gary Larson is reprinted by permission of Chronicle Features, San Francisco.

"Wait a minute here, Mr. Crumbley... Maybe it isn't kidney stones after all."

Venereal Diseases

See Sexually Transmitted Diseases

Urology (cont.)

tube through the urethra to the prostate gland. The tube contains three tiny antennas that emit microwaves, which raise the temperature of the prostate to about 108°F. (42°C).

Boyd said that the treatment improved the condition of 24 of the 25 patients on whom he tested the procedure. Zerbib also reported good results with the treatment.

Balloon treatment. Urologist Jerome Ludwig of Lutheran Hospital in Fort Wayne, Ind., reported at the AUA meeting that a balloon treatment relieved compression of the urethra in most patients tested. In

this technique, the urologist inserts a tube through the urethra to the level of the prostate. Mounted on the end of the tube is a balloon, which the urologist then inflates with a clear fluid. The balloon presses against the prostate gland, relieving the obstruction. When the balloon is deflated and the tube removed, the urethra remains open.

In most cases, the patient is treated as an outpatient and receives local anesthesia and a sedative. By contrast, a TURP requires admission to the hospital and a general anesthetic.

Incontinence treatment. *Incontinence* (involuntary passing of urine) is a frustrating problem for both urologist and patient, especially after surgical attempts have failed. Bhalchandra G. Parulkar of the Mayo Clinic, Rochester, Minn., has reported results of a new treatment for incontinence in women. The technique involves surgically implanting an artificial *sphincter* called the AS-800. (A natural sphincter is a ring of muscle that contracts to partly or completely close a bodily orifice, such as the anus.) Parulkar reported definite improvement in 83 per cent of the patients studied.

☐ Dennis A. Pessis

In World Book, see Prostate Gland.

Veterinary Medicine

Diabetes in animals continued to be an important focus of research in 1988 and 1989, with encouraging results reported by Rodolfo Alejandro and his colleagues at the Diabetes Research Institute at the University of Miami in Florida. Diabetes, the most common hormonal disorder in dogs, also occurs in cats, horses, and cattle. In many animals, the disease is the result of damage to *islet of Langerhans cells* (pancreas cells that produce the hormone insulin). Like some human diabetics, diabetic animals may need daily insulin injections.

Alejandro and his co-workers attempted to cure a group of diabetic dogs by giving each an islet-tissue

transplant. The researchers then administered the drug cyclosporine, which weakens the immune system, to prevent rejection of the transplanted cells.

The transplants were so successful that the treated dogs no longer needed injections of insulin. But cyclosporine's effect on the dogs' immune system may have made the animals more susceptible to a variety of other diseases.

An improved rinderpest vaccine was reported in November 1988 by researchers in California and New York. Frequently referred to as *cattle*

Veterinary Medicine (cont.)

plague, rinderpest is the most severe infectious viral disease of cattle. The virus causes pneumonia, diarrhea, and death in more than 2 million cattle and buffalo in developing countries each year.

Researchers in Plum Island, N.Y., vaccinated 15 cattle with the new vaccine and then exposed them and a group of unvaccinated cattle to the rinderpest virus. All the vaccinated cattle survived, while all the unvaccinated cattle died.

The new vaccine, which was produced using genetic engineering techniques, is an improvement over the previously used preparation because it is easier to produce, transport, and administer, and it does not require refrigeration. For these reasons, the new vaccine will be of special importance to the control of rinderpest by nomadic herders in developing countries.

A breakthrough in flea control
was reported by researchers in California, Texas, Australia, and Denmark in January 1989. An insect hormone called methoprene was found to be useful for killing fleas by interfering with their normal growth cycle. The advantage of this type of flea control is that fleas can be destroyed without the use of insecti-

Vitamin E and zoo animals
Nutritionist Ellen Direnfeld of New York City's Bronx Zoo offers vitamin E enriched food to a tamandua, or collared anteater. Through a worldwide research project, Direnfeld discovered that many zoo animals suffer from a dietary deficiency of vitamin E.

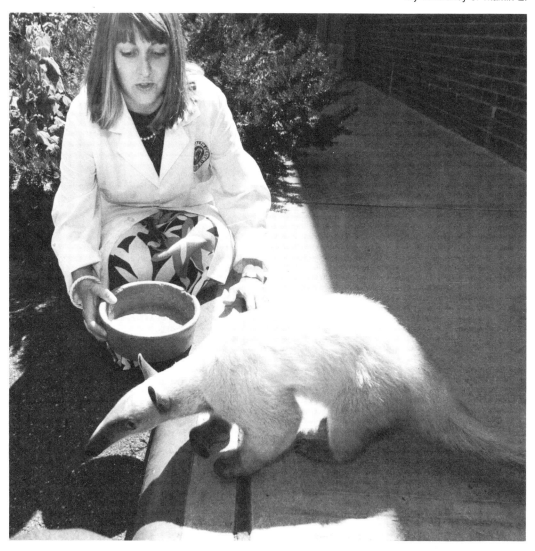

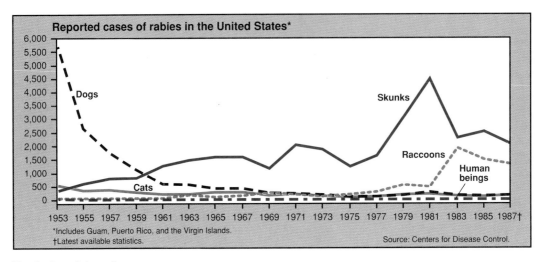

Reported cases of rabies in the United States*

*Includes Guam, Puerto Rico, and the Virgin Islands.
†Latest available statistics.

Source: Centers for Disease Control.

Vaccination of domestic animals has made rabies uncommon among people and pets despite an increase in the reported number of rabid wild animals.

Veterinary Medicine (cont.)

cides, which may have harmful side effects for animals and people.

Help for poisoned swans. A technique to treat trumpeter swans suffering from lead poisoning was developed in late 1988 by veterinarians at the University of Minnesota's Raptor Rehabilitation Center in St. Paul and a *gastroenterologist* (specialist in disorders of the digestive system, liver, and pancreas) from the Hennepin County Medical Center in Minneapolis.

Trumpeter swans, whose population has been slowly increasing after a brush with extinction in the early

1900's, fall victim to lead poisoning after swallowing spent lead shot that has settled to the bottom of lakes and ponds. The problem intensified during the drought of 1988, when low water levels made the lead shot more readily accessible.

To treat a poisoned swan, the team anesthetized the bird and flushed its *gullet* (a saclike part of the esophagus used for grinding food) with water. To locate lead pellets still trapped in folds in the gullet after the flushing, the team used an *endoscope*, a long, flexible tube equipped on the end with a light and a tiny camera. The endoscope was threaded through the swan's throat and the image recorded through the camera was viewed on a computer screen. The team used remote-controlled forceps to remove any lead discovered in the folds in the gullet.

Because lead quickly dissolves and enters the bloodstream, the team then gave the swans a chemical called calcium EDTA, which chemically alters the dissolved lead so that it can be excreted by the kidneys. By mid-February 1989, the team had used the technique on more than 20 poisoned swans with satisfactory results.

☐ Thomas J. Lane

In WORLD BOOK, see VETERINARY MEDICINE.

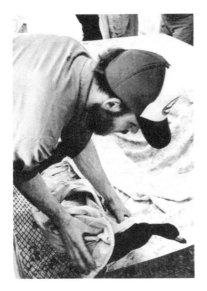

Duck clean-up
A volunteer tries to clean oil from the feathers of a duck at an Alaskan animal rescue center after a large March 1989 oil spill endangered wildlife in Prince William Sound.

Scientists have long suspected that the digestive system sends messages to the brain, which in turn controls appetite and the body's use of food. Now two groups of scientists have reported findings on chemical messengers connecting gut with brain.

For years, researchers have sought a means by which *adipocytes* (fat cells) might influence the brain's control of appetite. In 1988, scientists at Harvard University Medical School in Boston reported research on the protein *adipsin*, the only fat cell product known to be released into the bloodstream—and thus able to reach the brain.

The Harvard team measured adipsin levels in normal, lean mice and rats as well as in three types of overweight mice and rats: some with hereditary obesity, some that became fat because of surgery that destroyed the appetite-controlling center in their brains, and normal rodents made fat just by overfeeding. Animals with a physiological cause for obesity—either heredity or altered brains—had only 0.5 to 1 per cent of the adipsin of normal ones, both lean and overfed.

The researchers said that mice and rats with low adipsin levels become obese on a diet that does not fatten normal ones. Earlier research showed that many obese people eat no more than lean people do. It may be that low adipsin levels help encourage weight gain in these people. If so, doctors may be able to use adipsin measurements to distinguish people who inherit a tendency to plumpness from those who simply overeat.

The Harvard researchers are now giving supplemental adipsin to mice to see if it makes them slim down. And Metabolic Biosystems Inc., a biotechnology company in Mountain View, Calif., is measuring adipsin levels in people. If the mouse pattern holds for human beings, the company will work toward marketing adipsin as an aid to weight loss.

When enough is enough. Scientists are also examining the role of an intestinal hormone called *chole-cystokinin* (CCK). Normally, when people or animals have eaten enough, they experience a feeling of fullness along with a rise in CCK. The CCK apparently tells the brain that it's time to stop eating.

Researchers at the United States Department of Agriculture, attempting to build bigger pigs, have developed a vaccine that blocks CCK's appetite-suppressing message. Vaccinated pigs gained 11 pounds (5 kilograms) more than their untreated litter mates in less than three months.

Now medical researchers, looking at CCK in human beings, are finding links between the hormone and the eating disorder *bulimia*. Bulimics, most of them young women, binge on huge quantities of food and then induce vomiting.

In a study reported in September 1988, scientists at the University of California in San Francisco and the National Institute of Mental Health in Bethesda, Md., compared CCK levels in 14 bulimic women and 10 normal ones. They found that all the women had similar CCK levels before eating. But after meals, CCK in bulimic women rose to only about half the normal level. These women didn't feel full and went on to eat abnormally large amounts.

The researchers treated five of the bulimic women with antidepressant drugs. After eight weeks they were secreting more CCK after meals and having more normal feelings of fullness. But the scientists do not know just how the drug relates to CCK and eating behavior.

Cholesterol and couch potatoes.
A study reported in October 1988 countered the common medical belief that exercise is the key to boosting levels of *high-density lipoprotein* (HDL) cholesterol—the so-called good cholesterol—in the blood. Researchers at Stanford University in Stanford, Calif., found that weight loss alone promotes HDL, which removes cholesterol from cells. Deposits of cholesterol can block arteries and promote heart disease.

The "Fast" Way to Lose Weight

When TV talk-show star Oprah Winfrey displayed her newly slender silhouette in November 1988, she single-handedly made liquid diet plans the hottest commodity in weight control. Winfrey announced that in less than four months she had shed 67 pounds (30 kilograms) thanks to a liquid-centered diet plan.

Liquid diets last made news in the late 1970's, when the Food and Drug Administration cited them as the cause of at least 60 deaths. Those products lacked essential nutrients, and some users died of heart irregularities after they lost heart muscle instead of fat.

The new generation of very-low-calorie (VLC) diets are more nutritionally sound and far safer, and liability-conscious manufacturers are dispensing them almost as carefully as prescription drugs. Companies distribute their products only through hospitals, clinics, and physicians, and they advise against use by people with certain health conditions—such as recent heart attacks or strokes, severe complications of diabetes, or stomach ulcers. Some require medical checkups before and during use, to make sure dieters start out healthy and stay that way.

Medical experts agree that today's programs can produce dramatic weight loss in obese people. The diets have drawbacks, however. They cost a great deal—usually between $2,500 and $5,000. They may cause temporary side effects ranging from bad breath and constipation to fatigue and hair loss. And the pounds often come right back.

The diets are not meant for people who want to lose a few pounds so they'll look better in their swimsuits. The programs usually accept only people who are at least 20 per cent above ideal weight for their height and age. Diet specialists not affiliated with VLC programs go further, saying that liquid diets are best for the 9 per cent of Americans who are at least 30 per cent above ideal weight and thus at risk for problems such as high blood pressure, diabetes, or heart disease.

Typically, the first 12 weeks of a VLC diet are a *modified fast*: The dieter consumes 400 to 800 calories daily, provided by a diet powder dissolved in water. Some programs add a very light meal as well. During the second phase, which might last 6 to 16 weeks, foods are gradually reintroduced until the dieter is eating 1,000 to 1,200 calories daily. Next comes a maintenance regimen aimed at permanent adjustment to a moderate calorie intake.

Throughout the process, some programs require participants to attend weekly counseling sessions on nutrition, exercise, and eating behavior. Independent experts agree that dieters are more likely to keep the weight off if they truly learn to change their ways.

Still, many dieters regress—and regain. Melbourne Hovell, a medical researcher at San Diego State University in California, followed 400 VLC dieters for several years. Based on his findings, he estimated that dieters in such programs regain an average of 50 per cent of their excess weight after one year and 80 per cent in two years. He noted that even a temporary loss can reduce health risks substantially. But dieters should realize that no program guarantees an easy, permanent solution to overweight. □ Patricia Thomas

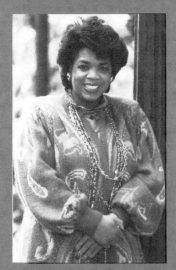
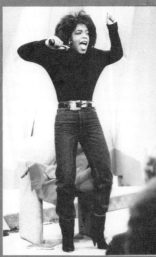

A fast change: Oprah before and after.

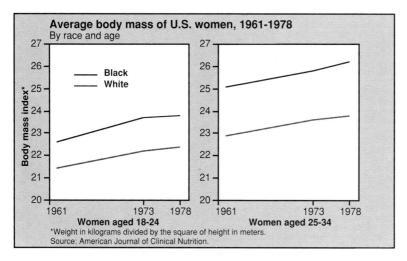

Average body mass of U.S. women, 1961-1978
By race and age

Body mass index*

— Black
— White

Women aged 18-24

Women aged 25-34

*Weight in kilograms divided by the square of height in meters.
Source: American Journal of Clinical Nutrition.

Women are getting fatter, a University of Michigan study shows. Researchers used height and weight data from federal surveys to compute *body mass index,* a measure of weight in proportion to height. Black women had higher indexes than white women—but all gained over time. Among men, however, body mass remained mostly constant and showed no strong differences by race.

Weight Control (cont.)

The researchers studied 155 men who were overweight and inactive but otherwise healthy. Some were put on a low-calorie diet without adding exercise. A second group began jogging regularly but didn't change eating habits.

After one year, the dieters lost an average of 7.2 kilograms (16 pounds), compared with a loss of 4 kilograms (9 pounds) among the exercisers. Some of that difference, however, reflected the fact that the exercisers gained muscle mass. In fat weight, both groups lost about 5 kilograms (11 pounds).

Both the dieters and the exercisers showed a rise in HDL levels of about 10 per cent. The researchers suggest that the increase in HDL was caused by fat loss specifically, regardless of whether the fat was lost by dieting or by exercise.

The researchers concluded that overweight people who can't or won't exercise can improve their cholesterol profiles by dieting to lose weight. Still, they cautioned that the study is not an excuse to abandon exercise. In fact, follow-up research is showing one drawback to being sedentary: The dieters tended to regain lost weight after the program ended, while most of the exercisers have stayed active and are keeping the weight off.

Where the pounds are. The National Academy of Sciences in Washington, D.C., reported in 1989 that 31 per cent of American men over age 18 are overweight, based on accepted statistical standards of weight and height. Only 25 per cent of women proved overweight.

But women aged 25 to 34 are gaining fast, according to a 1988 report by researchers at the University of Michigan in Ann Arbor. They computed *body mass index* (a measure that accounts for both weight and height) from data gathered on 6,850 women in government surveys from 1960 to 1980.

Women's body mass rose consistently over the years (see the graph on this page). So did the frequency of obesity, which the researchers defined as body mass greater than that of 85 per cent of all women in the same age group in 1960. In 1960, 13.3 per cent of white women and 28.8 per cent of black women age 25 to 34 were obese. By 1980, those numbers had risen to 17.1 per cent and 31 per cent.

The researchers considered the data on black women especially troubling, as those women already have more weight-linked health problems than do whites. Studies show that obesity increases the risks for heart disease, diabetes, high blood pressure, and many other problems.   □ Patricia Thomas

In WORLD BOOK, see WEIGHT CONTROL.

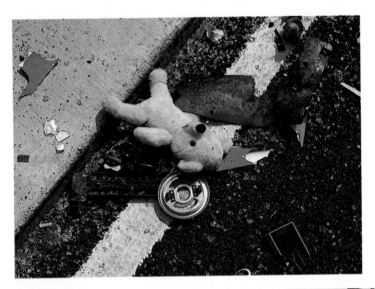

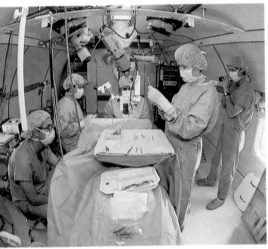

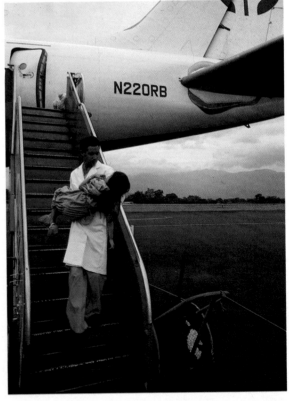

People in Health Care

Two articles provide a glimpse of health care professionals in action.

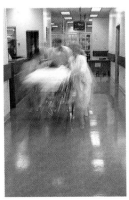

Rescuing Young Lives: Inside a Trauma Center
by Alan Doelp   340

They Fly to Save Sight
by Mary Krier   354

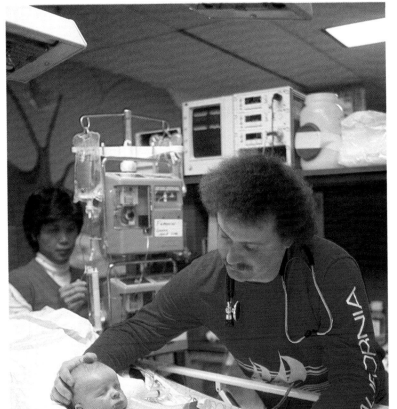

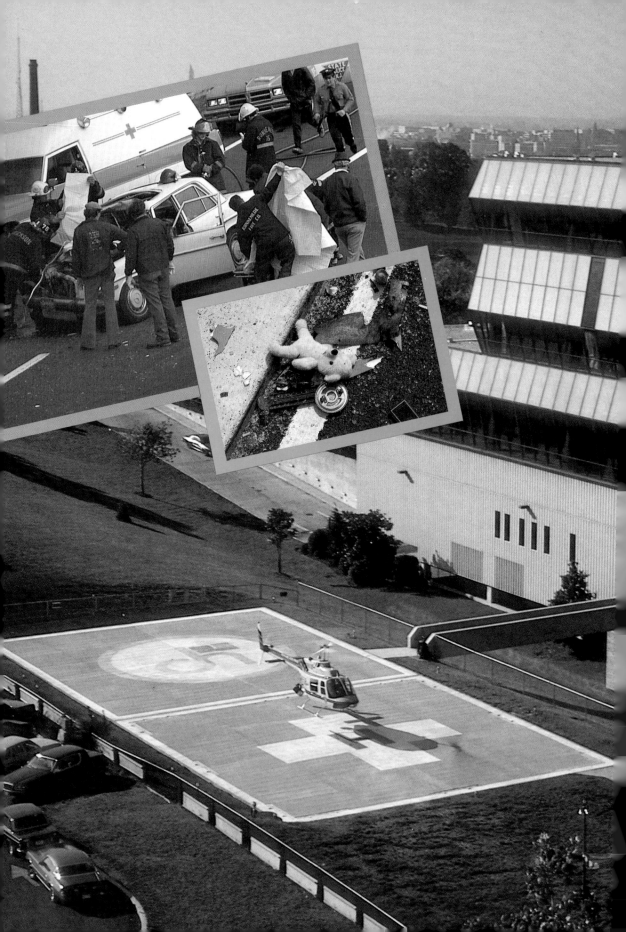

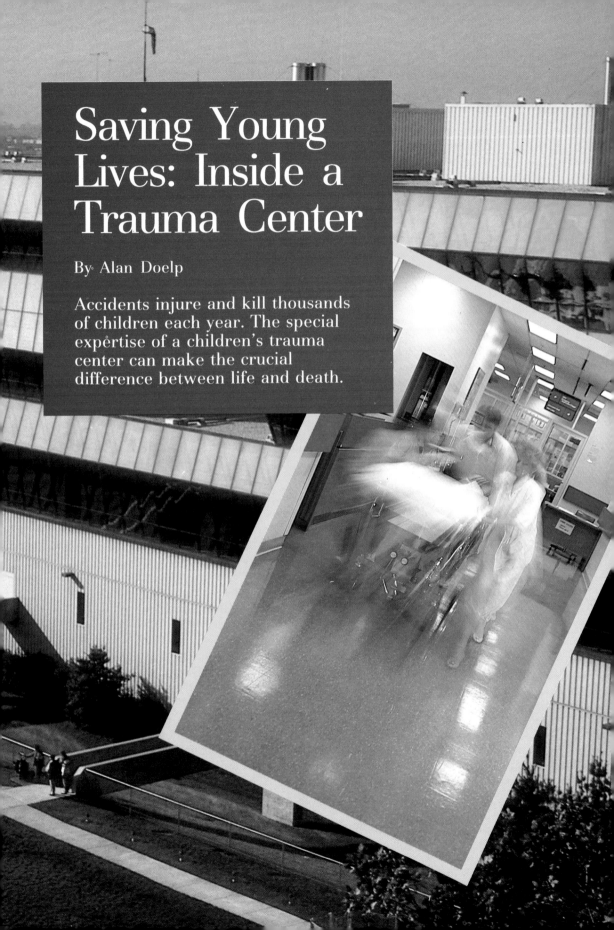

Saving Young Lives: Inside a Trauma Center

By Alan Doelp

Accidents injure and kill thousands of children each year. The special expertise of a children's trauma center can make the crucial difference between life and death.

Standing up in the back seat was a spanking offense, but 3-year-old Lisa Burnett had figured out that mommy couldn't drive and spank at the same time, so occasionally she would jump up, clinging for support to the kiddy seat she detested, and have a quick look at the world flashing by. Often, she would sit back down in the seat before mommy noticed. The threat of being strapped into the hated kiddy seat was real, but sometimes the view was simply irresistible.

So as it happened, little Lisa actually saw the garbage truck as it lumbered out of a side street directly into the path of the Burnetts'* car. She felt, for a single frozen instant, a sensation of lightness as her mother hit the brakes. Then, at almost precisely the same instant that the car smashed into the garbage truck, Lisa slammed face first into the dashboard.

As car crashes go, it was a comparatively minor one. The hood of the automobile was crumpled, the right fender buckled, and the front wheel flattened. Mrs. Burnett had the wind knocked out of her when she hit the steering wheel, and she spent what seemed like an eternity just sitting, gasping for breath, before she could even move toward her daughter, who now lay crumpled on the floor of the front seat.

Fortunately, the accident occurred less than half a block from the Bethesda-Chevy Chase, Md., fire company. Even before Mrs. Burnett had recovered enough breath to begin screaming, two fire fighters had raced on foot to the accident scene. The first one to reach the car yanked open the driver's door, glanced inside, then pointed an arm toward the firehouse. "Get the ambulance," he shouted to his partner. "There's a kid in here."

Moments later, at a nearby hospital, the red pagers came to life with a screeching whine. There was no ignoring it, or the message that followed: "Trauma stat. E.R. ETA four minutes. Trauma stat. ETA four minutes." (E.R. stands for emergency room; ETA for estimated time of arrival.)

The word *stat* is a medical term. It means now. This instant. This is top priority. The word *trauma* is the medical term for injury. At the phrase "trauma stat," 18 key employees at Children's Hospital National Medical Center in Washington, D.C., drop what they're doing and head for the emergency room. They are the 18 members of the hospital's trauma team.

Trauma is a disease unlike any other. Infections, cancer, and heart disease strike only those people who are vulnerable. The progress of one of these diseases in the body is often measured in days—perhaps months or even years. Trauma, on the other hand, can strike anyone anywhere. No one is immune. The disease hits randomly and without warning. Its onset is measured in milliseconds, its critical course in minutes. Its aftereffects can last a lifetime—and without proper treatment, that can be a very short time indeed.

The author:

Alan Doelp, a free-lance writer based in Baltimore, is author of the 1989 book *In the Blink of an Eye: Inside a Children's Trauma Center.*

*Lisa and Elizabeth Burnett are composites drawn from several different cases at the Children's Hospital National Medical Center. Their names are fictitious.

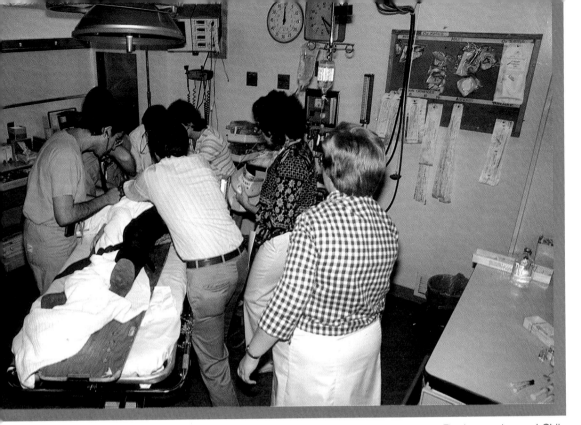

The trauma team at Children's Hospital—a group of doctors and nurses trained to treat injured children—surround an injured youngster who has just arrived at the hospital. The team will work to stabilize the child's condition before determining the extent of injuries. To minimize frightening young patients, most doctors and nurses at Children's do not wear hospital garb.

Accidents affect the lives of many people. According to the National Safety Council (NSC), accidents are the fourth major cause of death in the United States, after heart disease, cancer, and stroke. Approximately 96,000 Americans died as the result of accidents in 1988. The death and injury toll among children is especially heavy. About 8,000 children age 14 years or younger die of accidental injuries each year. The American Academy of Pediatrics estimates that about 50,000 children are permanently disabled each year as a result of accidents.

It was in the late 1950's that physicians first began to describe trauma as a disease—as something with recognizable symptoms and a predictable clinical course, or sequence of physical events. Before that, the approach was simply to patch up the patient and hope for the best. To describe trauma as a disease carried with it the implication that its symptoms and course could be managed clinically, and that with proper management, the outcome could be improved.

The result was the growth of highly specialized trauma centers. As of 1988, there were 403 trauma centers in the United States, according to the American College of Surgeons (ACS). Although each state sets its own requirements for trauma centers, the ACS has established guidelines for different levels of trauma centers depending on the type of treatment available.

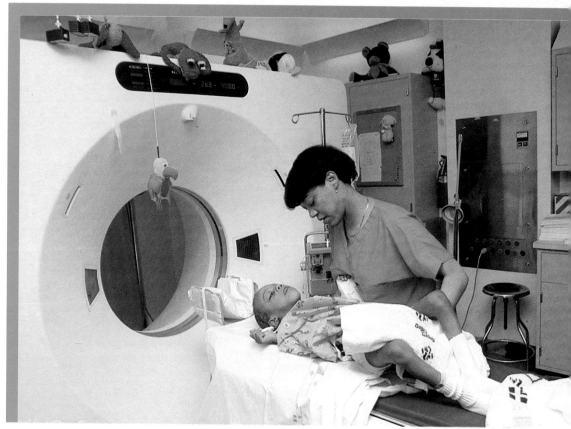

A menagerie of stuffed animals stands by as a Children's radiology technician gently places an injured child on the table of a computerized tomographic (CT) scanner. A CT scanner provides detailed X-ray images of the body, allowing doctors to pinpoint any damage to internal organs.

Trauma centers like the one at Children's Hospital, which are staffed with surgical experts and intensive-care nurses and are equipped with the latest state-of-the-art machinery, earn the highest level rating. These centers have helped increase the survival rate from serious accidental injury from about 40 per cent (in the late 1950's, before specialized trauma centers) to more than 90 per cent 20 years later, in the late 1970's.

But around that time, Marty Eichelberger, a young pediatric surgeon, took a hard look at the statistics and realized that as far as children were concerned, the survival rate figures weren't as good as they ought to be. Looking beyond the numbers, Eichelberger dug into the medical literature and discovered the reason, astonishing if only for its simplicity: Kids are different. Browsing through the medical journals, he read case report after case report concerning death or disability in children whose injuries would have been treatable in a trauma center properly equipped to handle kids.

Children, for one thing, come in all sizes, and to treat an injured child, a hospital must have equipment appropriate to that particular child's size. An adult-sized blood pressure cuff is useless when the patient is 3 years old. An adult-sized airway tube is worse than useless. In a desperate situation, it can be used to save a child who has stopped breathing, but the oversized tube will destroy the vocal cords, and though the child may survive, he or she will never speak again.

When, in 1980, Eichelberger joined the staff of the Children's Hospital National Medical Center, one of his first suggestions was to start a pediatric trauma service. Children's pediatric trauma center was not the first such service in the United States, but the unit Eichelberger set up became the national standard by which the other U.S. pediatric trauma centers are judged.

The ambulance crew that first reached the Burnetts' car had carefully strapped Lisa to a plywood backboard and placed a pink plastic collar around her neck. If her neck and back were seriously injured, the backboard and collar would give them necessary support. They also would prevent Lisa from moving suddenly and injuring herself further. Because Lisa had not regained consciousness, the ambulance crew decided to transport her to Children's Hospital in the fastest way possible—by helicopter. Lisa's mother, however, did not join her. Because her injuries appeared less serious—and because there is room for only one patient in the helicopter—she was driven by ambulance the 8 miles (13 kilometers) to the Washington Hospital Center, located next door to Children's Hospital.

As soon as the helicopter touched down on the concrete pad, the pilot adjusted the giant rotor blade so that it no longer bit into the air. This changed the sound that the chopper made and lessened the blast of wind coming from it, signaling the hospital's waiting trauma team to move forward, knees bent, heads ducked, pulling an empty stretcher.

Four sets of hands gently lifted the girl out of the helicopter and onto the waiting stretcher. The right side of Lisa's face was bruised and had begun to swell. A gauze compress bandage covered part of her forehead; her blond hair was matted with dried blood. A green plastic oxygen mask lay loosely over her mouth and nose. Her eyes were closed; she made no sound.

One of the scrub-suited figures bent close to the girl's head, and with a fingertip opened Lisa's eyelids one at a time. Then he nodded to the team. Crouching again, the trauma team turned and wheeled the stretcher rapidly toward the hospital. The helicopter medic jogged along behind.

Just inside the doorway are two fully equipped trauma bays.

At Children's Hospital these are called *code rooms*. Code room number two is nearer the helipad door by a few feet, so for helicopter admissions it is always the code room of choice.

Inside code room number two, the rest of the trauma team was already waiting. As the stretcher slid into place, the "inner core" team of eight medical professionals moved into position around the child. Among them were two physicians, one a surgical resident; a respiratory technician, and an anesthesiologist. There also was a surgical nurse, an intensive care nurse, a medications nurse, and a nurse responsible for recording all the activity occurring in the room. One of the nurses quickly removed the straps that held Lisa to the backboard; another began cutting the child's clothes off with large blunt-nosed scissors. A third wrapped a small blood pressure cuff around the child's left arm. In a corner of the room, a nurse noted the time of admission—10:23 a.m.

The helicopter medic appeared in the doorway. "This is Lisa," he announced to the trauma team. "She's 3 years old and was unrestrained in the back seat when mom hit a garbage truck at moderate speed, maybe 25 miles per hour. Lisa hit the dashboard and was found on the floor of the front seat. She has been unconscious since the accident.

"Vital signs have been okay. Her blood pressure has been stable at 110 over 75, her pulse is about 80, respiration a little jerky. Pupils slow but responsive and equal. She has not showed any sign of regaining consciousness so far. Scalp lacer-

In Children's operating room, doctors perform surgery to save the life of an injured child. Each year, 1 out of 4 children in the United States is injured severely enough to need medical attention.

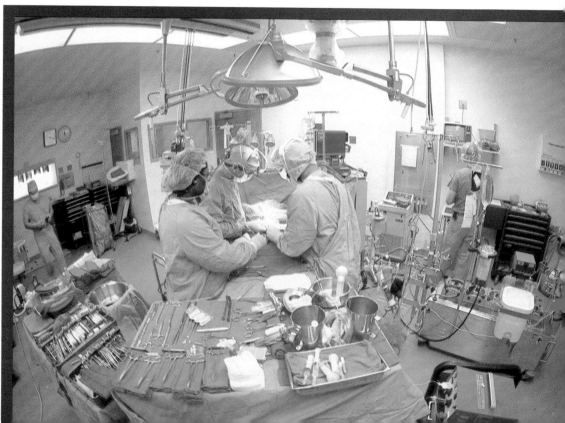

ation [a jagged wound] and minor blood loss," the medic added, pointing to the bandage on Lisa's head.

The resident looked at the bandage, thinking hard. What sort of blow could knock a child unconscious for—how many minutes? "When was the accident?" he asked the medic.

"10:06."

The resident glanced at a nurse standing just outside the code room door. "Did you call neurosurgery?" he asked.

The nurse nodded. A simple scalp wound, the surgeon and the nurse both knew, would not keep a child unconscious for almost 20 minutes. If Lisa had suffered a serious brain injury, a *neurosurgeon* (a surgeon who specializes in surgery on the brain and nervous system) should be prepared to operate.

"110 over 70," announced the nurse with the blood pressure cuff. Then, to the medic, "How's Lisa's mother?"

"Her mother hit the steering wheel," the medic reported. "She's probably okay. The ambulance crew has taken her to Washington Hospital so she'll be close by."

Even as the medic was speaking, members of the trauma team were busy, each with a check list of tasks. One of the first tasks was to set up an *intravenous injection* (IV) in which medicines and other fluids are injected directly into a vein. On Lisa's right, the surgical resident examined her inner arm closely, then swabbed it with antiseptic and expertly inserted a hypodermic needle into the vein just below the skin. The nurse standing next to him attached the needle to a slender tube that was hooked up to a bag of clear fluid. There was no reason yet to suspect that Lisa was bleeding internally, but just in case, the fluid flowing through the IV into the child's bloodstream would help keep her blood pressure close to normal.

On Lisa's left, a medical resident drew three small vials of blood, which he handed one by one to a nurse standing beside him. The nurse labeled the vials, then handed them to a waiting lab technician, who turned and ran down the hallway toward the laboratory. If Lisa were bleeding internally, her blood chemistry would begin to change, subtly at first, but enough to show up in lab tests. As long as the blood tests looked good, and Lisa's blood pressure remained stable, the trauma team could go on with the rest of the check list.

The first priorities of trauma care are as simple as ABC: airway, breathing, and circulation. If the airway—the pathway from the nose and mouth to the lungs—is blocked, then the patient will strangle. If the airway is open but the patient is not breathing, the patient will suffocate. The trauma team knew that Lisa's breathing had been steady since the accident, and at the head of the bed, a respiratory technician held a

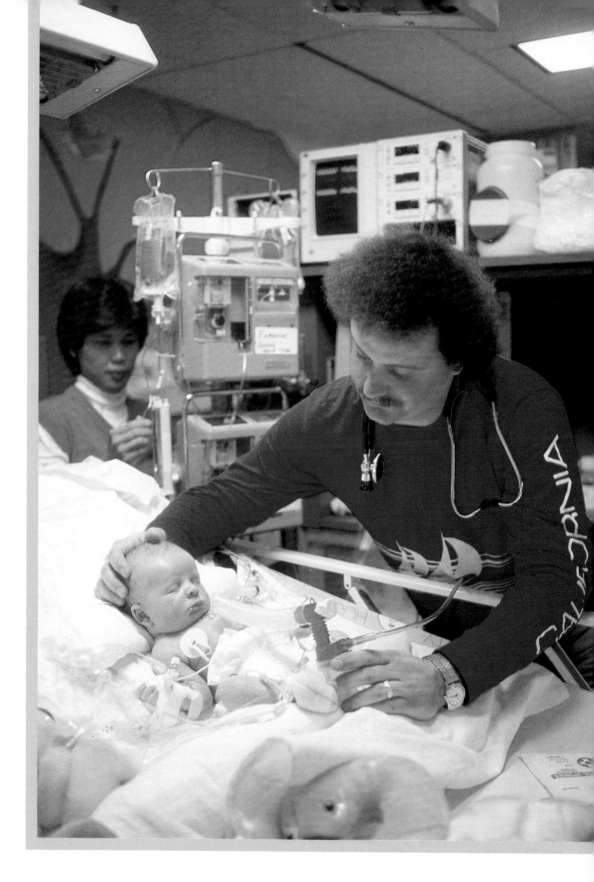

mask near her mouth and nose, feeding extra oxygen into her lungs. So much for A and B.

Now the trauma team was concentrating on item C—circulation. If a patient loses too much blood, the body will go into *shock*, a condition in which the blood pressure drops and becomes too low to maintain an adequate supply of blood to the tissues. If the lost blood is not replaced, then the organs and tissues of the body, deprived of life-giving oxygen, slip deeper into shock. At some point, usually after about an hour, the condition becomes irreversible and the patient will die.

Opposite page: Cradling the head of an infant, a respiratory therapist at Children's Hospital prepares to administer medication through a *nebulizer,* a device that converts medicine into a mist that is inhaled.

Having drawn his blood sample, the resident on Lisa's left stepped back to let the surgical resident start a second intravenous line. If Lisa's blood pressure were to drop suddenly, the team could quickly replace the blood she was losing through the two lines. If her blood tests showed that blood loss had robbed her body of too many oxygen-carrying red blood cells, the trauma team could give her blood transfusions. Now A, B, and C were under control. The patient was alive, stable, and likely to stay that way for a while. The trauma team could begin to worry about Lisa's injuries.

"X ray," the surgical resident called out. "Ready for X ray." The radiology technician wheeled her portable X-ray machine into the code room. One nurse donned a lead-lined apron and stayed to assist the technician. The rest of the team waited outside while she made films of Lisa's neck, chest, and pelvis.

When the technician left, the trauma team returned to continue working down the check list. A nurse took a urine specimen and checked it for blood: There was none. The laboratory phoned with the results of the blood tests: They were normal. Near the bed, a blood pressure machine continued to register a steady 110/70. Above the bed, Lisa's heartbeat traced a steady rhythm across a glowing monitor screen.

The beauty of trauma medicine is its simplicity. Trauma medicine is done "by the book." Because accidental injury is so unpredictable, *traumatologists*—physicians who specialize in treating trauma—make no attempt to guess the nature or extent of an injury. Instead, they follow a check list that assumes the worst, and in descending order of urgency, they rule out injury after injury. The operative phrase is "rule out." The trauma team assumes that the patient has every injury in the book, and they proceed on that assumption until, one by one, the tests prove them wrong.

In Lisa's case, less than five minutes after she arrived in the code room, the trauma team had learned a great deal about her, even though she was still unconscious. She obviously had head injuries. The team had removed the bandage and discovered several cuts, and from the bruising and swelling the team

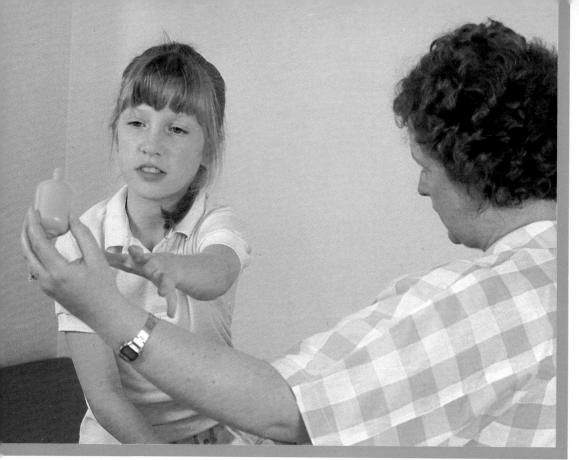

Under the supervision of a physical therapist at the John F. Kennedy Institute in Baltimore, a girl performs an exercise to strengthen her injured arm. Children treated at Children's Hospital who require long-term rehabilitation, such as physical therapy, are often sent to the nearby Kennedy Institute for treatment.

could guess that she might have broken bones in her face. But as for the full extent of the damage, they could only guess.

The X rays arrived in the code room at the same time as the neurosurgeon, and the three doctors stood around a lighted display board and took turns counting the vertebrae in Lisa's neck. If all seven *cervical* (neck) vertebrae are not visible, it can mean the neck is broken.

While the two residents counted the neck bones on the X ray, the neurosurgeon stepped to the head of the bed. Because Lisa had not regained consciousness, he was concerned that she might have seriously injured her brain. He tried to rouse her. "Lisa," he called sharply. "Lisa! Can you hear me? Squeeze my finger. Can you squeeze my finger, Lisa?" The girl's hand rested limply around the surgeon's forefinger. She made no response. Pulling a small flashlight from his pocket the surgeon opened each eyelid, in turn, and shined the bright light across first one eye, then the other. The response of her pupils to light—their size and how quickly they contract—is a clue to brain injury. He repeated the procedure twice, then turned to the two residents. "How were her pupils when she came in?"

"Slow, but equal," the surgical resident answered.

"Well, the left one's bigger now," replied the neurosurgeon.

"How fast can we get her up to the CT scanner?"

Medicine has enjoyed many technological advances in the last three decades, but one of the most important has been the development of the *computerized tomographic*, or CT, *scanner*. A CT scanner is a large metal machine resembling a square doughnut. Inside the doughnut hole, an X-ray emitter and a set of sensors that can detect X-ray beams are mounted on a rotating ring. As a patient lies on the examining table inside the hole, the ring rotates and takes X-ray images from many different angles. Instead of exposing a piece of film, the X-ray beam and sensors generate millions of bits of electronic information, which a computer then assembles into a remarkably accurate picture of the inside of the patient.

Before the CT scanner, physicians had only a few ways to find out what was going on inside a patient. One was the conventional X ray. But standard X-ray pictures do not provide a very clear image of the brain, lungs, or other soft tissues. Another common way to check what was happening inside the body was to perform exploratory surgery. Now, the amazing scanners can pinpoint the location of an injury and also help doctors gauge the seriousness of the problem, thus preventing the need to "explore" the patient with a knife.

In Lisa's case, the neurosurgeon ordered a CT scan of the child's head because he suspected she had a brain injury. Shining a bright light in a person's eye will cause the pupil of the eye to contract immediately. If the pupils contract slowly, it means the brain is functioning slowly. If the left pupil is dilated and contracts more slowly than the other, for example, it usually means that the left side of the brain is functioning less well than the right.

The CT scanner at Children's Hospital is one of the latest models, but even so it takes several seconds to build up each image of the brain. The neurosurgeon fidgeted impatiently as each successive two-dimensional "slice" scrolled onto the computer screen. The fourth image showed the beginnings of a shadow on the left side, and the fifth and sixth confirmed it: Inside Lisa's head a blood vessel had broken, and a pool of blood was collecting underneath the tough leathery membrane that lines the inside of the skull. The pool of blood was pressing directly on Lisa's delicate brain tissues.

The neurosurgeon let out a long breath. He looked at the resident standing beside him. "We're going to need an operating room," he said. "If they don't have one, get the schedule and bump somebody. I want to operate in 20 minutes."

When the Bethesda-Chevy Chase ambulance got to the Washington Hospital Center with Lisa's mother, they used their radio to advise Children's Hospital. Lisa's mother was found to be bruised but otherwise uninjured, so the ambulance crew used the radio again to tell Children's that they were bringing her over. When the ambulance arrived at the hospital, the social worker who was assigned to the emergency room was waiting to greet Elizabeth Burnett.

In the 10 minutes that followed, the social worker acted as friend, counselor, and tour guide for Mrs. Burnett. She gave her a summary of what had happened so far and escorted her to the second floor to see Lisa, who was being readied for surgery. Then she took Mrs. Burnett to her office so she could make phone calls, helped her fill out the admission forms, and consoled her when, finally, she began to cry.

No brain surgery is ever considered minor, but Lisa's operation was at least straightforward and uncomplicated. The neurosurgeon bored a small hole through the side of Lisa's head, drained off the blood that had accumulated there and, after he had closed the surgical wound, sent Lisa back to the CT scanner to make sure there was no additional bleeding.

By afternoon, Lisa had been admitted to the intensive care unit. At the neurosurgeon's recommendation, she remained attached to a respirator, a device that artificially maintains a patient's breathing. The next morning, when the medications were allowed to wear off, Lisa responded by immediately attempting to pull the respirator tube out of her mouth. The neurosurgeon made note of that encouraging sign, but also noted that in her struggles, she used only her left hand.

Shortly afterward, one of Lisa's doctors removed the respirator tube from her windpipe. She coughed and tried to speak, but the words made no sense. What did make sense, at least to Lisa, was when, a few minutes later, she tried to bite a nurse who pricked her finger for a blood sample.

Lisa's mother was aghast, but the nurse was reassuring. "For a child with a head injury, that is a perfectly appropriate response," the rehabilitation coordinator told Mrs. Burnett. "If Lisa were an adult, she'd probably be cursing instead. Consciousness comes back in stages; right now she has awareness, but without any inhibitions. She's doing fine."

The doctors seemed to agree. By the end of the day, they decided that Lisa was well enough to be moved into a general care bed. Although she could move them when asked, her right arm and leg were noticeably weaker than her left. This was because her injury was to the left side of her brain, which controls the movement of her right arm and leg.

Six days after the accident, Lisa left the hospital and moved to the nearby rehabilitation center, where specially trained nurses and technicians kept her busy with a long list of specific activities and exercises. In the institute's playroom, Lisa participated in games designed to strengthen the use of her right arm and leg. As her brain healed, the part that "knew" how to operate these limbs had to be retrained.

Six weeks after the accident, Lisa's parents arrived at the rehabilitation center to reclaim their daughter. Lisa cried when she saw her parents, then cried again when she realized she would have to say good-by to all her new-found friends.

She did not, however, cry when mommy strapped her snugly into the kiddy seat. In fact, she smiled.

For further information:

Child safety information is available from the National Safe Kids Coalition, Children's Hospital National Medical Center, 111 Michigan Avenue NW, Washington, DC 20010.

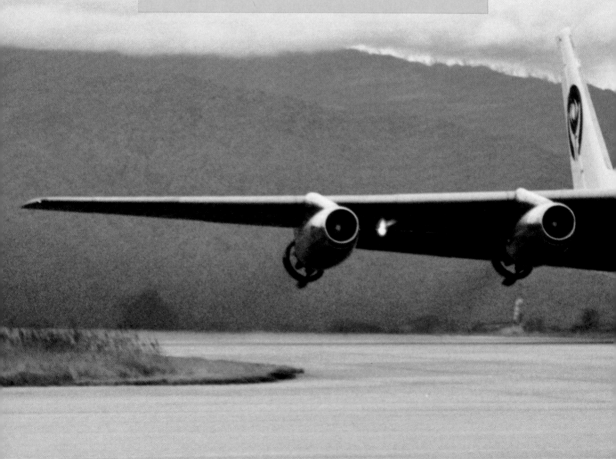

They Fly
to Save Sight

By Mary Krier

Aboard Project Orbis' airplane,
eye doctors share their skills
to help fight world blindness.

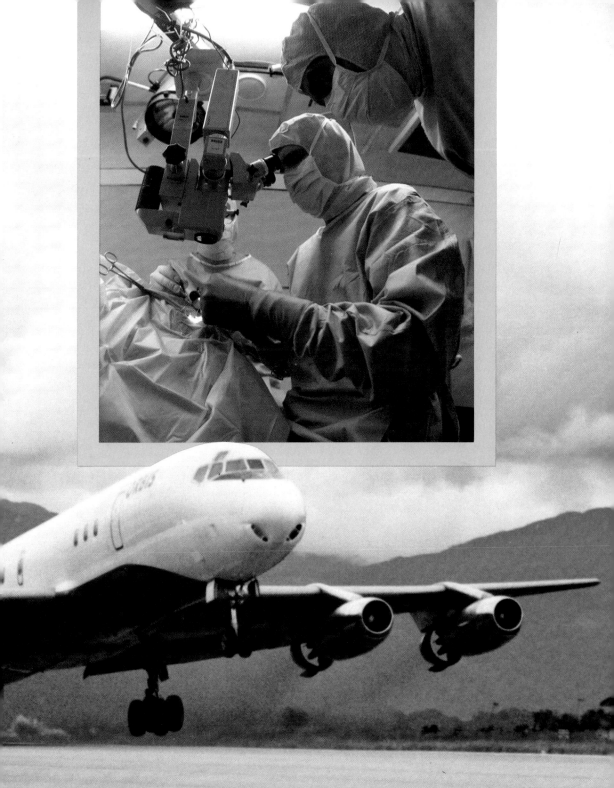

Project Orbis' flying eye hospital takes off after completing a mission in Nepal, *above*. While visiting host countries, volunteer physicians perform delicate eye surgery in the jet's fully equipped operating room, *inset*.

Hundreds of miles away from home, Jay Fleischman, a 40-year-old surgeon from Montefiore Medical Center in New York City, cheerfully waits for his last patient of the day. The setting for this operation, like the others Fleischman has performed that day, is one of the most sophisticated facilities for eye surgery in the world—a high-tech operating room tucked into a compartment of a jet aircraft.

This is obviously no ordinary airplane. It is, in fact, the center of activity for Project Orbis, a nonprofit international organization that is dedicated to fighting blindness. Just now, the jet is parked in a corner of the airport in Kingston, Jamaica.

Inside the plane, a staff nurse settles the patient, an elderly Jamaican man, onto the operating table. The man, a diabetic who is blind, came to the airport to seek help from the Orbis physicians. Eye disorders are common among people with diabetes; in Fleischman's patient, the disease had destroyed the *retina* (the part of the eye that absorbs light rays) in one eye. Two years ago, the man lost the sight in his other eye because of bleeding in the *vitreous humor* (the clear, jellylike substance that fills the eyeball). Fortunately, the Jamaican man is in good hands. Jay Fleischman is an *ophthalmologist*, a physician who specializes in the diagnosis and treatment of eye diseases. His task is to try to remove the blood and restore some sight to the Jamaican's eye.

Before surgery begins, 11 video cameras swivel into place around the operating table. The cameras, remote-controlled from an on-board audio-visual room, will transmit every step of the delicate operation to dozens of physicians watching the surgery on television monitors.

As the cameras move into position, the patient is given a general anesthetic to put him to sleep, and Fleischman begins the operation. Peering through an operating microscope, which magnifies the small, delicate structures of the eye, he works to restore the elderly man's vision by removing the blood that has leaked into the vitreous humor.

As Fleischman labors over his patient, several dozen Jamaican physicians—some in an adjacent compartment on the plane that has been transformed from a first-class passenger section into a classroom, others in an unused terminal at the airport—watch the surgery intently on the television monitors. A camera mounted on the operating microscope gives them the same close-up view of the eyes as the surgeon; a two-way audio hookup allows them to ask Fleischman questions about the surgery in progress.

Although the operation is a simple one, Fleischman suspects that diabetes has damaged the retina of this eye as well and that surgery may not restore vision to the eye. But when he removes the blood, he is amazed to see a healthy retina. This

The author:

Mary Krier is a senior editor of *The World Book Health & Medical Annual.*

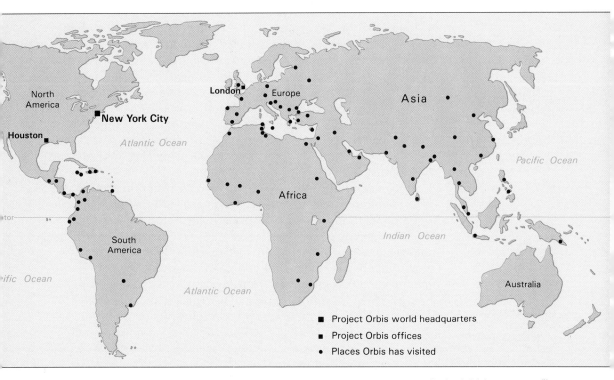

North America

London

Europe

Asia

New York City

Houston

Atlantic Ocean

Pacific Ocean

Africa

Indian Ocean

South America

ific Ocean

Atlantic Ocean

Australia

■ Project Orbis world headquarters
■ Project Orbis offices
• Places Orbis has visited

man will be able to see tomorrow, he says excitedly to the surgical team and the Jamaican ophthalmologist assisting him.

According to the World Health Organization, 42 million people in the world are blind, a number that is growing at the rate of 3 million people a year. And few of them are as lucky as Fleischman's patient. Despite the fact that blindness is a largely preventable medical problem, prevention has been difficult to achieve, especially in developing countries.

Although injury to the eyes or to the part of the brain that controls sight can cause blindness, most blindness is the result of disease, infection, or malnutrition—factors that often go hand-in-hand with poverty. Thus, it is not surprising that easily 80 per cent of all blind people live in developing countries.

Some of the more common eye disorders that Orbis physicians such as Jay Fleischman encounter include *cataracts*, a clouding of the eye's natural lens; *corneal opacity*, a scarring of the *cornea* (the clear tissue covering the eye); and *diabetic retinopathy*, a complication of diabetes in which blood vessels in the retina rupture, causing bleeding in the eye. Often, such eye conditions can be corrected by surgery. Other eye disorders can be prevented by teaching people sanitation practices, improved personal hygiene, and better nutrition. But in very

Project Orbis, a nonprofit organization based in New York City, has completed 93 missions to 55 countries since its inception in 1982. It has provided surgical demonstrations for about 9,000 physicians and has restored sight to more than 8,000 people.

poor countries, there is often an insufficient supply of food to help improve nutrition and not enough ophthalmologists and health-care workers to treat all those who need help or to teach people prevention practices. The problem is further compounded by the fact that the surgical and diagnostic equipment that would best help these doctors and health workers is not readily available to them. Hospitals either cannot afford the sophisticated equipment or are unable to properly operate and maintain it.

To David Paton, an ophthalmologist from Houston, such a situation in his own professional backyard seemed all wrong. Why should millions of people be blind when the means are available to prevent or treat most cases of blindness? It was Paton who, in the mid-1970's, first got the idea for an airborne teaching hospital that would circle the world and provide a place where eye doctors from different countries could exchange skills and technological know-how. Aware that many countries do not permit foreign doctors to perform operations in local hospitals or allow their doctors to travel to other countries to learn new techniques, Paton envisioned an operating room right in the plane, where volunteer ophthalmologists and local eye surgeons could operate side-by-side without any legal restrictions.

It was not until 1982 that Paton's idea was realized as Project Orbis. (The word *orbis* means, appropriately, *of the eye* in Latin and *around the world* in Greek.) United Airlines Incorporated donated the plane, a Douglas DC-8 built in 1960. Tiger Air Modification Center, a subsidiary of Flying Tigers

People with eye problems who have been preselected by host country doctors wait to be evaluated by the Project Orbis staff at a clinic in Hyderabad, India, *below.* From this group, the staff will select those who require surgical procedures that host country doctors have a particular interest in seeing demonstrated.

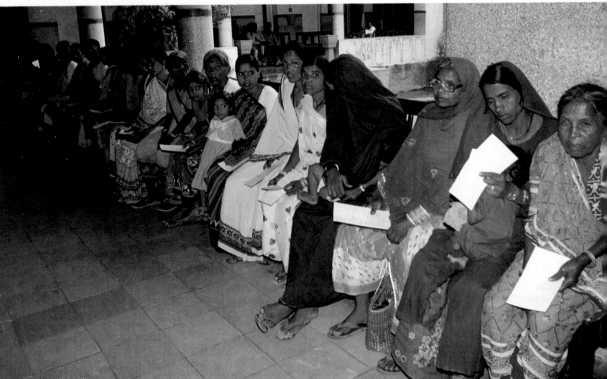

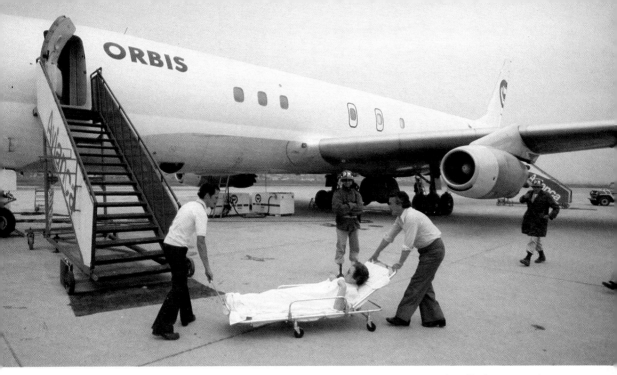

International, an air transportation equipment company, helped transform the jet into a hospital, building an operating room in the center of the plane and fitting an examination area, a laser-treatment room, an audio-visual control room, and a classroom around it. Examination and recovery areas were installed in the rear of the plane. Sony USA Incorporated contributed and installed $1 million worth of state-of-the-art audio-visual equipment, which links the operating room and the classroom.

To staff the plane on its year-round missions, Project Orbis hired a crew of 20 medical professionals—ophthalmologists, nurses, engineers, and technicians—as well as a flight mechanic. The organization also recruited ophthalmologists to donate a week of their time to teach on the plane. Pilots from United Airlines and Delta Air Lines volunteered to fly the plane from place to place. With its world headquarters and a small executive staff set up in New York City and grants coming in from dozens of organizations, Project Orbis took off.

Since 1982, the Orbis plane has circled the globe 2½ times on 93 missions to 55 countries. It visited the Soviet Union for the first time in 1987; in 1988, it made its first mission to India. A world map hanging in Project Orbis' New York offices is peppered with little yellow flags marking the sites of the plane's past visits. A red flag shows the location of Orbis' current mission.

Today, Project Orbis operates with an annual budget of $6-million. One-third of this budget comes to the organization as gifts from airlines, fuel companies, hotels, and manufacturers of medical, aviation, and computer equipment. Another one-

The flying eye hospital

Snugly fit into a DC-8 jet is a sophisticated teaching eye hospital. As the diagram below shows, the jet has everything from a laser treatment area to an operating room.

The eye operating suite

Video cameras above the operating table capture the moves of the surgical team during cataract surgery. Local doctors usually participate in such operations.

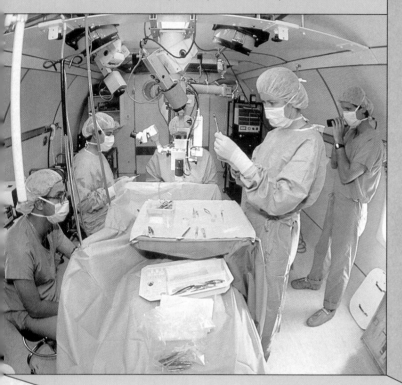

The audiovisual control center

Oswald Font, Orbis audiovisual produ runs the video control center linking the operating room and the classroc

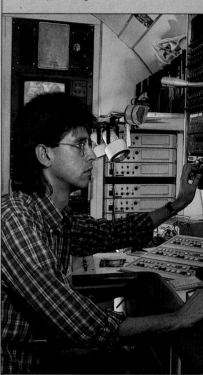

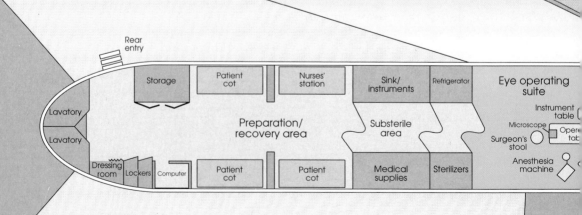

Rear entry

Lavatory

Lavatory

Dressing room | Lockers | Computer

Storage

Patient cot

Patient cot

Nurses' station

Preparation/ recovery area

Patient cot

Sink/ instruments

Substerile area

Medical supplies

Refrigerator

Sterilizers

Eye operating suite

Instrument table

Microscope

Surgeon's stool

Opera tab

Anesthesia machine

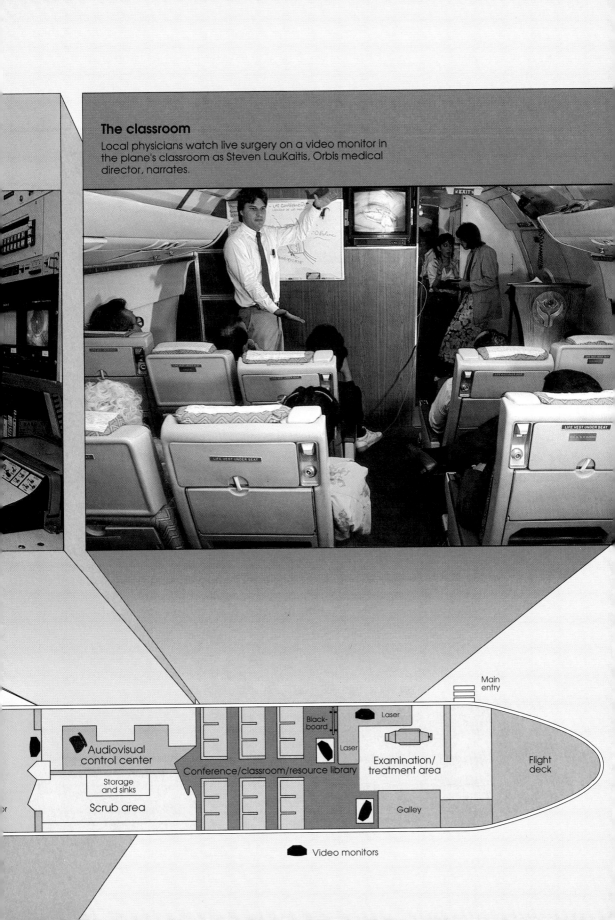

The classroom

Local physicians watch live surgery on a video monitor in the plane's classroom as Steven LauKaitis, Orbis medical director, narrates.

Main entry

Blackboard

Laser

Laser

Audiovisual control center

Examination/ treatment area

Flight deck

Conference/classroom/resource library

Storage and sinks

Galley

Scrub area

Video monitors

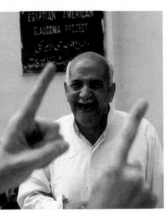

An Egyptian man whose sight was restored by Orbis physicians gives a wide grin as his vision is tested in a clinic, *above.* In San José, Costa Rica, *below,* Patrick Versace, an Orbis physician, carries a girl who has undergone surgery to an ambulance that will take her to the local hospital for recovery.

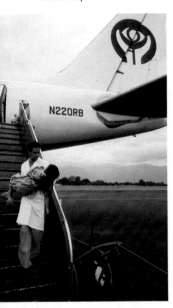

third comes from the United States Agency for International Development (a federal agency that administers programs designed to improve the quality of life in developing countries), and the rest is from foundations and corporate and private donors. This support—as well as the time donated by more than 300 ophthalmologists since 1982—has allowed Project Orbis to restore sight to more than 8,000 people and to help train some 9,000 ophthalmologists.

For the plane's crew of 20, any Orbis mission is part crusade, part adventure, and part ordeal. Logistically, Project Orbis is a kind of medical road show, visiting remote spots on a tight schedule, with high drama in almost every act. The plane usually makes 12 three-week missions a year. This fast pace is broken only three times a year, when the plane—and the crew—take a well-deserved break. During these breaks, which last several weeks, some crew members turn tourist, visiting the sights in whatever country the plane happens to be in at that time. Other members of the crew opt to fly home to visit family and friends.

Around the jet's crew, the cast of characters changes weekly, as different volunteer doctors and pilots fly in and a procession of local eye surgeons and patients visit the plane. Holding the entire show together is the Project Orbis medical director, Steven LauKaitis, an ophthalmologist who joined Project Orbis four years ago. Energetic and articulate, LauKaitis seems to thrive on the challenge of being Project Orbis' medical ringmaster.

On his crew, LauKaitis has three ophthalmologists; an *anesthesiologist* (a physician who specializes in administering anesthetics); a nurse anesthetist and five registered nurses; two biomedical engineers responsible for setting up and maintaining the plane's medical equipment; and a flight engineer. There is also a public affairs director, a mission coordinator, and an assistant to the coordinator, all of whom are responsible for organizing each mission's work schedule, arranging accommodations in the host city for the crew and visiting doctors, and other vital duties. An assistant to the medical director, a flight mechanic, and an audio-visual technician complete the roster. The Orbis crew is truly international, currently comprised of people from Canada, Great Britain, the United States, India, Yugoslavia, Thailand, Singapore, and the Philippines.

Those who know what an Orbis mission is like say that crew members must be special individuals—people who are able to work hard for weeks on end while keeping up their energy level. One crew member described his job as "having life experiences coming at you [as fast as water out] of a firehose."

But although the job can be intense, Steven LauKaitis says it is worth it. "The intensity is eclipsed by the goodness you feel in your heart by helping another person to see."

When the plane sets down at an airport, everyone, including the volunteer surgeons, will pitch in to unpack medical gear, set up audio-visual equipment, and start working with local doctors to screen patients. Even with a workday that can stretch from 7 o'clock in the morning to 11 o'clock at night, only about five operations a day can be performed.

Project Orbis will visit a country only at the invitation of the government and the local ophthalmological association. Nowadays, more invitations are offered than the organization can accept. Oliver Foot, Orbis executive director, emphasizes that each mission tries to be responsive to the needs of the local medical community by teaching the skills that local doctors say are most needed. Cataract operations are nearly always on the day's operating list. Treatment of some eye diseases with *lasers* (intense and narrow beams of light) is also often demonstrated, because lasers are becoming more affordable for many large hospitals in developing countries.

For obvious reasons, Project Orbis concerns itself with the level of ophthalmological treatment available in the cities with airports where it can land. These cities usually have hospitals that already have some modern equipment. But the problem of blindness is felt more acutely in smaller cities where hospitals lack modern surgical equipment and may even have no ophthalmologists on their modest staffs. The situation is even more desperate in rural areas, where there are few health-care workers of any kind, let alone hospitals, lasers, or surgical microscopes.

Increasingly, Project Orbis is trying to reach these small cities and rural areas through off-the-plane programs. Teaching nurses, medical assistants, and other health-care workers from these areas how to prevent eye diseases is a crucial part of Orbis' activities. Almost every evening and some afternoons, Orbis staff members and volunteer ophthalmologists give workshops, lectures, or informal talks in local hospitals.

Although the heart of Project Orbis is fighting blindness by sharing technological know-how and, in some cases, equipment, the sharing is not one-sided. The crew and volunteer doctors learn much from their local counterparts. Ironically, the greatest lesson has been just how well doctors in developing countries fight medical wars with only limited technology. Doctors from the United States and Europe often learn simple surgical techniques devised by local doctors that can be as ef-

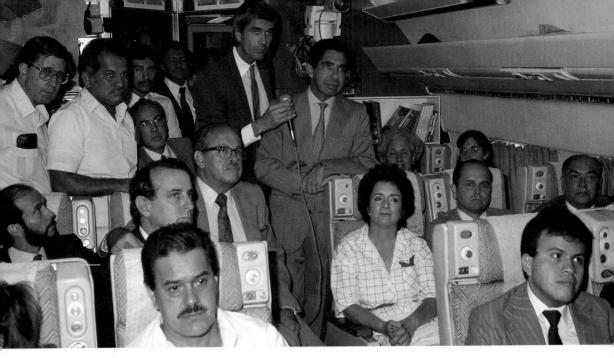

To introduce Project Orbis to a host country's government leaders and medical community, the staff invites them to tour the plane. Standing in the plane's classroom, *above,* Costa Rican President Oscar Arias Sánchez, at right, and Orbis Executive Director Oliver Foot, observe surgery on a TV monitor. In Dakar, Senegal, *below,* a local healer peers into an operating microscope.

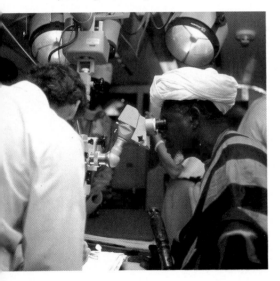

fective as the more sophisticated techniques practiced in other countries.

"It [has been] an eye opener for me," says Fleischman, who has volunteered for several Orbis missions. "I'm learning to see how people cope with much less." Fleischman and the other volunteer doctors often take the techniques they have learned from doctors on one mission and share them with doctors in other countries.

A conspicuous presence wherever it lands, the flying hospital helps make local leaders more aware of the problem of blindness in their countries. This diplomatic component of Project Orbis is where the organization's executive director excels. Oliver Foot is the son of Lord Caradon, a British diplomat and former ambassador to the United Nations. The younger Foot fully appreciates the use of artful publicity and the value of cultivating the interest of influential people who may be interested in joining Project Orbis' fight against blindness.

During each mission, Foot makes sure that the country's leaders are invited aboard the plane for a tour. While the dignitaries get the chance to witness the technological "miracles" being performed on board, they also learn what their country realistically needs to fight blindness. In some cases, this may be better surgical equipment, or a public campaign on eye care, or the establishment of an *eye bank* (a facility that supplies donated corneas for transplants).

During Project Orbis' visit to the Philippines in January and February 1989, President Corazon Aquino went aboard and announced her support of a new eye bank that Project Orbis is helping to set up in Manila. In Bangladesh, tradition has prevented the donation of eyes, but in January 1989, during Orbis' visit to Dhaka; Bangladesh President Hussain Muhammed Ershad publicly pledged his eyes for donation.

In cities without an eye bank, Orbis personnel will promote the idea by demonstrating the effectiveness of corneal transplants. In these cases, the Orbis doctors will be in close touch with nurse Risa Kory, who is Project Orbis director of medical coordination in New York City. Kory has the difficult task of finding available corneas through the network of eye banks in the United States and Canada and then figuring out how to rush them, on ice, to the plane. The job can be time-consuming, and Kory often finds herself making countless telephone calls in the middle of the night to smooth the long trip the precious corneas will have to make.

Often, a country's health ministry will give visiting surgeons the opportunity to operate in a local hospital. In these situations, host-country doctors are able to learn the most efficient way to use the equipment they already have.

One measure of the success of Project Orbis is the impact that a single mission can have on physicians in the host country. During a 1989 mission to the Philippines, Fleischman operated on a diabetic man who was blind in one eye. Assisting him at the operating table was a Philippine ophthalmologist. Although she was well trained, a lack of equipment—and confidence—had prevented her from performing operations like the one Fleischman was demonstrating.

A month after Fleischman returned to New York, he received a letter from the Philippine doctor. After Fleischman left, the patient needed a second operation, the doctor wrote. Where before she would not have attempted the surgery, the coaching she received from Fleischman gave her the confidence to perform it. Experiences such as these are what keep Orbis volunteers returning. Says Fleischman, "It's a humbling—and inspirational— experience to see people striving to improve the quality of their lives and to realize that you can make a difference."

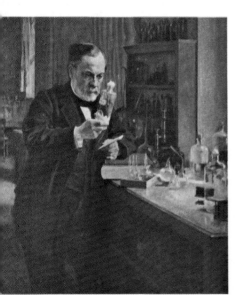

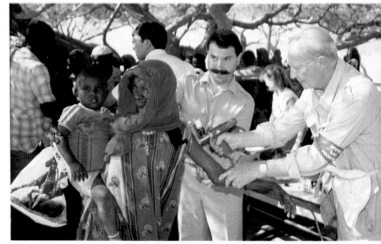

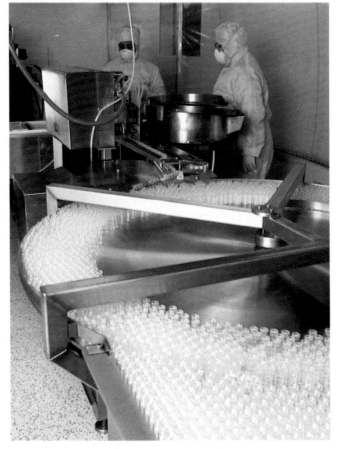

Health Studies

The World Book Health & Medical Annual takes a wide-ranging, in-depth look at a crucial issue related to personal health and fitness.

Vaccines and Your Health
by Boyce Rensberger

Vaccines have nearly eliminated a dozen common diseases that, only a generation ago, killed thousands of people every year. This report looks at how vaccines work, how they're made, and how their use is changing today.

The power of vaccines	368	Risks of vaccines	379
What is a vaccine?	369	Vaccine use worldwide	380
How vaccines are made	373	Trends in vaccine use	381
Who should be vaccinated?	378		

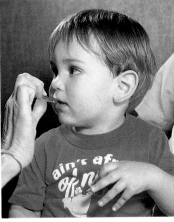

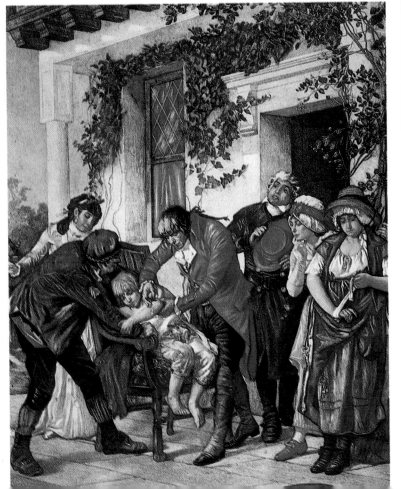

Vaccines and Your Health

By Boyce Rensberger

Read the tombstones in an old graveyard and the horrifying evidence leaps out. So many stones are for babies. And stones for older children and adults often bear similar death dates, down to the month.

Mass murders? Massacres? Yes, in a way, but worse. Before medical scientists developed vaccines, epidemics of smallpox, measles, and other diseases swept like wildfire through cities and countrysides. Sometimes whole families died together.

The power of vaccines

In this age, when health concerns focus on diet, exercise, and cancer-causing chemicals, it is easy to forget the horrors that infectious diseases—illnesses caused by "germs," or disease-causing microorganisms—have visited upon humanity. Infectious viruses and bacteria, not heart disease and cancer, were the great feared killers early in this century.

To many people over age 40, today's hysteria over AIDS is but a reminder of another epidemic that terrified the United States beginning in the late 1940's: polio. In 1950 alone, more than 33,000 Americans—mostly children—came down with "infantile paralysis," as polio was called then. The virus destroyed the nerves that controlled muscles. Paralyzed legs and arms withered. Victims whose breathing muscles were stilled gasped harder and harder for air. Some faced a lifetime of dependency on "iron lungs"—respirators that encased the body. Many stopped breathing altogether.

The mysterious epidemic spread during the 1950's, seeming to surge fastest in the summer. Children at camps were stricken in groups, and panicked parents blamed swimming pools or just contact between children. Summertime became a season of terror and, for children, confinement indoors.

But by 1955, a polio vaccine was in use. A grateful nation hailed its developer, medical researcher Jonas E. Salk, who—though only the most visible member of a large scientific program—personified the seemingly miraculous powers of vaccines. Thanks to the historic Salk vaccine and a second polio vaccine introduced a few years later by researcher Albert B. Sabin, the annual rate of new polio cases plummeted within a decade from tens of thousands to around 100 or fewer.

Polio became one in a long list of diseases tamed by vaccines. Until a vaccine for smallpox—the world's first vaccine—was developed nearly 200 years ago, nearly everyone in many parts of the world caught the disease at some point in their lives, and 20 per cent of them died of it. Even as recently as 1967, smallpox struck some 15 million people a year.

Now, thanks to a modern version of that first vaccine and a concerted effort by the World Health Organization to use it worldwide, smallpox is utterly absent from the earth. Measles, diphtheria, whooping cough, and other scourges once common in the United States are also rare today, thanks to the same two factors—an effective vaccine and a program to encourage its use.

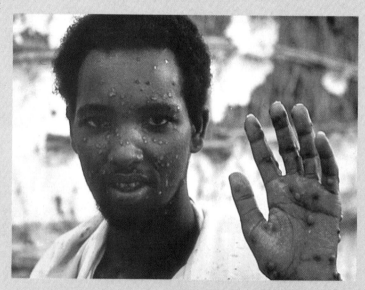

Thanks to worldwide vaccination, the centuries-old chain of smallpox infection ended in 1977 with Ali Maalin of Somalia.

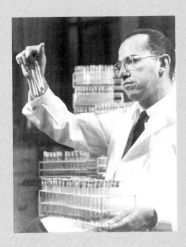

Medical researcher Jonas E. Salk became a national hero in the 1950's after he developed the first polio vaccine.

What is a vaccine?

The power of a vaccine lies not so much in the vaccine itself as in the way the human body naturally responds to it. A vaccine mimics a real disease, and in doing so, it prompts the body to defend itself. Then if the body is infected with the real disease later, it is already prepared to fight back.

To understand how a vaccine works, we must first know what types of agents cause disease—and how the body responds to them.

Agents that cause disease

Vaccines in use today work against two types of infectious microbes: viruses and bacteria. To date, no vaccines have proven fully effective against a third type of infectious agent, parasites.

Viruses cause such diseases as polio, hepatitis, measles, mumps, rabies, influenza, rubella (sometimes called German measles), and yellow fever. Vaccines exist for all these. (For more information on these diseases and their vaccines, see SOME VACCINE-PREVENTABLE DISEASES

on page 372.) Virus-caused diseases for which there are no vaccines yet include chicken pox, herpes, and AIDS.

Viruses, which are thousands of times smaller than body cells, consist of a core surrounded by an outer shell. The core contains several *genes*—coded chemical messages that all cells can read. Encasing the genes is a shell consisting of protein molecules or of a membrane in which protein molecules are embedded. These viral proteins act as *antigens*—substances (usually proteins) that the body regards as foreign and potentially dangerous.

Cells in your body also have protein molecules on their outer surfaces. These proteins are called *receptors*, and each has a particular shape. When another protein comes along with the right shape to fit onto a receptor, the combination acts like a lock and key.

When a virus enters the body, it circulates in body fluids until one of its surface proteins comes into contact with a matching type of cell receptor.

Like a key, the viral protein unlocks the receptor, and the receptor takes the virus into the cell. Receptors don't exist to take in viruses; their purpose is to take in proteins necessary to the body's functioning. It just happens that some viral proteins mimic the useful protein and thus are able to fool the cell into accepting the virus.

Cells can't tell the difference between their own genes and those of an invading virus. The cell obeys the viral genes' commands, which tell the cell to make more viruses that are exact copies of the original. Within hours, the new viruses break out of the cell, usually killing it, and go on to infect other cells, repeating the process. As more and more cells are destroyed, the body becomes ill.

Bacteria cause cholera, pertussis (also known as whooping cough), tuberculosis, pneumococcal pneumonia, diphtheria, tetanus, plague, and typhoid. Vaccines exist for all these, but not for the bacteria that cause botulism, gonorrhea, or Legionnaires' disease, among others.

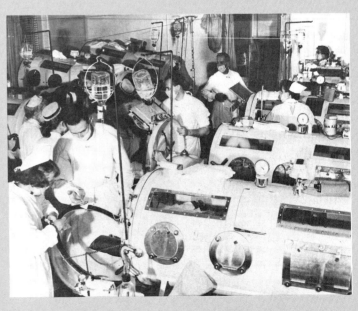

As polio spread in the 1950's, hospital wards filled with rows of iron lungs, respirators that kept victims alive but immobile.

Bacteria are living, one-celled organisms, bigger than viruses but still much smaller than human cells. Like viruses, bacteria have protein antigens embedded in their outer walls.

Many types of bacteria live harmlessly on the skin or in the body. Some, however, may cause disease under certain circumstances. Sometimes bacteria produce *toxins* (poisons) that kill cells so that they may feed on the cells' remains. The destruction of cells causes illness. Bacteria may also release toxins as waste products; these spread through the body and poison various organs.

Parasites, which are more complex than either viruses or bacteria, are microscopic animals whose natural habitat is the bodies of larger animals. Some examples are the amebas that cause dysentery, the protozoans that cause malaria, and the trypanosomes that cause sleeping sickness.

Each parasite goes through its own complex life cycle, often developing through several stages in different parts of the body or in different animals. Parasites also have protein antigens on their surfaces. Although there are experimental vaccines against some parasites, none so far are effective enough for general use.

The immune response

The immune system is the body's natural defense mechanism. Its job is to distinguish harmful agents from the body's own substances and then to attack the invaders. Two types of white blood cells, *B cells* and *T cells*, carry out these tasks. Like other cells, B cells and T cells have receptors shaped to fit various antigens. This allows the cells to recognize the characteristic antigens on a microbe's surface.

For example, when a virus enters the body, certain T cells may match its antigen and thus be able to bind onto it. Those T cells then begin dividing, making an army of T cells with the same receptor. If the virus has already invaded a body cell, the infected cell will begin producing viral antigens on its surface. The matching T cells can spot these antigens, bind to the infected cell, and kill it along with its viral inhabitants.

As a second line of defense, the infection-activated T cells also stimulate B cells. The B cells' job is to manufacture *antibodies*—protein molecules that roam the bloodstream as free-floating receptors. When these antibodies bind to viral antigens, they have two effects. First, by occupying all the virus's antigens, they prevent the virus from attaching to a cell. Second, a microbe covered with antibodies becomes an attractive morsel for another kind of immune system cell, a *macrophage*. The hungry macrophages engulf and digest anything covered with antibodies.

For many years scientists were baffled by how the immune system could have enough different kinds of antibodies to fit the millions of possible antigens that might show up on invading microbes. Research has shown that the cells of the immune system have an amazing ability to evolve, randomly creating new shapes of antibodies and receptors. When stimulated by a new antigen, the cells with the best fit reproduce faster than others. Over a period of days or weeks after an infection, the immune system "learns" to make the most effective antibody. This is why it may take some time before the immune system gains the strength to knock out a new kind of infection.

Once the microbes are defeated, the body maintains low levels of specialized T cells, B cells, and antibodies in the blood for years. If the same microbe should invade again, the immune system is ready and waiting to knock it out before it

can cause symptoms. The body has become *immunized* against that particular microbe.

How vaccines work

Most infections are highly effective at protecting a person from catching the disease again—assuming they don't kill the victim first. Vaccines induce immunity, too, though not always as powerful as the immunity from a real infection.

Vaccines work by tricking the immune system into thinking the body is being infected. When it enters the body, a vaccine—though generally harmless—has some of the features of a particular invading microbe. The immune system responds to the vaccine by making T cells, B cells, and antibodies tailored to it. These defenses, which the body continues to maintain, are equally effective against the real disease agent. Should a real infection occur, the immune system is prepared and can destroy the microbes before they can cause illness.

In most cases, a vaccine carries out its masquerade by adopting the microbe's chief identifying characteristic: its surface antigens. Some vaccines contain the microbe itself, treated so that it cannot reproduce and thus cannot destroy body cells. Such vaccines are said to use "killed" or *inactivated* viruses or bacteria.

Other vaccines contain live, *attenuated* microbes—viral or bacterial strains, developed in the laboratory, that are weakened so that they cannot cause disease. The first vaccine ever developed, the smallpox vaccine, is a special case of a live vaccine: It is simply a different, relatively harmless virus whose surface proteins are so similar to those of the smallpox virus that it prompts immunity to smallpox as well as to itself.

Not all vaccines use microbes. Some are designed to attack the toxic proteins produced by certain bacteria. The

How vaccines work

When a virus invades the body, the body fights back. Vaccines work by mimicking an infection, prompting the body to prepare a defense before the real disease strikes.

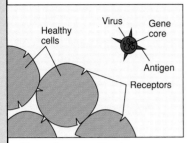

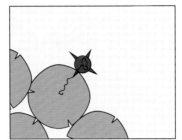

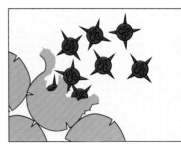

How viruses attack
A virus has a core of genes surrounded by a shell. On the shell are proteins called antigens, which are shaped to fit proteins called receptors on certain body cells.

The virus infects a cell by entering through a receptor. The virus then passes to the cell its coded genetic message, which instructs the cell to produce more viruses.

The cell begins to manufacture new viruses just like the original. Within hours, the viruses break out of the cell, killing it, and go on to infect other cells.

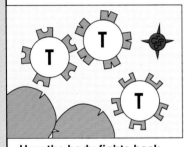

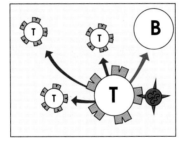

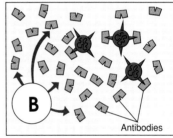

How the body fights back
The body's chief defender is the T cell, a type of white blood cell that also has receptors. A T cell with the right shape of receptor will bind to the virus.

Activated by the virus, the T cell makes more T cells, which hunt more viruses. The T cell also sends a message to another type of white blood cell, the B cell.

The B cell then produces proteins called antibodies. The antibodies, which are shaped to match and bind to viral antigens, prevent the viruses from infecting cells.

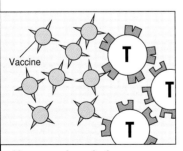

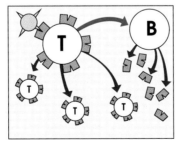

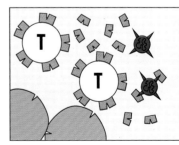

How vaccines help
Some vaccines are made of viruses that have been weakened so that they cannot harm body cells. But T cells still react to the antigens on the weakened viruses.

The T cells see the vaccine as an invading virus and bind to it. As with a real infection, the body produces more T cells and antibodies to match the virus's antigen.

Matching T cells and antibodies may be maintained in the body for years, or even for life. If a real virus of this type appears, the body is ready to defend itself.

Some vaccine-preventable diseases

Cholera, an often fatal bacterial disease that attacks the digestive system, is commonly transmitted by contaminated food or water. The vaccine is given mostly to travelers visiting places where cholera is common.

Diphtheria, a bacterial disease, usually attacks the tonsils and throat and may cause death from suffocation or heart damage. The vaccine, developed in the 1920's, is given routinely to children, its most frequent victims.

Hepatitis B, a viral disease that attacks the liver, is transmitted through blood or sexual contact. The first hepatitis vaccine was licensed in 1981; it was replaced with the first genetically engineered vaccine in 1986. It is given to people whose jobs or habits put them at high risk for the disease.

Influenza infects the respiratory tract, causing chills, weakness, aches and pains, and fever. In the elderly, it may lead to more serious diseases, such as pneumonia. A vaccine was first developed in 1943, but a new variation must be produced each time the influenza virus mutates, about once a year.

Measles, a viral disease, is characterized by a rash of small red spots; it can be fatal to very young or undernourished children. The vaccine, licensed in 1963 and improved over the years, is routinely given to children.

Meningitis, a sometimes fatal disease that attacks the protective membranes around the brain or spinal cord, causes a wide variety of symptoms including fever, vomiting, or convulsions. Vaccines exist for two forms caused by bacteria. The vaccine for *hemophilus influenzae* (sometimes called bacterial meningitis) is routinely given to children. The *meningococcal meningitis* vaccine—effective only for a short time in children—is given to certain adults, such as military recruits.

Mumps, a viral disease, causes swelling of the salivary glands and difficulty swallowing. In adults, mumps may cause sterility. The vaccine, developed in 1967, is routinely given to children.

Pertussis (whooping cough), a bacterial disease that mostly affects children, attacks the air passages, causing loud, gasping coughing. The disease can affect the brain, causing mental retardation, paralysis, or death. The vaccine, developed in the 1920's, is given routinely to children.

Pneumococcal pneumonia, a sometimes fatal bacterial disease of the lungs, causes fever, pain, and coughing. The vaccine is given to the elderly or the chronically ill, in whom the disease is most dangerous.

Polio, a viral disease, attacks the spinal cord, sometimes causing paralysis or death. Children, polio's primary victims, routinely receive either the Salk vaccine, approved in 1955, or the Sabin oral vaccine, approved in 1961.

Rubella (German measles), a viral disease resembling measles, is most dangerous in pregnant women; it can cause birth defects or death of the fetus. Since 1969, the vaccine has been given routinely to children.

Smallpox, a highly contagious viral disease, killed many of its victims and left others scarred or blind. In 1796, physician Edward Jenner discovered that the milder cowpox virus would protect a person against smallpox. Routine vaccination with cowpox continued in the United States until 1971; the last known naturally occurring smallpox case in the world was 1977.

Tetanus, a disease characterized by muscle stiffness and spasm (including lockjaw), and sometimes death, is usually caused by contamination of a wound with dirt in which the bacteria live. The vaccine, developed in the 1920's, is given routinely to children and should be repeated throughout life.

Tuberculosis, a bacterial disease that usually affects the lungs, causes coughing, pain, fatigue, and many other symptoms. The vaccine is not always effective, and is generally reserved for people in contact with victims.

Typhoid, a sometimes fatal intestinal disease, is spread by contaminated food. The vaccine is given to some travelers and people exposed to patients.

Yellow fever, a viral disease spread by infected mosquitoes, causes chills, fever, and liver disorders, and sometimes coma and death. The vaccine is given to people traveling to tropical areas where the disease is common.

Above are the best-known diseases for which vaccines are available in the United States. Other vaccines, mostly for rarer diseases, are restricted to high-risk populations or experimental uses.

vaccines contain similar proteins that are just different enough not to be toxic. Antibodies to these harmless *toxoids* will also attack the real toxins, preventing them from harming the body.

Still other vaccines focus not on the proteins of a microbe or its toxins but on other identifying molecules on the surfaces of the invading agents. And researchers continue to seek new ways to trick the immune system into a defensive response.

Types of immunization

When a person develops immunity either from having a disease or in response to a vaccine, the process is called *active immunization*. This means the immune system has developed cells on its own to fight the infection.

Another kind of immunity can be created through *passive immunization*. This is done by injecting a person with *serum* (the liquid part of the blood left after the blood cells are removed) from a person or animal that is already immune to the disease. Serum contains antibodies that the donor developed earlier through active immunization. This procedure is used to treat infections in which victims without immunity might suffer or die before they develop their own antibodies. For example, some serums provide antibodies against fast-acting toxins from snake bites and spider bites. Other serums work against the viruses that cause hepatitis, measles, chicken pox, rabies, and tetanus.

A natural form of passive immunization takes place in a woman's womb during pregnancy, when some of the mother's antibodies enter the fetus's bloodstream. After birth, the mother can pass on even more antibodies in her milk. This is why doctors stress the value of breast-feeding newborn babies. Antibodies from the mother can protect a baby for the first few months of its life, as its own immune system develops.

How vaccines are made

History books credit the English physician Edward Jenner (1749-1823) with developing the first vaccine in 1796. But Jenner's achievement was based on a folk tradition reaching back thousands of years.

The oldest records of immunization refer to Chinese and Indian civilizations of around the year 1000. These peoples would take tiny bits of scab or pus from the sores of a smallpox victim and administer them to a healthy person, either by inhalation or through a cut in the skin. The latter method was later called *variolation* (from *variola*, the Latin word for smallpox). We know now that material from smallpox sores contained smallpox viruses. The small quantity passed in variolation would usually cause only a mild case of smallpox. After that, the person would be protected from the disease.

In 1721, an English author named Mary Wortley Montagu, who had learned of variolation while living in Turkey, introduced the technique into England. Variolation worked most of the time, but it was dangerous; about 2 to 3 per cent of the people who received it developed a bad case of smallpox and died before their immune systems could respond fully. Jenner found a safer method.

The first vaccines

Jenner noticed that people who worked with cattle—milkmaids in particular—seemed to be immune to smallpox. He also found that many milkmaids had at some point had a case of *cowpox*. This cattle disease can infect people who come

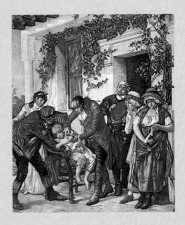

Physician Edward Jenner tested his theory of smallpox prevention by inoculating an 8-year-old boy with cowpox in 1796.

into contact with sores on an infected cow. In human beings, cowpox produces only a minor, passing illness, typically caus-

The impact of vaccines on three childhood diseases

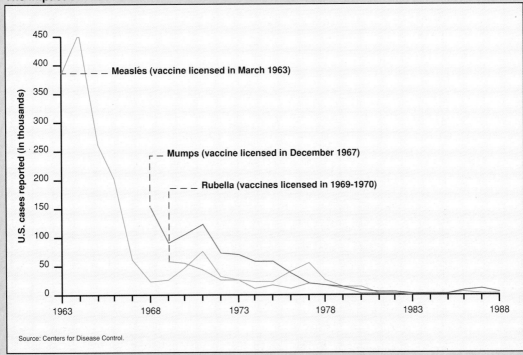

In the last 25 years, vaccines have reduced the incidence of measles, mumps, and rubella — three once-common childhood diseases — to fewer than 5,000 cases of each in most years since 1981.

ing some sores on the hands.

Jenner reasoned that if people could be deliberately infected with cowpox, they might be protected against smallpox. To test this theory, he collected the pus from a milkmaid's cowpox sores and rubbed it into scratches in the skin of an 8-year-old boy. The boy developed cowpox. Seven weeks later, Jenner tried to infect the boy with smallpox. He was immune.

We know now that cowpox virus has surface proteins so similar to those of smallpox that antibodies against these antigens also attack smallpox viruses. Thus, a person who has developed immunity to cowpox becomes immune to smallpox. Jenner did not know about viruses or antigens. But his procedure worked and was eventually used widely. It was called *vaccination*, from *vacca*, the Latin word for cow.

The next step in vaccine science would not come for almost 100 years. In 1878, the great French microbiologist Louis Pasteur (1822-1895) was studying

chicken cholera, an often fatal disease of chickens. Pasteur found that chicken cholera was caused by bacteria that he could grow in bottles. When he injected healthy chickens with the bacteria, they became ill.

His chief discovery, however, came as the result of an accident. A batch of chicken cholera bacteria was inadvertently left standing in a laboratory over a long, hot summer. When Pasteur injected these bacteria in chickens, the chickens suffered only a mild form of the disease, from which they recovered. Pasteur wondered whether these chickens might now be immune to ordinary, virulent cholera bacteria. Further experiments showed that they were. Apparently the heat-damaged bacteria were too weak to cause severe illness but were still able to trigger immunity. Pasteur had inadvertently made a vaccine of attenuated live bacteria.

Pasteur went on to produce, in 1881, an attenuated vaccine for *anthrax*, a disease of hoofed animals that can also infect human beings. To honor Jenner,

he adopted the term *vaccine* to cover all his immunizing preparations. Most notable of all was his vaccine for *rabies*, a viral disease of the nervous system often transmitted through bites from infected animals.

One day in 1885, word reached Pasteur of a 9-year-old boy who had been bitten by a rabid dog. Rabies does most of its damage before the immune system can respond sufficiently, and in Pasteur's day most victims died. Pasteur, who had been developing attenuated rabies virus strains in his laboratory, reasoned that a vaccine might provoke an immune response in time to fight the infection. He gave the boy 13 injections over a 10-day period. The youngster lived.

Pasteur's work launched modern vaccine science on a spectacular course. Vaccines for typhoid, cholera, and plague followed by 1900. The 1920's saw the development of vaccines for diphtheria, tetanus, and pertussis. Some of the other important vaccines developed since then are listed in SOME VACCINE-PREVENTABLE DISEASES on page 372.

Making modern vaccines

Today, vaccines are made by five main methods. For some diseases, different vaccines have been developed using different techniques.

Related live-microbe vaccine. The oldest method is Jenner's approach: Find an existing virus that causes little or no disease but which is so similar to the disease agent that antibodies for one will work on both. To date, the smallpox vaccine— made from cowpox—is the only vaccine of this type.

The cowpox virus is grown in the laboratory in *tissue culture*. This technique involves introducing a virus to animal or human cells grown in bottles with a nutrient fluid. As the infected cells multiply in the container, the fluid surrounding the cells

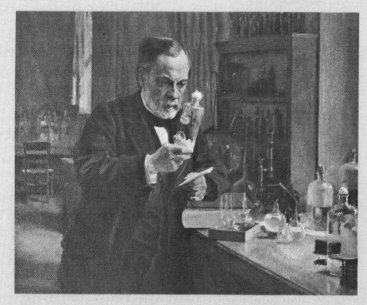

French microbiologist Louis Pasteur, building on Jenner's discovery, developed vaccines for rabies and other diseases.

fills with viruses, which are separated out for the vaccine.

Attenuated live-microbe vaccines. In this approach, scientists work to produce a new strain of a virus or bacterium. To be useful, the new strain must retain the original's surface proteins and multiply in the human body, but must cause little or no illness. Vaccines were developed this way from the viruses that cause measles, mumps, polio (the Sabin vaccine), rubella, and yellow fever.

For virus-based vaccines, the first step is to grow the virus in the laboratory. Since viruses need living cells to reproduce, scientists look for a kind of animal cell that can live in a test tube and can harbor the virus. The virus for the Sabin polio vaccine, for example, is grown in cultures of monkey kidney cells. The mumps virus used in that vaccine is grown in chicken embryos.

Not all copies of a given virus are alike; when the virus reproduces, normal mutations frequently create individual viruses with slightly different genes. Because the cells in a laboratory culture are a different type from those the virus normally infects, only a few of these variant viruses will also happen to possess the ability to live in the culture. These survivors are then tested on animals. The goal is to find a strain of the virus that retains the original antigens (and thus creates immunity) but which has lost the genes that make it cause disease. This hit-or-miss process usually requires many attempts before a suitable strain can be found.

The tuberculosis vaccine is the only attenuated bacterial vaccine. It was bred from active tuberculosis bacteria in the early 1900's, through a painstaking process that took 13 years of careful culturing of altered strains. The resulting vaccine strain—named *bacille Calmette-Guerin*, or BCG—has continued to evolve in the many laborato-

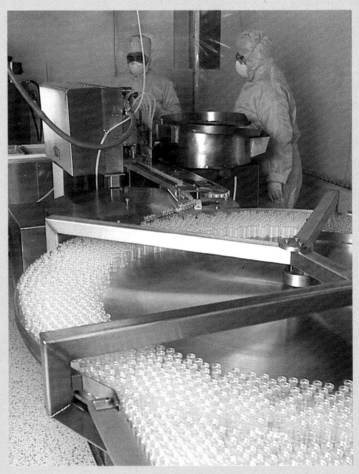

Vials are filled with a combined vaccine for measles, mumps, and rubella at a pharmaceutical plant in Pennsylvania.

ries that grow it for use. Thus, the current tuberculosis vaccine is actually a family of dozens of related vaccine strains.

Killed-microbe vaccines. If no effective live vaccine can be produced, an alternative is to use chemicals or ultraviolet light to inactivate or "kill" the microbe—that is, to damage it so that it can no longer reproduce. This method is used for the Salk polio vaccine, as well as for vaccines for influenza, cholera, pertussis, plague, and typhoid. The rabies vaccine used today is a killed-virus vaccine; it is the latest of several new vaccines developed since the 1950's to

replace Pasteur's original live-virus vaccine.

Killed-microbe vaccines generally do not create as long-lasting an immunity as those containing live microbes. That is because the number of antigen molecules available to stimulate the immune system is limited to those in the vaccine dose itself. These antigens can prompt the body to make only a small number of antibodies. With live-microbe vaccines, the microbes continue to multiply in the body for a while, creating more copies of the antigen—which in turn stimulate the production of special T cells and B cells.

Thus, to maintain a person's immunity, killed-microbe vaccines must be repeated at intervals. For example, children getting their first dose of pertussis vaccine at 2 months of age typically also receive four booster doses by age 6. The vaccines for cholera and plague, which are given only to certain people who risk exposure to the disease, last only about 6 months and must be repeated if additional exposure is expected.

Toxoid vaccines. An entirely different method uses not the organism itself, but rather protein molecules closely related to the toxins produced by the infecting bacteria. These *toxoids* are made by purifying an extract of real toxins and then chemically treating them to alter their structure. Toxoids are enough like toxins to stimulate antibody production, but different enough that they are not harmful. Tetanus and diphtheria vaccines are toxoids.

Like killed-microbe vaccines, toxoid doses need to be repeated periodically to be effective. In children, the diphtheria and tetanus toxoids are usually combined with the pertussis vaccine into a preparation called DTP. After age 6, the two toxoids should be repeated every 10 years throughout life.

Polysaccharide vaccines. While most vaccines work by dosing the immune system with protein antigens, others use different molecules that also act as antigens and can stimulate antibody production. These molecules, called *polysaccharides*, are sugars that certain bacteria carry on their outer surfaces. A vaccine is produced by growing the bacteria in the laboratory and chemically treating them to break off the polysaccharides. These are then purified and given as a vaccine.

Vaccines for pneumococcal pneumonia, hemophilus influenzae (a form of bacterial meningitis), and meningococcal meningitis are made this way.

Immunity from these vaccines can wear off, but this varies from person to person.

New vaccine techniques
Classic vaccine-making procedures, which contain a form of the disease agent itself, work well for microbes that can be altered to make them unable to cause illness. But new methods of alteration have to be invented for each microbe, and a great many infectious agents have not yet succumbed to any method.

A new set of techniques, however, offers hope for fighting many diseases that still plague humanity. These approaches use the powerful new methods of genetic engineering.

The most promising approach is based on the fact that immunity is not a response to the entire microbe but to a particular part, or *subunit*, of it—specifically, an antigenic surface protein. This approach seeks to manufacture only the required subunit, apart from the disease agent itself.

To do this, molecular biologists extract from the virus the gene that carries the instructions for producing its antigen. This gene is placed inside yeast cells, which can be grown easily in large vats. The yeast cells follow the gene's instructions and churn out large quantities of the antigen—but not the rest of the virus.

The vaccine made from these antigens is called a *subunit vaccine.* One subunit vaccine—the vaccine for hepatitis B—was approved for U.S. use in 1986. This vaccine replaced an older vaccine produced in a difficult and costly process from the blood of living human carriers.

An even newer idea calls for bringing Jenner's highly successful *vaccinia* (cowpox) virus out of semiretirement. Its general use as a smallpox vaccine ended when smallpox was declared eradicated in 1980. Now, however, scientists are experimenting with inserting genes

from other viruses into vaccinia. Thus, for example, when vaccinia virus bearing the gene for hepatitis B antigen is grown in cell cultures, it emerges bearing not only its own surface proteins but also those of hepatitis B. Researchers think that a person vaccinated with this enhanced virus might become immune to hepatitis B.

Some researchers think it may be possible to insert genes from more than one disease-causing virus into the same vaccinia virus. This "supervaccine" would theoretically immunize people against several different diseases at once. Such a vaccine might take another 5 to 10 years to develop, but the idea is considered promising because vaccinia is generally safe and methods for producing vaccines from it were established long ago. Similar "piggybacking" experiments are being done with the BCG bacterium, used in the vaccine for tuberculosis.

While these methods involve inserting genes from a dangerous microbe into a harmless carrier, another approach seeks to alter the disease agent itself. To do this, scientists identify a gene crucial to the microbe's harmful abilities and use gene-altering techniques to remove or disable it. In effect, they attenuate the microbe by reprogramming its genes.

This approach eliminates a major problem with live-microbe vaccines. Attenuated strains bred in the laboratory can continue to mutate over time and may sometimes return to a disease-causing form. A genetically attenuated microbe cannot return to a harmful state because it lacks the genes it would need to do so. And since researchers can design their own strains, they need not rely on random breeding in hope of isolating one that works. This method has produced successful vaccines for animal diseases, and researchers hope to apply it to human diseases.

Vaccines for children

Vaccines for the following eight diseases are given routinely to children in the United States.

Diphtheria. Prevalent before the first vaccine was developed in the 1920's, diphtheria is now rare, with only 23 cases reported in the United States from 1980 through 1988. The vaccine is usually given along with tetanus and pertussis vaccines in a combination called DTP. A series of four DTP doses is recommended for babies. A fifth dose is recommended upon starting school, unless the fourth dose was given after age 4. Children age 7 and older who have not been immunized should have three doses of an adult vaccine, called Td, which includes only the tetanus and diphtheria vaccines. Immunity usually lasts 10 years; everyone should be revaccinated periodically throughout life.

Tetanus. Incidence of the disease does not follow a pattern because the bacteria are transmitted through contaminated wounds, not from person to person in epidemics. The number of cases has declined steadily since the first vaccine was developed in the 1920's. The vaccine is usually given in combination with diphtheria and pertussis vaccines, as described above. Everyone should be revaccinated every 10 years for life.

Pertussis (whooping cough). Once fairly common, pertussis has generally declined over the last 40 years. In 1988, however, there were about 3,000 U.S. cases, up significantly from an average of 1,600 a year in the early 1980's. The rise may be due to a decline in vaccination, as several widely publicized instances of severe reactions to the vaccine have led many parents to avoid vaccinating their children. Since the mid-1940's, a vaccine has been given in combination with diphtheria and tetanus vaccines, as described above. Pertussis vaccine is not usually given to people over age 7 because the disease is milder in older people and because adverse reactions to the vaccine are more common. The duration of immunity is not well established.

Polio (poliomyelitis, infantile paralysis). Epidemics struck as many as 15,000 Americans a year until the Salk killed-virus vaccine and the Sabin live-virus vaccine were introduced in the late 1950's. Incidence of the disease fell dramatically; between 1980 and 1988 there was an average of eight cases a year. The Salk vaccine confers immunity for five years. The Sabin vaccine grants lifelong immunity. Given in four doses throughout childhood, the Sabin vaccine is the only generally available vaccine administered orally.

Measles (rubeola). Before the single-dose vaccine was licensed in 1963, measles was so common that 90 per cent of the population was infected before age 20, causing nearly 500,000 cases per year. Many of the few thousand cases that still occur annually are among children who have not yet been vaccinated. To remedy this, the ACIP in 1989 lowered the recommended age of vaccination from 15 months to 9 months for children in areas of measles outbreaks; a booster dose is given at 15 months. The vaccine used today usually gives lifelong immunity; earlier versions were less reliable, leaving some young adults at risk.

Mumps. Before the vaccine was licensed in 1967, mumps struck about 150,000 Americans a year. By the mid-1980's, the number had declined to around 3,000. The number rose to nearly 13,000 cases in 1987, largely as the result of lax enforcement of vaccination in several states, but has since fallen again. A single dose of the vaccine, usually given in combination with measles and rubella vaccines, is recommended for children 15 months old.

Rubella (German measles). Before the vaccine was licensed in 1969, epidemics every few years produced waves of handicapped children, born to women who caught the disease while pregnant. Vaccination caused the number of rubella cases to drop from around 50,000 cases a year in the 1960's to fewer than 300 today. The vaccine is given as a single dose to all children at age 15 months, often in combination with measles and mumps vaccines. Boys as well as girls are vaccinated to prevent epidemics of disease that may spread to pregnant women. Immunity is lifelong.

Hemophilus influenzae. About 12,000 cases occur annually in the United States, mostly in children under age 5. About 5 per cent die; many others suffer permanent nerve damage. The vaccine, licensed in 1985, is highly effective in children older than 18 months. It is now given to children around their second birthday. Its effectiveness in reducing the number of cases will not be known for several years.

Recommended vaccination schedule for children

These are general recommendations from the Advisory Committee on Immunization Practices (ACIP), which operates under the U.S. Public Health Service. Individual circumstances may vary according to such factors as geographic region, current epidemics, missed or late doses, and special health considerations of the child. In addition to these vaccines in the first two years of life, ACIP recommends additional doses of diphtheria/tetanus/pertussis vaccine (DTP) and oral polio vaccine at or before school entry.

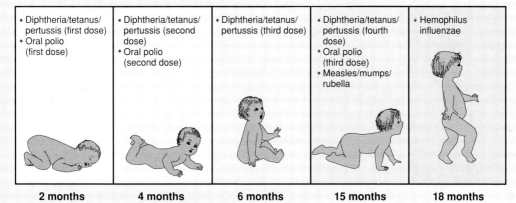

2 months	4 months	6 months	15 months	18 months
• Diphtheria/tetanus/ pertussis (first dose) • Oral polio (first dose)	• Diphtheria/tetanus/ pertussis (second dose) • Oral polio (second dose)	• Diphtheria/tetanus/ pertussis (third dose)	• Diphtheria/tetanus/ pertussis (fourth dose) • Oral polio (third dose) • Measles/mumps/ rubella	• Hemophilus influenzae

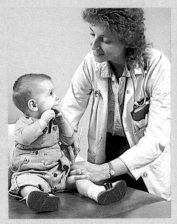
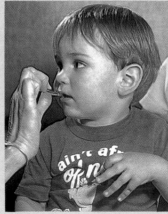

Children routinely receive vaccines for eight diseases. Most are injected, left; *only polio vaccine is given orally,* right.

Who should be vaccinated?

Although vaccination is simple in principle, many factors make it impossible or unwise to give all vaccines to anybody at any time. Some vaccines are more effective than others. Some are effective for only a short time. Some are too expensive or too scarce for mass use.

And not all vaccines are completely safe. Some may cause side effects or, rarely, even the disease they are supposed to prevent. Use of these vaccines is thus justified only among people for whom the risk of contracting the disease itself outweighs the risks of the vaccine.

To help with these decisions, the U.S. government has set up a panel of experts to monitor vaccination practices and recommend standards for use. This group is the Immunization Practices Advisory Committee, which meets regularly under the auspices of the Centers for Disease Control (CDC), a branch of the U.S. Public Health Service (PHS) based in Atlanta, Ga.

When most people think of vaccines, they think of the routine "shots" most children get early in life. (The Sabin polio vaccine is the only oral vaccine in common use.) Most children should be vaccinated for diphtheria, tetanus, pertussis, polio, measles, rubella, mumps, and hemophilus influenzae. Details on childhood vaccinations appear in VACCINES FOR CHILDREN, page 377.

Vaccinated children carry most of their immunities into adulthood. But special groups of adults should also be vaccinated on certain occasions.

Vaccines for the elderly

In younger people, influenza— or "flu"—is a relatively minor viral disease. But it can be fatal for the elderly or for people with *chronic* (ongoing) illnesses that reduce their natural ability to fight off infection.

Influenza poses a special problem for scientists, however. The virus mutates rapidly, producing new types with different antigens every year or so. As a result, a vaccine effective on one type will be useless against a new type. A new vaccine must be created and distributed as each new strain arises.

Because vaccine makers must repeatedly develop new flu vaccines, there is usually not enough of a given type to immunize everyone. Moreover, frequent revaccination is inconvenient both for patients and for the health professionals who must keep track of them. For these reasons, the vaccine is recommended chiefly for those threatened most by the disease: the elderly and people of any age with chronic diseases.

Pneumococcal pneumonia is often fatal for the elderly, but a single dose of the vaccine will usually prevent the disease. The version of the vaccine in use since 1983 includes the polysaccharides of 23 types of bacteria, which among them cause about 90 per cent of all bacterial pneumonias.

Still, immunity may last as little as five years, and some studies suggest that a second dose may cause a severe reaction. Thus, only a single dose is recommended in a lifetime—and that dose is usually reserved for late in life, when the disease poses its greatest threat.

About half of all cases of tetanus—an often-fatal disease typically caught through a contaminated wound—occur in people over age 60. About half of the people in this age group carry few or no antibodies to the tetanus toxin, either because they were never immunized or be-

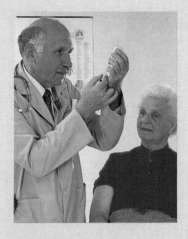

One of the most important adult vaccines is for influenza. Most older adults should receive an annual "flu shot."

cause their immunity has disappeared over time.

All people, regardless of age, should be revaccinated for tetanus every 10 years. But if a severe or contaminated wound occurs more than 5 years after the last immunization, another dose is recommended.

Vaccines for travelers

Residents of the United States who travel abroad may need vaccinations, depending on the countries they plan to visit. No special immunizations are recommended for travel to western Europe, Canada, Australia, or Japan. Many other countries require official documents proving vaccination against cholera or yellow fever or both. By contrast, the United States requires no vaccination for Americans returning home.

It is generally recommended that travelers be adequately immunized against measles, tetanus, diphtheria, polio, typhoid, and meningococcus if visiting areas where the level of sanitation is poor. Hepatitis B vaccine is recommended if sexual contact is expected in Southeast Asia or certain parts of Africa. Smallpox vaccination is no longer required anywhere, because the only existing smallpox viruses left on earth are laboratory specimens.

Because the advisability of various vaccinations varies widely with the traveler's plans and personal circumstances, travelers should consult a physician for guidelines. General recommendations are available in the annual *Health Information for International Travel Supplement*, a CDC booklet available from that agency as well as from passport offices and many travel agents.

Other high-risk groups

Several vaccines are available only to people who face high risk of exposure through jobs, hobbies, or habits.

Some types of diseases

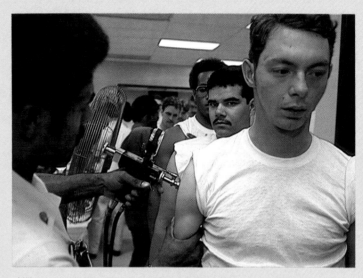

Military recruits receive several special vaccines, including those for meningococcal meningitis, adenovirus, and smallpox.

spread particularly rapidly among new military recruits, who come from many different backgrounds and regions and live in large communal groups. Especially troublesome have been epidemics of meningococcal meningitis as well as of respiratory diseases caused by adenoviruses. New recruits are now routinely vaccinated for both. Recruits are also vaccinated for smallpox, to protect against any reappearance of this deadly disease—and because of fear that it may be used in biological warfare.

Tuberculosis vaccine often confers lifelong immunity, but results have varied widely; it is given only to people in close, prolonged contact with infected patients. Hepatitis B vaccine is recommended only for members of groups shown to be at high risk, such as intravenous drug abusers, homosexual men, families of carriers, and certain health-care professionals.

Some vaccines are available only to people who may be exposed to the animals that carry certain diseases. Rabies vaccine is recommended for veterinarians, kennel workers, and others who may come in contact

with infected wildlife, as well as for people bitten by possibly rabid animals. People who handle imported animal hides and hair may be vaccinated for anthrax, which infects hoofed animals outside the United States. Some laboratory and animal workers may be vaccinated for plague, which is carried by some wild animals in the Southwest. And vaccine for *tularemia* (rabbit fever), a sometimes fatal bacterial disease often transmitted by tick bites, is available only for people who work with wild animals in which the disease is common.

Risks of vaccines

The extraordinary success of vaccines has not come without high costs and occasional public opposition. The most devastating setbacks have resulted from health threats caused by the vaccines themselves.

One of the worst episodes occurred at the height of one of the greatest successes of vaccine development—in 1955, when the first lots of the much-heralded Salk polio vaccine were being given to children. Beginning within days after their vaccinations, 94 of the recipients came down with polio. They, in turn, passed the disease to 166 others. Of those 260 victims, 192 were permanently paralyzed. Eleven died.

As it turned out, certain lots of the vaccine contained active polio virus instead of the intended killed virus. Salk's method of inactivating the virus worked for small batches of vaccine produced in the laboratory, but it did not work at one of the six pharmaceutical companies producing the vaccine in large batches. Public trust of vaccination was severely damaged, and rebuilt only after years of official reassurance that more stringent manufacturing methods were being enforced.

All vaccinations pose some risk of side effects. Most common are relatively mild soreness and inflammation at the site of the injection. Sometimes temporary fever and *malaise* (a general ill-feeling) result. These reactions are all part of the immune system's natural response to the foreign proteins.

Specific problems vary with each particular vaccine. Repeated immunizations with diphtheria and tetanus vaccines often cause increasingly severe soreness, but this goes away on its own. Rubella vaccine can cause a temporary inflammation and soreness of the joints. And in rare cases, the ingredients in a vaccine—or in a particular manufacturer's formulation— may prompt an allergic reaction in a sensitive person.

Perhaps the most serious side effects come from pertussis vaccine, which on rare occasions causes fever, excessive crying, seizures, or—even rarer—brain damage or death. The severest side effects are so infrequent that studies often cannot measure their incidence; the accepted estimate is that 1 in 310,000 pertussis vaccinations produces permanent brain

damage. Some researchers even suggest brain damage or death after vaccination may have resulted from an underlying disease that was triggered by the vaccination, not caused by it. Whatever the case, researchers are seeking a safer pertussis vaccine.

Live-microbe vaccines pose their own risks. They should not be given to pregnant women unless there is an immediate threat from an ongoing epidemic. This is because researchers do not know how the virus might affect the fetus. Similarly, live vaccines are not recommended for people with deficient immune systems, which might be caused by AIDS or other illnesses, radiation therapy, or certain drug treatments.

Live-microbe vaccines also pose the risk that some of the microbes may mutate back to their disease-causing form. This problem is most notable with the Sabin polio vaccine, which sometimes contains viruses that can cause polio. Vaccine-caused polio is extremely rare— less than one case for every million doses of vaccine, according to figures from the CDC. Still, the vaccine has been so successful in eradicating polio that the 5 to 10 vaccine-caused cases each year now account for virtually all new polio cases in the United States.

Vaccine use worldwide

The availability and effectiveness of vaccines is not the same throughout the world. In addition, the risks for certain diseases vary widely from place to place. Because of these variations, public health experts around the world often differ on the best ways to use vaccines.

The industrialized world

Like the United States, other industrialized countries have seen vaccine use dramatically

reduce disease during recent decades. But policies and practices vary greatly from one country to another, and so do the resulting benefits.

For example, most of the Communist countries of Europe—including Albania, Bulgaria, Czechoslovakia, East Germany, Hungary, and the Soviet Union—have enforced vaccination so completely that some diseases are nearly eradicated there. But the same diseases may still be problems in other countries, including the United States.

One example is measles, the largest remaining cause worldwide of vaccine-preventable illness and death. The European Communist countries report that an estimated 98 or 99 per cent of children were immunized as of 1984. But only 58 per cent of British children were. The measles immunization level among U.S. children entering school has been 95 per cent or more since 1981.

Albania has already declared measles eradicated within its borders. Other European countries have set a goal of eradicating measles by 1995. The European Regional Committee of the World Health Organization (WHO) has set a goal of eliminating measles, polio, and diphtheria—as well as tetanus and rubella in newborns—in Europe by the year 2000.

In some aspects, the European countries differ as a group from the United States in their immunization policies. For instance, the vaccine for tuberculosis is not routinely given in the United States, but it is recommended or required in most European countries.

The rubella vaccine offers another example of different views. Rubella is a minor disease for adults, but if a pregnant woman catches the disease, her baby may be born with such birth defects as mental retardation or heart malformations. Two European countries—Great Britain and Ireland—have chosen to vaccinate only females. The other European countries, like the United States, vaccinate both sexes. Officials in these countries maintain that vaccination of all women is probably impossible to achieve, and if rubella is common among boys and men, an unvaccinated woman might contract it from them. Vaccinating males, therefore, protects females.

Developing countries

Vaccine use in developing nations also varies greatly from country to country. Some of the more advanced nations in this category—such as India and several countries in Latin America—have followed U.S. vaccination standards or guidelines prepared by WHO.

WHO estimates that as of 1988 just over half of the children in developing countries were immunized against diphtheria, tetanus, pertussis, and polio in the first year of life. This figure, however, is an average that obscures a highly spotty distribution of vaccine. Vaccination rates are highest among affluent and urban classes. The poor, especially in rural areas, are woefully lacking in the most basic protection.

The situation is especially bad in poorer countries. Polio, for example, is still a problem in much of Africa, and people with withered limbs are a common sight in many parts of the continent. In Latin America, however, polio vaccine has been so successful that the Pan American Health Organization expects to eliminate polio in that region by the end of 1990.

Three major problems hinder delivery of vaccines to developing countries. First, many developing countries do not require children to be vaccinated for entry into school—or at any other time. That means health professionals may have no way to find or reach the children who need vaccination.

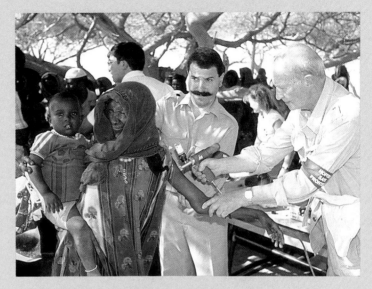

French and African health officials work together to carry out the World Health Organization's vaccination program in Djibouti.

Second, because many vaccines require continuous refrigeration from the point of manufacture to the patient, it has proven impossible to get them to remote regions that lack electricity or even roads over which refrigerated trucks can travel. One hope for overcoming this problem lies in some of the new subunit vaccines, which do not have to be kept cold.

But the biggest stumbling block is cost. As inexpensive as vaccines are for those in more affluent countries, their cost in the poorest regions can amount to a month's income. For families with several children, vaccination is out of the question. To help remedy this, industrialized countries often donate vaccines to poorer ones.

For all the problems, vaccines have prevented great suffering in developing countries. WHO's smallpox eradication program, for example, banished one of the great scourges of the poor countries. And WHO estimates that its Expanded Program on Immunization, which began sending health-care workers and vaccines into underdeveloped countries in 1974, has saved the lives of 1.5 million children every year since.

Trends in vaccine use

There's no doubt of vaccines' immense contribution to the health of Americans. But health officials cite several disturbing trends of the 1980's that may hamper the success of vaccines in the years to come.

Undervaccination

Immunization has been overwhelmingly successful in driving down rates of disease and death. Still, officials say sizable minorities of children remain unvaccinated against the seven major vaccine-preventable childhood infections—diphtheria, tetanus, pertussis, rubella, measles, mumps, and polio. In addition, a large majority of the elderly are unprotected against the two main vaccine-preventable illnesses of adults—influenza and pneumococcal pneumonia—and many are also unprotected against tetanus.

Children. In 1980 the PHS established a goal of immunizing at least 90 per cent of the nation's 2-year-olds against the seven basic vaccine-preventable diseases by 1990. (An eighth childhood vaccine, for hemophilus influenzae, was added to the recommended list in 1985.) But in the following years, the proportion of fully immunized 2-year-olds showed little or no improvement—from an estimated 70 per cent to 80 per cent in 1979 to about 77 per cent by 1985, the last year in which data were collected. Significant outbreaks of measles were still occurring—chiefly among children in lower-income families, whose levels of immunization are lowest. According to a 1988 report by the CDC, the 1990 goals are not likely to be met.

Statistics show, however, that immunization levels improve considerably by the time youngsters enter school. Another PHS goal was to vaccinate at least 95 per cent of children attending licensed day-care facilities and grade schools. In the 1986-1987 school year, immunization levels in day care exceeded 90 per cent; for children entering kindergarten or first grade, the level was 97 per cent.

Mumps poses the worst problem; in 1987, it accounted for nearly twice the number of cases of illness as the other six childhood vaccine-preventable diseases combined. After a long-standing downward trend, reports of mumps jumped from a record low of 2,982 in 1985 to 7,790 in 1986 and 12,848 in 1987—the highest level since 1979. Many of the cases reflected outbreaks among high school and college students, who probably were never immunized. Researchers at the CDC also attributed the rise to the lack of, or lax enforcement of, immunization requirements in schools in some states. Illinois and Tennessee, for example, had the highest mumps rates in

1986 and 1987; both states began requiring vaccination for schoolchildren shortly thereafter. Early statistics for 1988 indicate that the national mumps rate has resumed its decline.

Studies indicate that certain children are more likely than others to go unvaccinated. These include those whose parents have less than a high school education; members of large families; poor children; those who depend on public clinics for immunizations; and those whose parents are young, single, and nonwhite.

Still, according to the CDC, many children remain unvaccinated out of carelessness. Some parents find a trip to the doctor inconvenient. And others simply forget to go.

Adults. By far the largest problem of undervaccination—and preventable disease—is among the elderly. Influenza and pneumococcal pneumonia kill about 60,000 Americans 65 and older each year. Yet both are preventable. Although the PHS recommends that all people 65 and over and those who suffer from chronic illnesses be immunized against both diseases, only about 20 per cent of these high-risk people are vaccinated annually for influenza, and as of 1985, less than 10 per cent had ever received pneumococcus vaccine.

Among people 60 and older, between 49 per cent and 66 per cent, depending on the survey, lack adequate protection from tetanus. And between 41 per cent and 84 per cent are not immune to diphtheria.

Many younger adults are also poorly protected. For example, up to 7 million young adults are vulnerable to measles. Some were never vaccinated. Some received a weak form of the vaccine used between 1963 and 1967. And others received the vaccine too young; in the mid-1970's, it was found that measles vaccination is most effective after 15 months of age.

Another potential problem disease is rubella. The disease does its worst damage to the unborn, but about 11 million women of childbearing age remain unvaccinated.

According to the CDC, the overwhelming reason for low levels of vaccination among adults is that health-care professionals too often fail to recommend and offer vaccination. For example, in a 1988 study, CDC researchers asked 716 people age 65 and older in the Atlanta, Ga., area whether they had been vaccinated in the previous year. Among those whose doctors had recommended influenza vaccine, 75 per cent followed that advice. Among those whose doctors did not suggest the vaccine, only 7 per cent were vaccinated. The figures for pneumococcus vaccinations were almost identical.

One key reason some doctors do not recommend vaccination, the CDC suggested, was that many hold unfounded concerns about the vaccines' safety and effectiveness. Another hindrance to adult immunization, CDC officials noted, is that although formal programs promote childhood vaccination, none exist to protect adults.

Cutbacks in vaccine making

Continued progress in conquering disease depends on research—by the pharmaceutical industry or in government and academic laboratories—to develop new vaccines and to improve existing ones. It also depends on the readiness of the pharmaceutical industry to make and distribute vaccines.

But the vaccine industry in the United States is dying. Despite the enormous benefits offered by vaccines, drug companies are gradually giving up the business. More than half the vaccine manufacturers of 20 years ago have abandoned the field.

Companies cite two reasons for discontinuing work on vaccines. One is the high cost of

Vaccines in the making

Researchers continue to work on developing vaccines for many human diseases. Here is a sampling of some areas of current research:

AIDS. The many scientists around the world who seek an AIDS vaccine face roadblocks never encountered with other diseases. A chief problem is that vaccines normally work by prompting the body's natural immunity, but the human body has no immune defense against AIDS. This may be because the AIDS virus—*human immunodeficiency virus* (HIV)—attacks T cells, the very heart of the immune system.

Researchers are experimenting with various vaccine approaches, ranging from traditional killed-virus methods to new genetic engineering techniques. Several studies suggest that it is possible to stimulate immune responses to the AIDS virus—though the strength and effects of such responses are still undetermined. At least four experimental vaccines were being tested as of early 1989.

Chicken pox. An experimental vaccine for chicken pox—the only remaining major childhood disease for which

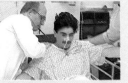

AIDS

no vaccine exists—has proved safe and effective in human tests and may be available in 1990. But some experts question the value of such a vaccine.

In healthy children, chicken pox is a relatively mild disease. It is more dangerous in adults, who can become seriously ill and suffer complications such as pneumonia or hepatitis. In pregnant women, chicken pox can harm or kill the fetus. And in people with severe health problems, such as cancer or immune disorders, chicken pox can be fatal.

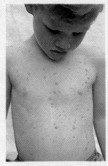

Chicken pox

If the vaccine turns out to provide only temporary protection, children who are protected from chicken pox while they're young might turn out to be susceptible to a serious case when they're grown. A vaccine might thus be appropriate only for seriously ill children, in whom chicken pox might be life-threatening, or for vulnerable adults who are in close contact with ill children.

Pregnancy. The principle that enables vaccines to prevent disease is now being studied as a method to prevent pregnancy. Several teams of researchers are testing vaccines that stimulate the body's natural defenses to block pregnancy—without causing side effects or premanent infertility.

One approach targets a hormone called *human chorionic gonadotropin* (HCG). When a human egg is fertilized, it produces HCG, which signals the woman's body to prepare for a pregnancy. Researchers in several countries are testing vaccines developed from the protein in HCG. Preliminary experiments show that vaccinated women make antibodies that attack HCG. It remains to be seen whether this can prevent the hormone's message from reaching the body, thus blocking pregnancy.

Another birth-control vaccine seeks to prevent the egg from being fertilized in the first place. In 1988, biologists at the University of Connecticut Health

Center in Farmington developed a vaccine from a surface protein on guinea pig sperm cells. Vaccinated guinea pigs produce antibodies that attack the protein and disable the sperm cells.

Tests show that the vaccine—used either in male or female guinea pigs—was 100 per cent effective for six months or more. Such a vaccine for human beings is still far off, however, because no comparable protein has yet been found on human sperm.

Melanoma. Cells of this deadly skin cancer produce antigens, just as viruses and bacteria do. Researchers have been working for about 20 years to develop vaccines that use these antigens. A successful vaccine might prevent melanoma from starting, spreading, or recurring.

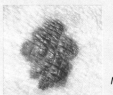

Melanoma

In December 1988, researchers at the New York University School of Medicine in New York City reported on preliminary tests of one vaccine. Of a group of melanoma patients given the vaccine, about half showed an immune response. Cancers progressed more slowly in these people than in those who did not respond. In mice, the vaccine has been able to prevent melanoma.

Scientists at the Merieux Institute in Lyon, France, have developed another melanoma vaccine from *vaccinia,* the virus used in smallpox vaccine. Preliminary trials have been promising, and the vaccine is now in large-scale tests involving six American health centers. In addition, several other melanoma vaccines are in early stages of development and testing.

---

developing and testing new vaccines. The second and more recent factor is soaring legal costs—the result of lawsuits filed by people claiming to have experienced bad results from vaccines. In a few cases, vaccines have caused the diseases they were supposed to protect against. In other cases, vaccination has caused serious side effects. Ironically, the number of

lawsuits and the sizes of the awards have been growing even as vaccines are generally becoming safer.

The most celebrated cases have involved the pertussis vaccine, which has caused brain damage in a small number of children who received it. As of 1986, claims in U.S. courts against vaccine manufacturers totaled more than $5 billion. To

protect themselves from litigation costs, the two DTP manufacturers remaining in the market have increased vaccine prices. The physician's cost for a dose of one company's DTP preparation was 23 cents in 1979; in 1989, it was $10.90.

Of that price, $4.56 goes to a new federal program designed to discourage lawsuits and control vaccine-makers' costs in the long run. The National Childhood Vaccine Injury Act of 1986 set guidelines for "no-fault" compensation for victims of vaccine injury. Under the program, which took effect in 1988, families of injured children can receive up to $250,000 in compensation, plus payments to cover medical expenses and other costs, without resorting to lawsuits. The money comes from the vaccine tax and government appropriations.

As of July 1989, 159 people had applied for compensation. The first award under the program was made that month.

The 1986 law that established the compensation program also created the National Vaccine Program, a broad-based effort to encourage the development and effective use of new and better vaccines. The law called for five government agencies—the National Institutes of Health (NIH), the CDC, the Food and Drug Administration, the Department of Defense, and the Agency for International Development—to develop a joint plan for creating, manufacturing, and distributing vaccines.

Although much vaccine research is done with federal funds, the government lacks the facilities to manufacture and distribute vaccines. The new law calls on the government to work with drug companies to ensure that manufacturers are available for needed vaccines. If no arrangement can be made, the law specifies that the government will be the manufacturer of last resort.

So far, much of the National Vaccine Program has not been put into action. The Administration of President Ronald Reagan, fighting budget deficits, requested no money from Congress to fund the program. In 1988 the program's advisory committee—a group of prominent scientists, manufacturers, parents' representatives, and public-health professionals—demanded that the program be fully funded at a level of $31 million in the 1990 federal budget. As of June 1989, the House of Representatives had requested a $10-million appropriation in its new budget; the Senate had yet to act, and the budget was still to be approved.

The cutback in vaccine development has come just as new research methods offer bright prospects for developing new vaccines to prevent more than a dozen major diseases that still run rampant. (For some examples, see VACCINES IN THE MAKING on page 383.) But such discoveries will be of little use if manufacturers decline to produce the vaccines—or if people refuse to use them.

Ironically, the very success of vaccines may be in part responsible for the troubles they face today. As more Americans grow up with no memory of how infectious diseases devastated the population only a few decades ago, fewer will understand the important role vaccines play in keeping these now-rare diseases at bay.

Researchers continue to work to make tomorrow's vaccines even safer and more effective. But in the meantime, the vaccines we have today are still a desirable alternative to the epidemics of the past.

Health officials scrambled to deal with a shortage of pertussis vaccine after liability costs led two manufacturers to drop out of the market in 1984. Meanwhile, some parents concerned about the vaccine's rare side effects did not immunize their children— and pertussis cases nearly doubled between 1982 and 1985.

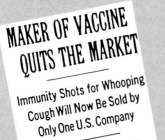

MAKER OF VACCINE QUITS THE MARKET

Immunity Shots for Whooping Cough Will Now Be Sold by Only One U.S. Company

By STEPHEN ENGELBERG
Special to The New York Times

WASHINGTON, Dec. 11 — Connaught Laboratories Inc. has stopped selling whooping cough vaccine, a company official said today. Health experts said the move would worsen shortages of the vaccine, which is used to protect nearly every infant in the country against the potentially fatal disease.

The company, one of two remainir American manufacturers of the va cine, said it was withdrawing ra than pay sharply higher rates for li ity insurance. Earlier this year, v Laboratories halted producti whooping cough vaccine, citi ... costs. ... manufac

Medical Panel Finds A Doubling of Cases Of Whooping Cough

WASHINGTON, Nov. 16 (AP) — Cases of whooping cough among American children, some of them fatal, have nearly doubled in three years as parents, wary of possible side effects of the vaccine against the disease, have apparently chosen not to immunize their children, medical experts say.

The American Academy of Pediatrics says 2,258 cases of whooping cough were reported to the Federal authorities from Jan. 1 through mid-October, as against 1,342 cases in all of 1982.

Dr. Martin H. Smith, the academy's president, also cited 10 local "near epidemic" outbreaks of whooping cough in the last year, some of them resulting in brain damage or death.

Dr. Smith called the out alarming and attributed among par

For more information:

For consumer information on vaccines, contact your state or local health department or the following offices:

Food and Drug Administration
Office of Consumer Affairs
HFE-88
5600 Fishers Lane
Rockville, MD 20857

American Academy of
 Pediatrics
Dept. C
141 Northwest Point Blvd.
Elk Grove, IL 60009

The author:
Boyce Rensberger is science editor of the *Washington Post*. He has written articles on scientific topics for newspapers and magazines nationwide for 25 years. His most recent book is *How the World Works: A Guide to Science's Greatest Discoveries* (1986).

Here are your

1990 WORLD BOOK HEALTH & MEDICAL ANNUAL Cross-Reference Tabs

For insertion in your WORLD BOOK

Each year, the WORLD BOOK HEALTH & MEDICAL ANNUAL will add a valuable dimension to your WORLD BOOK set. The Cross-Reference Tab System is designed especially to help students and parents alike link the HEALTH & MEDICAL ANNUAL's Special Reports and other major articles to the related WORLD BOOK articles they update.

How to Use These Tabs

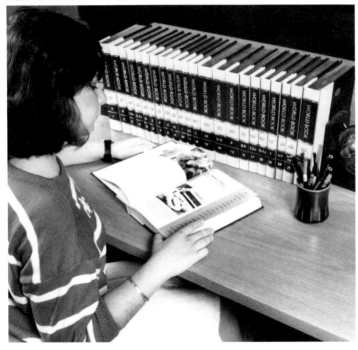

The top Tab on this page is AIDS. Turn to the A volume of your WORLD BOOK and find the page with the AIDS article on it. Affix the AIDS Tab to that page. If your WORLD BOOK is an older set without an AIDS article in it, put the AIDS Tab in the A volume in its proper alphabetical sequence. For most older sets, the AIDS Tab would go on the same page as the article about AIKEN, CONRAD POTTER.

Put all of the remaining Tabs in your WORLD BOOK volumes, and your new HEALTH & MEDICAL ANNUAL will be linked to your encyclopedia.

Special Report
AIDS
1990 Health & Medical Annual, p. 112

Close-Up Article
ALLERGY
1990 Health & Medical Annual, p. 237

Special Report
ANXIETY
1990 Health & Medical Annual, p. 10

Special Report
ASTHMA
1990 Health & Medical Annual, p. 182

Special Report
BACKACHE
1990 Health & Medical Annual, p. 198

Special Report
BURNS AND SCALDS
1990 Health & Medical Annual, p. 212

Special Report
CANCER
1990 Health & Medical Annual, p. 26

Health Studies
IMMUNIZATION
1990 Health & Medical Annual, p. 366

Special Report
LEAD POISONING
1990 Health & Medical Annual, p. 168

Special Report
LEGIONNAIRES' DISEASE
1990 Health & Medical Annual, p. 154

Close-Up Article
MILK
1990 Health & Medical Annual, p. 310

Special Report
MONONUCLEOSIS
1990 Health & Medical Annual, p. 126

Close-Up Article
PHYSICAL FITNESS
1990 Health & Medical Annual, p. 278

Special Report
STEROID
1990 Health & Medical Annual, p. 42

Special Report
STROKE
1990 Health & Medical Annual, p. 56

People in Medicine
TRAUMA CENTER
1990 Health & Medical Annual, p. 340

Special Report
TUBERCULOSIS
1990 Health & Medical Annual, p. 140

Special Report
ULCER
1990 Health & Medical Annual, p. 70

Special Report
VEGETARIANISM
1990 Health & Medical Annual, p. 98

Close-Up Article
WEIGHT CONTROL
1990 Health & Medical Annual, p. 336

Index

This index covers the contents of the 1988, 1989, and 1990 editions of *The World Book Health & Medical Annual.*

Each index entry gives the edition year and a page number—for example, 90-123. The first number, 90, indicates the edition year, and the second number, 123, is the page number on which the desired information begins.

There are two types of entries in the index.

In the first type, the index entry (in **boldface** type) is followed immediately by numbers:

Dentistry, 90-261, 89-263, 88-248

This means that *The Health & Medical Annual* has an article titled Dentistry and that in the 1990 edition the article begins on page 261. In the 1989 and 1988 editions, the Dentistry article begins on pages 263 and 248, respsectively.

In the second type of entry, the **boldface** title is followed by a clue word instead of by numbers:

Public health: AIDS, Special Report, 90-116; Health Professions, 88-363; People in Medicine, 89-340

This means that there is no *Health & Medical Annual* article titled Public health, but that information about this topic may be found in a Special Report of the 1990 edition on page 116. Earlier editions also contain information on the pages cited.

Sometimes information appears only as an illustration:

Spirometer: il., 90-192

This means that there is a picture of a spirometer on page 192 of the 1990 edition.

The "See" and "See also" cross-references direct the reader to other entries within the index:

Deoxyribonucleic acid. See **DNA.**

A

A, Vitamin: nutrition, 88-296

Abortion: birth control, 90-243; People in Medicine, 89-346; prenatal diagnosis, Special Report, 88-66; Soviet medicine, Special Report, 90-94

Abuse-reactive behavior: child abuse, Special Report, 89-359

Acanthamoeba infection: eye and vision, 90-283

Accidents: pediatric trauma, Special Report, 90-342, safety, 90- 318

Acetaminophen: kidney, 90-303

Acetylcholine: aging, 90-228, 88-212; Alzheimer's disease, Close-Up, 89-229

Acid rain: environmental health, 88-263

Acquired immune deficiency syndrome. See **AIDS.**

Acromegaly: steroids, Special Report, 90-53

Actinic keratosis: skin cancer, Special Report, 89-36

Acupuncture: back problems, Special Report, 90-209

Adenomas: cancer, 90-255

ADHD (attention deficit hyperactivity disorder): hyperactivity, Special Report, 89-185

Adipsin: weight control, 90-335

Administrative nurse: Health Professions, 88-359

Adolescence: Health Studies, 89-381; hyperactivity, Special Report, 89-186; mental and behavioral disorders, 88-291; osteoporosis, Special Report, 89-65; weight control, 89-337. See also **Alcohol and drug abuse.**

Aerobic exercise: exercise and fitness, 88-265

Aerosolized pentamidine: AIDS, Special Report, 90-125

Aesthetic surgery: cosmetic surgery, Special Report, 89-147

Affective disorder: depression, Special Report, 88-70

Age-related macular degeneration (AMD): aging eyes, Special Report, 88-190

Agent Orange: environmental health, 90-275

Aggressive behavior: child development, 90-258; mental and behavioral disorders, 90-307; steroids, Special Report, 90-48

Aging, 90-228, 89-228, 88-212; aging eyes, Special Report, 88-180; books of health and medicine, 90-248; caring for the aged, Special Report, 89-199; Health Studies, 89-373; nutrition, 89-311; osteoporosis, Special Report, 89-56. See also **Alzheimer's disease.**

Agoraphobia: anxiety disorders, Special Report, 90-12

Agricultural society: cholesterol, Special report, 88-29

AIDS, 90-230, 89-231, 88-214; alcohol and drug abuse, 89-238; allergies and immunology, 90-239; books of health and medicine, 90-248; brain and nervous system, 88-234; drugs, 88-254; health care facilities, 90-294; health fraud, Special Report, 89-177; health policy, 90-295, 89-292; hospitals, 88-285; infectious diseases, 90-300, 89-303; kidney, 88-290; mental and behavioral disorders, 89-308; mononucleosis, Special Report, 90-137; People in Medicine, 89-348; polio, Special Report, 89-114; sexually transmitted diseases, 89-324; skin, Special Report, 88-10; Soviet medicine, Special Report, 90-92; Special Report, 90-112; tuberculosis, Special Report, 90-153

Air pollution: asthma, Special Report, 90-189; ear and hearing, 89-274; environmental health, 90-276; lead poisoning, Special Report, 90-173; Legionnaires' disease, Special Report, 90-167

Airbag: safety, 89-321

Airplane: emergency medicine, 90-274; safety, 90-321; 89-319; smoking, 89-329

Al-Anon: alcohol, Health Studies, 88-378

Alar: Close-Up, 90-320

Alcohol: brain and nervous system, 88-237; breast cancer, Special Report, 90-30; Health Studies, 88-368; insomnia, Special Report, 88-172; mental and behavioral disorders, 88-293; ulcer, Special Report, 90-76

Alcohol and Drug Abuse, 90-233, 89-235, 88-217; alcohol, Health Studies, 88-368; Soviet medicine, Special Report, 90-86; stroke, 88-312

Alcohol tolerance: alcohol, Health Studies, 88-374

Alcoholics Anonymous (A.A.): alcohol, Health Studies, 88-378

Allergies and Immunology, 90-236, 89-238, 88-220; asthma, Special Report, 90-184; drugs, 90-270

Allograft: burns, Special Report, 90-222; skin, 88-308

All-terrain vehicle (ATV): Close-Up, 89-320; safety, 88-303

Alpha interferon: AIDS, 90-232

Alprazolam: anxiety disorders, Special Report, 90-20

Altitude sickness: emergency medicine, 90-274

Aluminum: kidney, 89-307

Alzheimer's disease: aging, 90-228, 89-228, 88-212; brain and nervous system, 90-250, 88-238; Close-Up, 89-229; drugs, 88-255; genetics, 88-273

Amenorrhea: glands and hormones, 89-291

American Hospital Association (AHA): Health Professions, 88-356; hospitals, 88-284

American Medical Association: health policy, 88-279

Amino acids: aging, 89-230; vegetarianism, Special Report, 90-106

Amish, Old Order: brain and nervous system, 88-238; depression, Special Report, 88-75

Amniocentesis: pregnancy and childbirth, 89-314; prenatal diagnosis, Special Report, 88-60

Amniotic fluid: prenatal diagnosis, Special Report, 88-61

Amyloid: kidney, 89-307

Amyotrophic lateral sclerosis (ALS): Health Policy, 88-279

Amyotrophic lateral sclerosis-Parkinson's dementia complex (ALS-PD): brain and nervous system, 89-253

Anemia: arthritis and connective tissue disorders, 89-242; glands and hormones, 88-276; kidney, 88-289; minerals, Special Report, 88-157

Aneurysm: drugs, 90-270; stroke, Special Report, 90-58

Angina pectoris: coronary artery disease, Special Report, 89-74

Angiography: coronary artery disease, Special Report, 89-79

Angioplasty: coronary artery disease, Special Report, 89-84

Anopheles mosquito: infectious diseases, 88-289

Antabuse: alcohol, Health Studies, 88-377

Antacids: ulcer, Special Report, 90-79

Antibiotic: burns, Special Report, 90-219; salmonella, Special Report, 89-136; tuberculosis, Special Report, 90-149

Antibodies: allergies and immunology, 89-239; Health Studies, 90-370; Lyme disease, Special Report, 89-47; mononucleosis, Special Report, 90-132; polio, Special Report, 89-105

Anticancer gene: genetics, 88-274

Anticoagulant drugs: stroke, Special Report, 90-58

Antidepressant drugs: anxiety disorders, Special Report, 90-20; depression, Special Report, 88-78; drugs, 89-273

Antigens: allergies and immunology, 89-240; kidney transplantation, Special Report, 88-117

Antihistamines: drugs, 90-270

Anti-inflammatory drugs: drugs, 90-267

Antral gastritis: digestive system, 89-268

Anxiety disorders: Special Report, 90-10

Aphasia: left-handedness, Special Report, 89-161; stroke, Special Report, 90-58

Appendicitis: digestive system, 90-266

ARC (AIDS-related complex): AIDS, Special Report, 88-15

Arch: foot problems, Special Report, 89-118

Arson: fire safety, Special Report, 89-218

Arteries: heart and blood vessels, 88-282

Arteriography: stroke, Special Report, 90-62

Arteriosclerosis: aging eyes, Special Report, 88-191

Arthritis and Connective Tissue Disorders, 90-240, 89-241, 88-224;

back problems, Special Report, 90-203; bone disorders, 89-247; caring for the aged, Special Report, 89-204; health fraud, Special Report, 89-174; knee, Special Report, 88-48; Lyme disease, Special Report, 89-40

Arthropod: Lyme disease, Special Report, 89-44

Arthroscopic surgery: bone disorders, 88-230; il., 88-49; knee, Special Report, 88-48

Artificial insemination: Health Policy, 88-277

Artificial knee: il., 88-49; knee, Special Report, 88-53

Artificial limbs, Health Professions, 88-326

Artificial pancreas: diabetes, 90-263

Artificial skin: burns, Special Report, 90-223

Asbestos: environmental health, 90-277, 89-277; safety, 89-323

Aspirin: asthma, Special Report, 90-189; Close-Up, 89-296; coronary artery disease, Special Report, 89-82; stroke, Special Report, 90-62; ulcer, Special Report, 90-74

Astemizole: drugs, 90-270

Asthma: allergies and immunology, 88-223; il., 89-240; respiratory system, 90-316; Special Report, 90-183

Astigmatism: aging eyes, Special Report, 88-193

Atherosclerosis: cholesterol, Special Report, 88-28; coronary artery disease, Special Report, 89-74; dietary fiber, Special Report, 89-97; drugs, 88-256; heart and blood vessels, 90-296, 88-282; stroke, Special Report, 90-58; vegetarianism, Special Report, 90-101

Athletes: foot problems, Special Report, 89-125; steroids, Special Report, 90-42

Atrial fibrillation: stroke, Special Report, 90-67

Aura: migraine, Special Report, 89-12

Autism: mental and behavioral disorders, 90-305, 89-311, 88-294

Autograft: burns, Special Report, 90-221

Autoimmune disease: allergies and immunology, 89-239; arthritis and connective tissue disorders, 88-225; bone disorders, 89-247; diabetes, 89-266; left-handedness, Special Report, 89-167. See also **AIDS.**

Autologous predeposit donation: blood, 90-246; 89-244

Automobile accidents: alcohol, Health Studies, 88-373, 381; pediatric trauma, Special Report, 90-342. See also **Safety.**

AZT. See **Zidovudine.**

B

B, Vitamin: alcohol, Health Studies, 88-374; vegetarianism, Special Report, 90-110

B cell: allergies and immunology, 90-240; Health Studies, 90-370; infectious diseases, 88-287

B lymphocytes: mononucleosis, Special Report, 90-136

B₆, Vitamin: nutrition, 89-311

Back problems: Special Report, 90-199

Bacteria: arthritis and connective tissue disorders, 90-241, 89-242; digestive system, 89-268; eye and vision, 90-283; Health Studies, 90-369; Legionnaires' disease, Special Report, 90-164; Lyme disease, Special Report, 89-44; salmonella, Special Report, 89-132

Baldness: Close-Up, health fraud, Special Report, 89-177; il., 90-270; skin, 89-327

Balloon angioplasty: coronary artery disease, Special Report, 89-84

Barbiturates: brain and nervous system, 88-237

Basal cell carcinoma: skin cancer, Special Report, 89-26

Behavior: anxiety disorders, Special Report, 90-18; child development, 90-259; Health Studies, 89-375, 378, 384; hyperactivity, Special Report, 89-185. See also **Mental and Behavioral Disorders.**

Benzodiazepines: anxiety disorders, Special Report, 90-20

Beta-blockers: aging eyes, Special Report, 88-187; anxiety disorders, Special Report, 90-22; coronary artery disease, Special Report, 89-81; migraine, Special Report, 89-23; steroids, Special Report, 90-53

Beta carotene: nutrition, 88-296

Bifocal lens: aging eyes, Special Report, 88-184

Bioethics: AIDS, Special Report, 90-114

Biofeedback: asthma, Special Report, 90-196; back problems, Special Report, 90-209; diabetes, 90-264; migraine, Special Report, 89-21

Biological rhythms: depression, Special Report, 88-76

Biologics: cancer, 88-240

Biomechanics: exercise, 88-265

Biopsy: breast cancer, Special Report, 90-36; checkup, Special Report, 88-206; ulcer, Special Report, 90-78

Biopty gun: urology, 89-333

Birth Control: 90-243, 89-243, 88-226; arthritis and connective tissue disorders, 90-241; breast cancer, Special Report, 89-30; migraine, Special Report, 89-16; Soviet medicine, Special Report, 90-94

Birth defect: alcohol, Health Studies, 88-379; birth control, 88-227; prenatal diagnosis, Special Report, 88-54

Birth trauma: mental and behavioral disorders, 88-291

Birthmark: skin, 90-327, 88-309

Bladder: cancer, 88-239; urology, 88-315

Blindness: AIDS, 90-232; eye and vision, 90-283, 88-268; veterinary medicine, 89-333

Blood, 90-244, 89-244, 88-228; AIDS, 89-234; Close-Up, 88-236

Blood alcohol concentration: alcohol, Health Studies, 88-373

Blood-brain barrier: lead poisoning, Special Report, 90-180

Blood clot: blood, 90-245; Close-Up, 89-296; heart and blood vessels, 89-297, 88-282; kidney transplantation, Special Report, 88-116; stroke, 89-331, Special Report, 90-58

Blood doping: steroids, Special Report, 90-53

Blood pressure: books of health and medicine, 90-249; checkup, Special Report, 88-202; coronary artery disease, Special Report, 89-75

Blood sugar: diabetes, 90-263, 88-250

Blood test: AIDS, 88-215; AIDS, Special Report, 90-115; alcohol and drug abuse, 90-234; infectious diseases, 90-301; lead poisoning, Special Report, 90-179; mononucleosis, Special Report, 90-138; pregnancy and childbirth, 90-314; prenatal diagnosis, Special Report, 88-59; respiratory system, 90-318

Blood transfusion: AIDS, Special Report, 90-116, 88-13; blood, 90-244; pregnancy and childbirth, 88-299

Blood type: kidney transplantation, Special Report, 88-118; ulcer, Special Report, 90-76

Body fat: Health Studies, 89-369; il., 89-336; heart and blood vessels, 90-299; smoking, 90-330. See also **Weight Control.**

Bone Disorders, 90-246, 89-247, 88-230; glands and hormones, 88-276; kidney, 89-307; osteoporosis, Special Report, 89-56

Bone fractures: aging, 90-228; bone disorders, 90-247; knee, Special Report, 88-45; minerals, Special Report, 88-164; osteoporosis, Special Report, 89-56

Bone marrow: blood, 90-244; bone disorders, 90-247; ils., 89-58, 246; radiation, Special Report, 88-148

Books of Health and Medicine, 90-248, 89-249, 88-232

Botulism: salmonella, Special Report, 89-141

Brace, Body: scoliosis, Special Report, 88-133

Braces, Dental: il., 89-263; orthodontics, Special Report, 88-91

Brain and Nervous System, 90-250, 89-251, 88-234; anxiety disorders, Special Report, 90-18; books of health and medicine, 90-248; child development, 88-144; Close-Up, 88-236; left-handedness, Special Report, 89-160; migraine, Special Report, 89-15; stroke, Special Report, 90-57

Brain disorder: left-handedness, Special Report, 89-165

Brain tissue: aging, 90-228

Bran: dietary fiber, Special Report, 89-89

Breast augmentation: breast cancer, Special Report, 90-33; cosmetic surgery, Special Report, 89-150

Breast cancer: cancer, 89-255, 88-242; cosmetic surgery, Special Report, 89-151; exercise and fitness, 88-267; Special Report, 90-26

Breast examination: breast cancer, Special Report, 90-38; checkup, Special Report, 88-206

Index

Breast milk: allergies and immunology, 89-238

Breast reconstruction: breast cancer, Special Report, 90-37

Bronchiolitis obliterans: respiratory system, 89-318

Bronchodilators: asthma, Special Report, 90-193

Bulk: dietary fiber, Special Report, 89-90

Bunion: foot problems, Special Report, 89-120

Burns: skin, 90-326; Special Report, 90-213

Bursitis: foot problems, Special Report, 89-120

Buspirone: anxiety disorders, Special Report, 90-20

By-pass surgery: coronary artery disease, Special Report, 89-82

C

C, Vitamin: vegetarianism, Special Report, 90-108

Caesarean section: pregnancy and childbirth, 90-313, 89-316, 88-297

Calcaneus: foot problems, Special Report, 89-118

Calcium: brain and nervous system, 90-251; glands and hormones, 88-276; minerals, Special Report, 88-154, 88-164; nutrition, 88-295; osteoporosis, Special Report, 89-63; vegetarianism, Special Report, 90-108

Calcium blocker: brain and nervous system, 90-252; coronary artery disease, Special Report, 89-82; drugs, 90-269; stroke, Special Report, 90-62

Calcium disodium edetate: lead poisoning, Special Report, 90-180

Callus: foot problems, Special Report, 89-123

Calories: Health Studies, 89-372

Campylobacter pylori: digestive system, 90-265; ulcer, Special Report, 90-75

Cancer, 90-254, 89-254, 88-239; allergies and immunology, 88-220; back problems, Special Report, 90-204; blood, 90-244; breast cancer, Special Report, 90-26; cosmetic surgery, Special Report, 90-151; dietary fiber, Special Report, 89-92; exercise and fitness, 89-281, 88-267; health fraud, Special Report, 89-175; Health Studies, 89-371, 88-375; mononucleosis, Special Report, 90-136; nutrition and food, 90-308; skin cancer, Special Report, 89-24; urology, 89-332. See also specific types of cancer.

Carbon monoxide poisoning: burns, Special Report, 90-214

Cardiovascular disease. See Heart disease.

Carotid endarterectomy: stroke, Special Report, 90-68

Carpal tunnel syndrome: kidney, 89-307

Cartilage: bone disorders, 88-231; knee, Special Report, 88-43

Cat: allergies and immunology, 89-238; pregnancy and childbirth, 89-315; veterinary medicine, 88-316

Cataracts: aging eyes, Special Report, 88-184; eye and vision, 90-283, 88-269; Project Orbis, Special Report, 90-357

Catastrophic disease costs: financing medical care, 88-272

Center for Pain Studies: Health Professions, 88-326

Centers for Disease Control (CDC): AIDS, 88-214, Special Report, 88-112; infectious diseases, 88-288; Legionnaires' disease, Special Report, 90-156; Lyme disease, Special Report, 89-41; sexually transmitted diseases, 88-306

Central nervous system: brain, 88-235

Cerebral embolism: stroke, Special Report, 90-58

Cerebral hemorrhage: stroke, Special Report, 90-58

Cerebral thrombosis: stroke, Special Report, 90-58

Cervical cancer: cancer, 89-258; Close-Up, 89-256; smoking, 90-328

Cervical cap: birth control, 89-244

Chancroid: sexually transmitted diseases, 89-325

Checkup, Medical: Special Report, 88-196

Chelating agents: lead poisoning, Special Report, 90-180

Chemotherapy: breast cancer, Special Report, 90-35; cancer, 90-257

Chernobyl nuclear accident: radiation, Special Report, 88-139

Child abuse: alcohol, Health Studies, 88-376; mental and behavioral disorders, 90-306; Special Report, 89-353

Child Development, 90-257, 89-259, 88-244; glands and hormones, 90-290; hyperactivity, Special Report, 89-185

Child Sexual Abuse Treatment Center: child abuse, Special Report, 89-353

Children: child abuse, Special Report, 89-353; Health Studies, 90-382, 89-381; hyperactivity, Special Report, 89-185; lead poisoning, Special Report, 90-170; mental and behavioral disorders, 90-305; pediatric trauma, Special Report, 90-342

Children's Hospital National Medical Center: pediatric trauma, Special Report, 90-342

Chiropractor: back problems, Special Report, 90-208; health policy, 88-279

Chlamydia: sexually transmitted diseases, 89-325, 88-307

Chlorine: skin cancer, Special Report, 89-35

Chlorofluorocarbons (CFC's): Close-Up, 88-262; environmental health, 88-261; skin cancer, Special Report, 89-35

Cholesterol: checkup, Special Report, 88-203; coronary artery disease, Special Report, 89-76; dietary fiber, Special Report, 89-97; drugs, 89-270, 88-256; exercise and fitness, 90-279;

glands and hormones, 90-289; Health Studies, 89-370; heart and blood vessels, 90-298, 89-295; nutrition and food, 90-309, 88-295; Special Report, 88-26; steroids, Special Report, 90-47; stroke, Special Report, 90-65; vegetarianism, Special Report, 90-101

Chorionic villus sampling (CVS): genetics, 90-288; pregnancy and childbirth, 89-314; prenatal diagnosis, Special Report, 88-56

Chromosomes: brain and nervous system, 88-238; cancer, 88-244; depression, Special Report, 88-75; prenatal diagnosis, Special Report, 88-61. See also Genetics.

Chronic cough: respiratory system, 90-317

Chronic fatigue syndrome: mononucleosis, Special Report, 90-137

Chronic open-angle glaucoma: aging eyes, Special Report, 88-186

Chronobiology: brain and nervous system, 89-252

Cigarette smoking. See Smoking.

Circulatory system: pregnancy and childbirth, 88-299

Circumcision: pregnancy and childbirth, 90-315

Cirrhosis: alcohol, Health Studies, 88-374

Classic migraine: migraine, Special Report, 89-12

Cleft lip: cosmetic surgery, Special Report, 89-149

Clinical ecology: allergies and immunology, 90-239

Clinical trial: health fraud, Special Report, 89-179

Clostridium: salmonella, Special Report, 89-141

Cocaine: exercise and fitness, 88-264; heart and blood vessels, 88-283. See also Alcohol and Drug Abuse.

Cochlea: ear and hearing, 88-257

Coffee: nutrition, 89-313

Cold, Common: allergies and immunology, 90-238; infectious diseases, 90-300, 89-306

Collagen: burns, Special Report, 90-223; cosmetic surgery, Special Report, 89-152; lead poisoning, Special Report, 90-177

Colon: checkup, Special Report, 88-207; dietary fiber, Special Report, 89-91; exercise and fitness, 88-267

Colorectal cancer: cancer, 90-255, 89-259; checkup, Special Report, 88-207; dietary fiber, Special Report, 89-92

Common migraine: migraine, Special Report, 89-12

Computer: arthritis and connective tissue disorders, 90-241; brain and nervous system, 90-252; dentistry, 90-261; emergency medicine, 89-275; Legionnaires' disease, Special Report, 90-161; il., 89-247

Computer-imaging system: cosmetic surgery, Special Report, 89-153

Computerized tomographic scanner (CT): back problems, Special Report,

90-206; ear and hearing, 90-272; pediatric trauma, Special Report, 90-351; stroke, Special Report, 90-61
Condom: AIDS, Special Report, 88-25; sexually transmitted diseases, 89-325
Conduct disorder: hyperactivity, Special Report, 89-187
Conductive hearing loss: ear and hearing, 89-273
Congestive heart failure: coronary artery disease, Special Report, 89-73
Congregate housing: caring for the aged, Special Report, 89-209
Constipation: dietary fiber, Special Report, 89-91
Constitutional delayed growth: glands and hormones, 90-290
Contact lens: aging eyes, Special Report, 88-184; eye and vision, 90-281, 89-285, 88-268
Contact tracing: AIDS, Special Report, 88-24
Continuing-care community: caring for the aged, Special Report, 89-209
Contraception. See Birth control.
Contraceptive sponge: sexually transmitted diseases, 88-307
Contraceptive vaccine: birth control, 90-243
Corn: foot problems, Special Report, 89-122
Cornea: aging eyes, Special Report, 88-182, 192; eye and vision, 90-281; Project Orbis, Special Report, 90-357
Coronary angiography: cholesterol, Special Report, 88-33; coronary artery disease, Special Report, 89-79; nutrition, 88-295
Coronary artery disease (CAD): exercise and fitness, 89-279; Health Studies, 89-371; nutrition, 88-295; Special Report, 89-72; vegetarianism, Special Report, 90-104
Coronary by-pass surgery: coronary artery disease, Special Report, 89-82
Corpus callosum: left-handedness, Special Report, 89-160
Corticosteroid: aging eyes, Special Report, 88-187; asthma, Special Report, 90-193; Close-Up, 88-221
Cortisol: alcohol and drug abuse, 90-234, 89-236; glands and hormones, 89-291
Cosmetic surgery: breast cancer, Special Report, 90-37; burns, Special Report, 90-224; Special Report, 89-144
Cosmic rays: radiation, Special Report, 88-143
Costs, Medical: AIDS, Special Report, 90-124; financing medical care, 89-286, 88-272
Crack: alcohol and drug abuse, 89-237, 88-218
Creosote: fire safety, Special Report, 89-217
Critical-care nurse: Health Professions, 88-359
Cromolyn sodium: asthma, Special Report, 90-193
Cross bite: orthodontics, Special Report, 88-84
Cryosurgery: skin cancer, Special Report, 89-37

Curvature of the spine: scoliosis, Special Report, 88-126
Cutaneous T-cell lymphoma: skin, 90-326
Cyclosporine: burns, Special Report, 90-222; diabetes, 89-265; kidney transplantation, Special Report, 88-119; skin, 90-327
Cyst: breast cancer, Special Report, 90-36
Cystic fibrosis: diabetes, 89-265; genetics, 90-288
Cytomegalovirus retinitis: AIDS, 90-232

D

D, Vitamin: minerals, Special Report, 88-162; osteoporosis, Special Report, 89-67; tuberculosis, Special Report, 90-142; vegetarianism, Special Report, 90-110
Death rates: Health Studies, 89-370
Debridement: burns, Special Report, 90-220
Deciduous teeth: orthodontics, Special Report, 88-87
Decongestant: Close-Up, 88-221
Defibrillation: emergency medicine, 90-273
Dementia: caring for the aged, Special Report, 89-205
Dendrites: aging, 90-228
Dentistry, 90-261, 89-263, 88-248. See also **Orthodontics.**
Deoxyribonucleic acid. See DNA.
Dependency: alcohol and drug abuse, 89-235
Depressant: alcohol, Health Studies, 88-373
Depression: aging, 90-229; alcohol and drug abuse, 89-237; caring for the aged, Special Report, 89-205; mental and behavioral disorders, 88-292; Special Report, 88-68
Dermatology: skin cancer, Special Report, 89-36
Dermatome: burns, Special Report, 90-220
DES (diethylstilbestrol): breast cancer, Special Report, 90-32
Desensitization: anxiety disorder, Special Report, 90-24; asthma, Special Report, 90-195
Detached retina: aging eyes, Special Report, 88-192
Diabetes, 90-262, 89-265, 88-249; aging eyes, Special Report, 88-192; dietary fiber, Special Report, 89-94; Health Studies, 89-370; left-handedness, Special Report, 89-168; stroke, Special Report, 90-65; veterinary medicine, 90-332
Diabetic retinopathy: aging eyes, Special Report, 88-192; Project Orbis, Special Report, 90-357
Diagnosis: asthma, Special Report, 90-190; back problems, Special Report, 90-204; brain and nervous system, 90-251; breast cancer, Special Report, 90-36; cancer, 88-242; coronary artery disease, Special

Report, 89-77; lead poisoning, Special Report, 90-170; Legionnaires' disease, Special Report, 90-167; Lyme disease, Special Report, 89-50; migraine, Special Report, 89-19; mononucleosis, Special Report, 90-130; pregnancy and childbirth, 88-298; prenatal diagnosis, Special Report, 88-54; respiratory system, 90-317; Soviet medicine, Special Report, 90-92; stroke, Special Report, 90-61; 88-54; tuberculosis, Special Report, 90-149
Diagnostic testing: checkup, Special Report, 88-196
Dialysis: kidney, 89-307, 88-289; kidney transplantation, Special Report, 88-113
Diarrhea: allergies and immunology, 89-239
Diastolic pressure: checkup, Special Report, 88-202
Diet: allergies and immunology, 88-223; books of health and medicine, 88-233; cancer, 88-239; cholesterol, Special Report, 88-26; coronary artery disease, Special Report, 89-79; diabetes, 88-251; dietary fiber, Special Report, 89-88; health fraud, Special Report, 89-174; Health Studies, 89-376, 382; hyperactivity, Special Report, 89-192; minerals, Special Report, 88-154; osteoporosis, Special Report, 89-63; ulcer, Special Report, 90-74; vegetarianism, Special Report, 90-99. See also **Nutrition and Food.**
Diet, Liquid: Close-Up, 90-336
Dietary fiber: nutrition and food, 90-309; Special Report, 89-88; vegetarianism, 90-104
Diethylstilbestrol. See DES.
Digestive System, 90-264, 89-268, 88-252; alcohol, Health Studies, 88-375; dietary fiber, Special Report, 89-90; ulcer, Special Report, 90-71
Digital hearing aid: ear and hearing, 89-274
Digitalis: heart and blood vessels, 88-280
Dioxin: environmental health, 90-275, 89-277
Disabilities: books of health and medicine, 90-248; brain and nervous system, 90-252
Discrimination: health policy, 89-292
Disease. See names of specific diseases.
Disease prevention: dietary fiber, Special Report, 89-88; Soviet medicine, Special Report, 90-97
Diskogram: back problems, Special Report, 90-206
Diuretic: heart and blood vessels, 88-280; steroids, Special Report, 90-53
Diverticulosis: dietary fiber, Special Report, 89-91
DNA (deoxyribonucleic acid): diabetes, 89-267; drugs, 88-254; infectious diseases, 88-287. See also **Genetics.**
Dog: veterinary medicine, 89-333
Dominance: left-handedness, Special Report, 89-160

Dopamine: brain and nervous system, 90-251

Double-blind study: health fraud, Special Report, 89-179

Double-major curve: scoliosis, Special Report, 88-128

Dowager's hump: il., 89-57

Down's syndrome: brain and nervous system, 88-238; genetics, 88-273; pregnancy and childbirth, 90-314; prenatal diagnosis, Special Report, 88-56

Drinking water: environmental health, 88-261; lead poisoning, Special Report, 90-181

Drug abuse: AIDS, 88-214; AIDS, Special Report, 90-118, 88-17; health policy, 90-295. See also **Alcohol and Drug Abuse.**

Drug resistance: Close-Up, 90-268

Drug testing: AIDS, Special Report, 90-123; alcohol and drug abuse, 88-219; safety, 90-324, 88-305; steroids, Special Report, 90-53

Drugs, 90-267, 89-270, 88-254; books of health and medicine, 90-248, 89-249, 88-232; Close-Up, 89-229; health fraud, Special Report, 89-178; health policy, 90-295; Health Studies, 89-378. See also specific disorders.

Dry eye: aging eyes, Special Report, 88-193

Duchenne muscular dystrophy: brain and nervous system, 89-251; il., 89-289

Duodenal ulcer: digestive system, 89-268; ulcer, Special Report, 90-72

Dyslexia: hyperactivity, Special Report, 89-190; il., 89-252; left-handedness, Special Report, 89-167

E

E, Vitamin: minerals, Special Report, 88-158; nutrition and food, 90-309, 88-296; veterinary medicine, 90-333, 89-333

Ear and Hearing, 90-271, 89-273, 88-257; veterinary medicine, 89-334

Ear infections: ear and hearing, 90-272

Eating disorders: alcohol and drug abuse, 90-235; books of health and medicine, 90-248; Health Studies, 89-371; weight control, 90-335

Echocardiography: stroke, 89-332

ECM (erythema chronicum migrans): Lyme disease, Special Report, 89-44

Egg donor program: pregnancy and childbirth, 88-299

Elderly persons. See Aging; Alzheimer's disease.

Electrocardiogram (ECG): checkup, Special Report, 88-208; coronary artery disease, Special Report, 89-77; emergency medicine, 90-274; heart and blood vessels, 88-282; pregnancy and childbirth, 88-298

Electroconvulsive therapy (ECT): depression, Special Report, 88-80

Electrodesiccation: skin cancer, Special Report, 89-36

Electroencephalogram (EEG): child development, 88-244; stroke, Special Report, 90-63

Electromagnetic waves: radiation, Special Report, 88-144

Emergency Medicine, 90-273, 89-275, 88-258; pediatric trauma, Special Report, 90-342; Soviet medicine, Special Report, 90-92

Emergency room nurse: Health Professions, 88-359

Emotions: child development, 88-245

Emphysema: respiratory system, 88-300

Encephalitis: lead poisoning, Special Report, 90-177

End stage renal disease: kidney, 88-289

Endoscopy: digestive system, 90-265; ulcer, Special Report, 90-72

Endurance training: knee, Special Report, 88-53

Enterobacteria: salmonella, Special Report, 89-133

Environmental Health, 90-275, 89-277, 88-260; brain and nervous system, 89-253; diabetes, 89-267; genetics, 89-290; weight control, 89-336

Environmental medicine: allergies and immunology, 90-239

Enzyme: alcohol, Health Studies, 88-371

Enzyme-linked immunosorbent assay (ELISA): AIDS, Special Report, 88-23

Epidemics: AIDS, Special Report, 88-10; polio, Special Report, 89-102

Epidemiology: AIDS, 88-214; Legionnaires' disease, Special Report, 90-156; Lyme disease, Special Report, 89-41

Epidermal growth factor: skin, 90-326

Epidermis: skin, 88-308

Epstein-Barr virus (EBV): infectious diseases, 88-286; mononucleosis, Special Report, 90-129, 136

Equilibrium: aging, 90-228

Erythropoietin: arthritis and connective tissue disorders, 89-243; blood, 90-245; glands and hormones, 88-276; kidney, 90-303, 88-289; kidney transplantation, Special Report, 88-112

Estrogen: minerals, Special Report, 88-164; nutrition, 88-295; osteoporosis, Special Report, 89-64. See also **Glands and Hormones.**

Estrogen replacement therapy (ERT): osteoporosis, Special Report, 89-68

Ethics: AIDS, Special Report, 90-114; books of health and medicine, 88-248, 89-249; health policy, 88-277

Evoked-response test: stroke, Special Report, 90-63

Exchange diet: Health Studies, 89-377

Exercise and Fitness, 90-277, 89-279, 88-264; aging, 90-229, 89-228; arthritis and connective tissue disorders, 90-242; brain and nervous system, 89-252; cholesterol, Special Report, 88-39; Close-Up, 88-266; glands and hormones, 88-277; Health Studies, 89-377, 383; knee, Special Report, 88-53; osteoporosis, Special Report, 89-63; respiratory system,

90-316; weight control, 88-321. See also **Running.**

Expert testimony: mental and behavioral disorders, 89-308

Extended-wear contact lenses: eye and vision, 90-282, 88-268

External electronic stimulator: scoliosis, Special Report, 88-132

Extracorporeal shock-wave lithotripsy (ESWL): digestive system, 90-266, 89-269, 88-252; urology, 88-314

Eye and Vision, 90-281, 89-282, 88-268; Project Orbis, Special Report, 90-356

Eye bank: Project Orbis, Special Report, 90-365

Eye cancer: genetics, 88-274

Eye charts: eye and vision, 90-283, 88-269

Eye surgery: Project Orbis, Special Report, 90-356; Soviet medicine, Special Report, 90-84

F

Face-lift: cosmetic surgery, Special Report, 89-148

Facial expression: child development, 88-246

Faith healing: books of health and medicine, 90-248

Fallen arches: foot problems, Special Report, 89-119

Familial hypercholesterolemia (FH): cholesterol, Special Report, 88-36; coronary artery disease, Special Report, 89-76

Family: alcohol and drug abuse, 89-236; alcohol, Health Studies, 88-375

Farming: salmonella, Special Report, 89-137

Fasting: Close-Up, 90-336; Health Studies, 89-379

Fat. See Body fat.

Fat, Dietary: breast cancer, Special Report, 90-32; vegetarianism, Special Report, 90-101

Fat deposit: cosmetic surgery, Special Report, 89-151

Fear: anxiety disorders, Special Report, 90-11

Fees: financing medical care, 89-287

Feingold diet: hyperactivity, Special Report, 89-192

Femur: knee, Special Report, 88-42

Fetal alcohol syndrome: alcohol and drug abuse, 90-234; alcohol, Health Studies, 88-379

Fetal tissue: brain and nervous system, 90-251; health policy, 90-294

Fetus: prenatal diagnosis, Special Report, 88-63. See also **Pregnancy and Childbirth.**

Fiber, Dietary: Special Report, 89-88

Fibrinogen: ear and hearing, 88-258

Fibroadenoma: breast cancer, Special Report, 90-36

Fibrocystic breast disease: breast cancer, Special Report, 90-32

Financing Medical Care, 90-284, 89-286, 88-271; Health Professions, 88-

357. See also **Health care costs; Health Care Facilities.**
Fingerprints: genetics, 90-287
Fingerstick test: coronary artery disease, Special Report, 89-77
Fire extinguisher: fire safety, Special Report, 89-219
Fireplace: fire safety, Special Report, 89-217
Fire safety: Special Report, 89-214
Fitness walking: Close-Up, 88-266. See also **Exercise and Fitness.**
Flashbacks: anxiety disorders, Special Report, 90-14
Flashover: fire safety, Special Report, 89-214
Floaters: aging eyes, Special Report, 88-194
Fluoride: dentistry, 88-248; osteoporosis, Special Report, 89-69
Food: migraine, Special Report, 89-17; safety, Close-Up, 90-320; salmonella, Special Report, 89-132
Food allergy: allergies and immunology, 88-223
Food groups: minerals, Special Report, 88-165
Food poisoning: infectious diseases, 88-288; salmonella, Special Report, 89-132
Foot drop: lead poisoning, Special Report, 90-177
Foot problems: bone disorders, 89-247; Special Report, 89-116
Fovea centralis: aging eyes, Special Report, 88-183
Framingham Study: heart and blood vessels, 89-295; smoking, 89-327
Fraud: health fraud, Special Report, 89-171
Fungal infection: foot problems, Special Report, 89-125

G

GABA receptor: brain and nervous system, 88-237
Gallstones: digestive system, 90-265, 89-269, 88-252; drugs, 90-271
Gamma globulin: polio, Special Report, 89-110
Gamma ray surgery: il., 89-253
Gamma rays: radiation, Special Report, 88-144
Ganciclovir: AIDS, 90-232
Gastric bubble: Health Studies, 89-380; weight control, 89-337, 88-320
Gastric ulcer: ulcer, Special Report, 90-72
Gastritis: digestive system, 89-268
Gastrointestinal disorder: dietary fiber, Special Report, 89-91
Gemfibrozil: heart, 89-299
Gene probe: genetics, 88-273
Gene splicing. See **Genetic engineering.**
Genetic code: Health Professions, 88-344
Genetic disorders: brain and nervous system, 88-235; depression, Special Report, 88-76; pregnancy and

childbirth, 89-314, 88-299; prenatal diagnosis, Special Report, 88-56
Genetic engineering: allergies and immunology, 90-239; blood, 90-245; 89-245; cancer, 90-254, 88-240; genetics, 90-286; heart and blood vessels, 89-298; kidney, 88-289; skin, 90-326
Genetics, 90-286, 89-288, 88-273; alcohol and drug abuse, 90-233; left-handedness, Special Report, 89-164; radiation, Special Report, 88-143
Genital sores: AIDS, 88-215
Genital ulcer: sexually transmitted diseases, 89-324
Genital warts: sexually transmitted diseases, 88-307
Geriatric care manager: caring for the aged, Special Report, 89-208
Gestational diabetes: prenatal diagnosis, Special Report, 88-60
Gingivitis: orthodontics, Special Report, 88-92
Glands and Hormones, 90-289, 89-291, 88-276; Health Studies, 89-374
Glaucoma: aging eyes, Special Report, 88-186
Glucose: checkup, Special Report, 88-204
Goiter: il., 88-157; minerals, Special Report, 88-159
Gonorrhea: sexually transmitted diseases, 88-306
Group A streptococcus: Close-Up, 89-304
Gum disease: dentistry, 90-261
Gun control: safety, 88-306

H

Hair cell: ear and hearing, 89-273
Hair loss. See **Baldness.**
Hairy leukoplakia: mononucleosis, Special Report, 90-137
Hammertoe: foot problems, Special Report, 89-121
Hamstrings: knee, Special Report, 88-45
Handicapped people: Health Professions, 88-326
Hangover: alcohol, Health Studies, 88-373
Harelip: cosmetic surgery, Special Report, 89-149
Head injury: safety, 90-321
Headache: migraine, Special Report, 89-11
Health care alternatives: books of health and medicine, 90-248; Special Report, 88-94
Health care costs: books of health and medicine, 90-248, 88-232; hospitals, 88-284. See also **Financing Medical Care.**
Health Care Facilities, 90-291
Health fraud: Special Report, 89-171
Health insurance: financing medical care, 88-272. See also **Insurance.**
Health maintenance organization (HMO): health care alternatives, Special Report, 88-96; health care facilities, 90-293
Health Policy, 90-294, 89-292, 88-277; books of health and medicine, 90-

248, 88-232; Soviet medicine, Special Report, 90-84
Health Studies: alcohol, 88-367; obesity, 89-368; vaccines, 90- 368
Hearing aid: ear and hearing, 89-273; veterinary medicine, 89-334
Heart and Blood Vessels, 90-296, 89-295, 88-280; aging, 89-228; coronary artery disease, Special Report, 89-72; dietary fiber, Special Report, 89-97; exercise and fitness, 88-265; glands and hormones, 89-291; Special Report, 90-58; stroke, 89-331; vegetarianism, Special Report, 90-104
Heart attack: alcohol and drug abuse, 88-217; cholesterol, Special report, 88-28; Close-Up, 89-296; drugs, 89-270; emergency medicine, 90-273
Heart defects: stroke, Special Report, 90-67
Heart disease: alcohol, Health Studies, 88-372; caring for the aged, Special Report, 89-205; cholesterol, Special Report, 88-28; coronary artery disease, Special Report, 89-72; dietary fiber, Special Report, 89-96; il., 89-73; smoking, 89-327; steroids, Special Report, 90-45; veterinary medicine, 88-316. See also **Heart and Blood Vessels.**
Heart palpitations: minerals, Special Report, 88-154
Heart valves: stroke, Special Report, 90-67
Heartworm disease: veterinary medicine, 88-316
Heavy metal: environmental health, 89-277
Height-weight tables: Health Studies, 89-368
Hemisphere, Brain: left-handedness, Special Report, 89-160
Hemodialysis. See **Dialysis.**
Hemophilia: AIDS, Special Report, 88-13; blood, 90-245; prenatal diagnosis, Special Report, 88-63
Hemorrhagic stroke: Close-Up, 89-297; coronary artery disease, Special Report, 89-82; stroke, Special Report, 90-58
Hepatitis: blood, 89-244; digestive system, 90-265; infectious diseases, 90-301
Herbal medicine: arthritis and connective tissue disorders, 88-225; books of health and medicine, 88-233
Hereditary disorder: alcohol and drug abuse, 89-236; arthritis and connective tissue disorders, 88-225; asthma, Special Report, 90-185; brain and nervous system, 89-251; breast cancer, Special Report, 90-31; coronary artery disease, Special Report, 89-76; depression, Special Report, 88-74; genetics, 89-288; Health Studies, 88-376; migraine, Special Report, 89-15; orthodontics, Special Report, 88-85; prenatal diagnosis, Special Report, 88-56
Heredity: alcohol and drug abuse, 90-233; anxiety disorders, Special

Report, 90-19; arthritis and connective tissue disorders, 90-240; cancer, 90-255; child development, 88-246; Health Studies, 89-374; ulcer, Special Report, 90-76; weight control, 89-336. See also **Genetics.**

Herniated disk: back problems, Special Report, 90-202

Herpesvirus: infectious diseases, 88-287; mononucleosis, Special Report, 90-132

High blood pressure. See **Hypertension.**

High-density lipoproteins (HDL's): cholesterol, Special Report, 88-36; coronary artery disease, Special Report, 89-76; dietary fiber, Special Report, 89-97; exercise and fitness, 90-280; heart and blood vessels, 89-295; weight control, 90-335

Highway accidents. See **Safety.**

Histamine: Close-Up, 88-221

Histamine antagonist: digestive system, 88-253; ulcer, Special Report, 90-80

Histamine releasing factor: allergies and immunology, 90-238

HIV. See **Human immunodeficiency virus.**

Hodgkin's disease: blood, 90-244

Holographic contact lens: eye and vision, 89-285

Home fire extinguisher: fire safety, Special Report, 89-219

Homeless people: Health Professions, 88-364

Homosexuality: AIDS, 90-230, 88-215; AIDS, Special Report, 90-123, 88-11

Hormone: alcohol, Health Studies, 88-375; arthritis and connective tissue disorders, 90-241, 88-225; breast cancer, Special Report, 90-31; migraine, Special Report, 89-16; osteoporosis, Special Report, 89-63; steroids, Special Report, 90-48. See also **Glands and Hormones.**

Hormone replacement therapy (HRT): osteoporosis, Special Report, 89-68

Hospitals, 89-300, 88-284; Soviet medicine, Special Report, 90-90. See also **Financing Medical Care; Health Care Facilities.**

House dust mite: allergies and immunology, 88-223

Human genome: genetics, 90-288

Human growth hormone (HGH): steroids, Special Report, 90-53

Human immunodeficiency virus (HIV): AIDS, 90-232, 89-233, 88-235; AIDS, Special Report, 90-113, 88-13; brain and nervous system, 88-235

Human leucocyte antigen (HLA): allergies and immunology, 89-240; diabetes, 89-267; kidney transplantation, Special Report, 88-118

Human papilloma-virus (HPV): sexually transmitted diseases, 88-307

Humidifiers: Close-Up, 90-237

Hydrocephalis: prenatal diagnosis, Special Report, 88-67

Hyperactivity: Special Report, 89-185

Hypertension: books of health and medicine, 90-249; checkup, Special Report, 88-202; coronary artery disease, Special Report, 89-75; drugs, 89-271; exercise and fitness, 90-279, 89-280; Health Studies, 89-370; kidney transplantation, Special Report, 88-113; minerals, Special Report, 88-154; prenatal diagnosis, Special Report, 88-56; stroke, Special Report, 90-65

Hypoglycemia: diabetes, 90-263; glands and hormones, 88-277

Hypothalamus: glands and hormones, 89-291; migraine, Special Report, 89-15

I

ICAM-1 cell receptor: allergies and immunology, 90-238; infectious diseases, 90-300

Ideal weight: Health Studies, 89-368

Imaginal flooding: anxiety disorders, Special Report, 90-24

Immune system: AIDS, Special Report, 88-11; alcohol, Health Studies, 88-375; allergies and immunology, 90-236, 89-239; arthritis and connective tissue disorders, 88-224; brain and nervous system, 90-252; breast cancer, Special Report, 90-28; Health Studies, 89-370; infectious diseases, 89-303; kidney transplantation, Special Report, 88-111; left-handedness, Special Report, 89-168; nutrition and food, 90-311, 89-311, 88-296; tuberculosis, Special Report, 90-146. See also **AIDS.**

Immune therapy: health fraud, Special Report, 89-175

Immunology. See **Allergies and Immunology; Vaccines.**

Immunosuppressive drugs: burns, Special Report, 90-222; diabetes, 89-266; kidney transplantation, Special Report, 88-119; mononucleosis, Special Report, 90-137

Impetigo: drugs, 89-273

Implant, Surgical: ils., 90-241, 251; cosmetic surgery, Special Report, 89-150

Incontinence: caring for the aged, Special Report, 89-205; urology, 90-332

Indian, American: Health Studies, 89-374; weight control, 89-336

Infant mortality: Soviet medicine, Special Report, 90-86

Infantile paralysis. See **Polio myelitis.**

Infarction: heart and blood vessels, 89-298

Infection: foot problems, Special Report, 89-124

Infectious Diseases, 90-300, 89-303, 88-286. See also specific diseases.

Inference: child development, 88-245

Infertility: il., 89-314

Influenza: Health Studies, 90-378; infectious diseases, 89-306

Ingrown toenail: foot problems, Special Report, 89-123

Inhalers: asthma, Special Report, 90-192

Insoluble fiber: dietary fiber, Special Report, 89-89

Insomnia: exercise and fitness, 88-264; Special Report, 88-166

Insulin: glands and hormones, 88-277. See also **Diabetes.**

Insulin pump: diabetes, 88-249

Insurance: health care alternatives, Special Report, 88-94; health policy, 89-293. See also **Financing Medical Care.**

Intelligence: child development, 90-258

Interferon: sexually transmitted diseases, 88-307

Interleukin-2: cancer, 90-255, 88-240

Intestinal by-pass surgery: Health Studies, 89-380

Intestine: salmonella, Special Report, 89-133

Intoxication: alcohol and drug abuse, 88-217; brain and nervous system, 88-237

Intracranial vasospasms: stroke, 90-331

Intraocular lens implant: aging eyes, Special Report, 88-185

Intravenous drug use: AIDS, 89-231; AIDS, Special Report, 88-17; alcohol and drug abuse, 89-238

Iodine: minerals, Special Report, 88-159

Iodization of salt: minerals, Special Report, 88-162

Ionizing radiation: radiation, Special Report, 88-140

IPV (inactivated poliovirus vaccine): polio, Special Report, 89-110

Iron-deficiency anemia: minerals, Special Report, 88-157; vegetarianism, Special Report, 90-108

Iron lung: polio, Special Report, 89-106

Ischemic heart disease: heart and blood vessels, 88-282

Ischemic stroke: stroke, Special Report, 90-58

Isolation: AIDS, Special Report, 90-117

IUD (intrauterine device). See **Birth Control.**

J

Jaundice: mononucleosis, Special Report, 90-134

Jaw: Close-Up, 89-264

Jews: depression, Special Report, 88-76; prenatal diagnosis, Special Report, 88-56

Jogging. See **Running.**

Johnson, Virginia E.: AIDS, 89-232

Joints: back problems, Special Report, 90-203; knee, Special Report, 88-40. See also **Arthritis and Connective Tissue Disorders.**

Juvenile acquired hypothyroidism: glands and hormones, 89-292

Juvenile rheumatoid arthritis (JRA): arthritis and connective tissue disorders, 90-240; Lyme disease, Special Report, 89-40

K

Kaposi's sarcoma: AIDS, 90-232, 88-214; AIDS, Special Report, 88-14
Keloid: cosmetic surgery, Special Report, 89-148
Keratinocyte: skin cancer, Special Report, 89-27
Keratotomy: eye and vision, 88-270
Kidney, 90-303, 89-307, 88-289; cancer, 90-254, 88-241; glands and hormones, 88-276
Kidney stones: glands and hormones, 90-290; minerals, Special Report, 88-165; urology, 89-333, 88-314
Kidney transplantation: Special Report, 88-108
Killed-virus vaccine: Health Studies, 90-370; polio, Special Report, 89-109
Knee: bone disorders, 89-247, 88-231; il., 89-281; Special Report, 88-40
Koop, C. Everett: AIDS, Special Report, 88-12; pediatric trauma, Special Report, 90-352; People in Medicine, 89-340
Kwashiorkor: vegetarianism, Special Report, 90-106

L

Labor monitor: il., 90–313
Lactose intolerance: Close-Up, 90-310; nutrition, 89-314
Laminectomy: back problems, Special Report, 90-209
Landfills: environmental health, 88-260
Laser: bone disorders, 89-247; coronary artery disease, Special Report, 89-85; eye and vision, 88-270; heart and blood vessels, 90-297; il., 89-332; skin, 90-327, 88-309; urology, 88-314
Laser Doppler blood profusion monitor: burns, Special Report, 90-218
Lateral arch: foot problems, Special Report, 89-118
L-dopa: brain and nervous system, 88-234
Lead poisoning: safety, 89-323; Special Report, 90-169; veterinary medicine, 90-334
Learning: child development, 89-260
Left-handedness: Special Report, 89-159
Legal issues: alcohol and drug abuse, 88-217; health policy, 88-277; mental and behavioral disorders, 89-308
Legionnaires' disease: Special Report, 90-154
Lens: aging eyes, Special Report, 88-182
Leprosy: drugs, 88-255
Leukemia: il., 89-245; radiation, Special Report, 88-150
Levamisole: cancer, 90-257
Licensed practical nurse (LPN): Health Professions, 88-354
Licensed vocational nurse (LVN): Health Professions, 88-354
Life expectancy: genetics, 89-290; Soviet medicine, Special Report, 90-87

Life style: coronary artery disease, Special Report, 89-79
Life-support systems: books of health and medicine, 88-232; health policy, 88-279
Ligament: back problems, Special Report, 90-200; knee, Special Report, 88-42
Lipoproteins: checkup, Special Report, 88-203; cholesterol, Special Report, 88-35; coronary artery disease, Special Report, 89-76; dietary fiber, Special Report, 89-97; exercise and fitness, 90-279; heart and blood vessels, 89-295; steroids, Special Report, 90-47
Liposuction: cosmetic surgery, Special Report, 89-151; weight control, 89-337
Lithium: depression, Special Report, 88-80
Liver: alcohol, Health Studies, 88-374; mononucleosis, Special Report, 90-134
Liver cancer: steroids, Special Report, 90-45
Livestock: Close-Up, 88-288; salmonella, Special Report, 89-136
Live-virus vaccine: Health Studies, 90-370; polio, Special Report, 89-109
Longitudinal arch: foot problems, Special Report, 89-118
Lou Gehrig's disease: health policy, 88-279
Lovastatin: cholesterol, Special Report, 88-39; drugs, 89-270, 88-256
Low-density lipoproteins (LDL's): cholesterol, Special Report, 88-36; coronary artery disease, Special Report, 89-76; dietary fiber, Special Report, 89-97; heart and blood vessels, 89-295
Low-impact exercise: Close-Up, 90-278
Low-level radiation: radiation, Special Report, 88-147
Lumbar curve: scoliosis, Special Report, 88-128
Lumpectomy: breast cancer, Special Report, 90-37
Lung cancer: cancer, 88-239; nutrition, 88-296; respiratory system, 90-318, 89-316, 88-302; smoking, 88-310
Lung disease: asthma, Special Report, 90-184; environmental health, 88-263; Legionnaires' disease, Special Report, 90-154; tuberculosis, Special Report, 90-146
Lyme disease: Special Report, 89-39
Lymphatic system: blood, 90-244; breast cancer, Special Report, 90-28; cancer, 89-257; mononucleosis, Special Report, 90-129; urology, 88-315
Lymphocyte: nutrition, 89-312. See also **White blood cell.**
Lymphoma: cancer, 88-240; kidney transplantation, Special Report, 88-120

M

Macrobiotics: vegetarianism, Special Report, 90-101
Macromineral: minerals, Special Report, 88-156

Macrophage: allergies and immunology, 89-240, 88-220
Macula: aging eyes, Special Report, 88-183; eye and vision, 89-283
Magnetic resonance imaging (MRI): back problems, Special Report, 90-206; bone disorders, 89-247; stroke, Special Report, 90-61
Major depressive disorder (MDD): caring for the aged, Special Report, 89-205; depression, Special Report, 88-70
Malaria: infectious diseases, 89-306, 88-289
Malignant melanoma: skin cancer, Special Report, 89-26
Malocclusion: orthodontics, Special Report, 88-84
Mammography: breast cancer, Special Report, 90-33; checkup, Special Report, 88-207; il., 90-27, 89-255
Manic depression: brain and nervous system, 88-238; depression, Special Report, 88-71; mental and behavioral disorders, 90-305
Manipulation technique: back problems, Special Report, 90-208
Marijuana: alcohol and drug abuse, 90-233, 88-220; respiratory system, 89-318
Mastectomy: breast cancer, Special Report, 90-31
Maternal age: prenatal diagnosis, Special Report, 88-63
Maternal antibodies: polio, Special Report, 89-105
Maternity leave: health policy, 89-293
Maximum aerobic capacity: aging, 89-228
MDphone: emergency medicine, 90-273
Measles: infectious diseases, 90-301
Meat processing: salmonella, Special Report, 89-140
Mechanical heart. See Artificial heart.
Medial arch. See Longitudinal arch.
Medicaid: financing medical care, 89-286, 88-271; health care alternatives, Special Report, 88-97
Medical tests: cancer, 89-254; checkup, Special Report, 88-197; Close-Up, 89-256; health policy, 89-293
Medical waste: health care facilities, 90-292
Medicare: books of health and medicine, 90-250; health care alternatives, Special Report, 88-97. See also **Financing Medical Care.**
Medullary cavity: il., 89-58
Megavitamin therapy: health fraud, Special Report, 89-176
Melanocyte: skin cancer, Special Report, 89-27
Melanoma: allergies and immunology, 88-222; cancer, 90-254; skin cancer, Special Report, 89-26
Meniscuses: bone disorders, 88-230; knee, Special Report, 88-45
Menopause: arthritis and connective tissue disorders, 88-225; bone disorders, 88-230; breast cancer, Special Report, 90-31; glands and

hormones, 90-289, 88-276; heart and blood vessels, 89-295; migraine, Special Report, 89-16; osteoporosis, Special Report, 89-63; stroke, 90-331
Menstruation: alcohol, Health Studies, 88-375; breast cancer, Special Report, 90-31; migraine, Special Report, 89-16; minerals, Special Report, 88-157
Mental and Behavioral Disorders, 90-304, 89-308, 88-291; anxiety disorders, Special Report, 90-10; brain and nervous system, 88-238; caring for the aged, Special Report, 89-205; child abuse, Special Report, 89-354; depression, Special Report, 88-68; genetics, 90-287; hyperactivity, Special Report, 89-185; Soviet medicine, Special Report, 90-94. See also **Psychological problems.**
Mental development: child development, 88-244
Mental imagery: health fraud, Special Report, 89-176
Metabolic therapy: health fraud, Special Report, 89-175
Metabolism: alcohol, Health Studies, 88-372; weight control, 89-336, 88-321
Metastasis: allergies and immunology, 88-220; breast cancer, Special Report, 90-28; smoking, 88-312
Metatarsal arch. See Transverse arch.
Metatarsal bone: foot problems, Special Report, 89-118
Methadone: alcohol and drug abuse, 90-234
Micromineral: minerals, Special Report, 88-156
Microvasectomy: birth control, 88-226
Migraine: Special Report, 89-10
Mine safety: safety, 88-306
Minerals: Special Report, 88-154
Minoxidil: drugs, 90-270; skin, 89-327
Misaligned jaw: orthodontics, Special Report, 88-82
Miscarriage: birth control, 88-227; lead poisoning, Special Report, 90-171; pregnancy and childbirth, 89-315; prenatal diagnosis, Special Report, 88-63
Mite: allergies and immunology, 88-223
Mobile hospitals: Project Orbis, Special Report, 90-359
Mobility problems: caring for the aged, Special Report, 89-204
Mole: skin cancer, Special Report, 89-36
Monoamine-oxidase inhibitors (MAOI's): anxiety disorders, Special Report, 90-20; depression, Special Report, 88-79
Monoclonal antibodies: kidney transplantation, Special Report, 88-121; respiratory system, 90-318
Mononucleosis: Special Report, 90-127
Monounsaturated oil: cholesterol, Special Report, 88-38; diabetes, 90-263

Mothers Against Drunk Driving (MADD): Health Studies, 88-382
Multipolar coagulation: ulcers, Special Report, 90-81
Muscle spasm: back problems, Special Report, 90-202; Close-Up, 89-264
Muscular dystrophy: brain and nervous system, 89-251; genetics, 88-274; il., 89-289
Mycobacterium avium: infectious diseases, 89-303
Myelin: brain, 88-235
Myelogram: back problems, Special Report, 90-206
Myopia. See Nearsightedness.

N

Narcotic analgesics: steroids, Special Report, 90-53
Nasal spray: Close-Up, 88-221
National Cholesterol Education Program (NCEP): cholesterol, Special Report, 88-39
National Institute of Allergy and Infectious Diseases (NIAID): AIDS, 89-232
National Institute of Mental Health (NIMH): alcohol and drug abuse, 88-217
National Institutes of Health: Health Professions, 88-339
Natural background radiation: radiation, Special Report, 88-147
Near-sightedness: eye and vision, 88-270
Needle aspiration: breast cancer, Special Report, 90-36
Nerve growth factors (NGF's): aging, 90-228
Nervous system: aging, 90-228; alcohol, Health Studies, 88-374; lead poisoning, Special Report, 90-177; polio, Special Report, 89-104. See also **Brain and Nervous System.**
Neural tube defects (NTD's): prenatal diagnosis, Special Report, 88-57
Neuritic plaques: brain and nervous system, 90-251
Neurofibrillary tangles: brain and nervous system, 90-251
Neurofibromatosis: cancer, 88-244
Neurological problems. See Brain and Nervous System; Brain disorder.
Neurotransmitter: aging, 88-212; alcohol and drug abuse, 90-235; brain and nervous system, 88-234; depression, Special Report, 88-76; hyperactivity, Special Report, 89-193; migraine, Special Report, 89-15
Neutrophils: cancer, 90-257
Nicardipine: drugs, 90-169
Nicotine: smoking, 89-329
Nimodipine: brain and nervous system, 90-251; drugs, 90-270
Nitrogen oxide: Close-Up, 88-262
Nitroglycerin: coronary artery disease, Special Report, 90-81
Noise pollution: ear and hearing, 90-273
Nonionizing radiation: radiation, Special Report, 88-140
Nonsteroidal anti-inflammatory drug (NSAID): drugs, 90-267

Norepinephrine: depression, Special Report, 88-76
Nuclear accelerators: cancer, 90-254
Nuclear accident: radiation, Special Report, 88-139
Nursing: Health Professions, 88-352. See also **Health Care Facilities.**
Nursing home: caring for the aged, Special Report, 89-209; financing medical care, 90-292, 89-287
Nutrition and Food, 90-308, 89-311, 88-295; books of health and medicine, 90-249, 88-233; minerals, Special Report, 88-154; vegetarianism, Special Report, 90-99. See also **Diet.**
Nutritional therapy: health fraud, Special Report, 89-174

O

Oat bran: dietary fiber, Special Report, 89-98; nutrition and food, 90-309
Obesity: arthritis and connective tissue disorders, 88-225; dietary fiber, Special Report, 89-98; Health Studies, 89-368; weight control, 88-319
Obstetrics. See Pregnancy and Childbirth.
Occult blood test: checkup, Special Report, 88-208
Ocusert: aging eyes, Special Report, 88-189
Opaque contact lenses: eye and vision, 90-283
Open bite: orthodontics, Special Report, 88-84
Operating room nurse: Health Professions, 88-362
Operation. See Surgery.
Opioids: alcohol and drug abuse, 90-236; mental and behavioral disorders, 88-294
Optic nerve: aging eyes, Special Report, 88-183
OPV (oral polio vaccine): polio, Special Report, 89-112
Oral cancer: cancer, 89-259, 88-239
Organ transplant: il., 89-268; kidney transplantation, Special Report, 88-108
Orphan drug: drugs, 88-255
Orthodontics: Special Report, 88-82. See also **Dentistry.**
Orthopedic nurse: Health Professions, 88-358
Orthotics: back problems, Special Report, 90-209; foot problems, Special Report, 89-120
Osteoarthritis: arthritis and connective tissue disorders, 88-225; back problems, Special Report, 90-203; caring for the aged, Special Report, 89-204; exercise and fitness, 89-281; knee, Special Report, 88-48
Osteoblast: orthodontics, Special Report, 88-90; osteoporosis, Special Report, 89-60
Osteoclast: orthodontics, Special Report, 88-90; osteoporosis, Special Report, 89-60

Osteomalacia: kidney, 89-307; vegetarianism, Special Report, 90-110

Osteopathy: back problems, Special Report, 90-208

Osteoporosis: back problems, Special Report, 90-203; bone disorders, 90-246, 88-230; books of health and medicine, 90-249; glands and hormones, 88-276; minerals, Special Report, 88-164; nutrition, 88-295; Special Report, 89-55

Outpatient surgery: cosmetic surgery, Special Report, 89-154

Overbite: orthodontics, Special Report, 88-84

Overweight: Health Studies, 89-368

Ovulation: glands and hormones, 89-291

Ozone: Close-Up, 88-262; environmental health, 88-261; skin cancer, Special Report, 89-35

P

Pacemaker: il., 90–298

Paget's disease: breast cancer, Special Report, 90-38

Pain: migraine, Special Report, 89-11

Pancreas: diabetes, 90-263

Panic disorders: anxiety disorders, Special Report, 90-12

Pap test: checkup, Special Report, 88-205; Close-Up, 89-256

Paralysis: polio, Special Report, 89-102

Parasite: Health Studies, 90-370; pregnancy and childbirth, 89-315

Parkinson's disease: brain and nervous system, 88-234

Passive smoking: environmental health, 88-263; smoking, 88-310

Pasteur, Louis: Health Studies, 90-374

Pathological left-handedness: left-handedness, Special Report, 89-165

Pediatric trauma: Special Report, 90-342

Pediatrics: allergies, 88-223; books of health and medicine, 88-232. See also **Child Development.**

Pelvic exam: checkup, Special Report, 88-205

Pentamidine: AIDS, 90-232

Pepsin: ulcer, Special Report, 90-71

Peptic ulcer: ulcer, Special Report, 90-71

Percutaneous diskectomy: back problems, Special Report, 90-209

Perilymphatic fistula: ear and hearing, 90-271

Periodontal disease: orthodontics, Special Report, 88-86

Peripheral vision: aging eyes, Special Report, 88-185

Peritoneal dialysis: kidney transplantation, Special Report, 88-115

Pertussis vaccine: Health Studies, 90-380

Pesticides: Close-Up, 90-320

Phalanges: foot problems, Special Report, 89-118

Phobia: anxiety disorders, Special Report, 90-12; mental and behavioral disorders, 90-306

Photoaging: skin, 89-325

Physical examination: checkup, Special Report, 88-196

Physical fitness. See **Exercise and Fitness.**

Physical therapy: back problems, Special Report, 90-207; burns, Special Report, 90-224; Health Professions, 88-330; stroke, Special Report, 90-63

Pima Indians: Health Studies, 89-374; weight control, 89-336

Pineal gland: mental and behavioral disorders, 88-293

Placebo: health fraud, Special Report, 89-180

Plant food: dietary fiber, Special Report, 89-88

Plantar arch. See **Longitudinal arch.**

Plantar warts: foot problems, Special Report, 89-124

Plaque (arterial): cholesterol, Special Report, 88-29; coronary artery disease, Special Report, 89-74; dietary fiber, Special Report, 89-97; heart and blood vessels, 90-296

Plasmid: arthritis and connective tissue disorders, 89-242

Plastic surgery: burns, Special Report, 90-224; cosmetic surgery, Special Report, 89-144

Platelet: coronary artery disease, Special Report, 89-74

Pneumococcal pneumonia: Health Studies, 90-378

***Pneumocystis carinii* pneumonia (PCP):** AIDS, 90-230, 88-214; AIDS, Special Report, 88-14

Pneumothorax: tuberculosis, Special Report, 90-148

Podiatrist: foot problems, Special Report, 89-127

Poisoning: Close-Up, 90-320; lead poisoning, Special Report, 90-170; safety, 90-321

Poliomyelitis: Health Studies, 90-368; Special Report, 89-102

Polycythemia: stroke, Special Report, 90-67

Polysaccharide vaccines: Health Studies, 90-376

Polyunsaturated oil: cholesterol, Special Report, 88-38

Portal vein: alcohol, Health Studies, 88-371

Postpolio syndrome: polio, Special Report, 89-115

Post-traumatic stress disorder (PTSD): anxiety disorders, Special Report, 90-12

Potassium: minerals, Special Report, 88-154

Poultry: infectious diseases, 88-288; safety, 88-304; salmonella, Special Report, 89-137

Preferred Provider Organization (PPO): health care alternatives, Special Report, 88-96

Pregnancy and Childbirth, 90-313, 89-314, 88-297; alcohol, Health Studies, 88-379; alcohol and drug abuse, 90-234; birth control, 88-226;

bone disorders, 89-248; il., 89-293; left-handedness, Special Report, 89-165; mental and behavioral disorders, 89-310; migraine, Special Report, 89-16; sexually transmitted diseases, 90-324; Soviet medicine, Special Report, 90-93; vegetarianism, Special Report, 90-105

Premarital screening: health policy, 89-295

Premature death: genetics, 89-290

Premature infants: eye and vision, 89-282

Prenatal diagnosis: pregnancy and childbirth, 90-314; Special Report, 88-54

Presbyopia: aging eyes, Special Report, 88-183

Pressure garments: burns, Special Report, 90-223; il., 90-327

Preventive medication: migraine, Special Report, 89-23

Progestagen: osteoporosis, Special Report, 89-68

Progesterone: birth control, 88-226

Programmable Implantable Medication System (PIMS): diabetes, 88-249

Project Orbis: Special Report, 90-354

Pronated arches. See **Fallen arches.**

Prostaglandins: respiratory system, 88-301; salmonella, Special Report, 89-135; ulcer, Special Report, 90-72

Prostate: cancer, 89-258; urology, 90-331, 89-332, 88-315

Protein: vegetarianism, Special Report, 90-106

Proton pump blockers: ulcer, Special Report, 90-81

Psittacosis: Legionnaires' disease, Special Report, 90-163

Psoriasis: skin, 90-327

Psychiatry: Health Professions, 88-327; Soviet medicine, Special Report, 90-95

Psychological problems: alcohol and drug abuse, 88-217; anxiety disorders, Special Report, 90-10; child abuse, Special Report, 89-354; depression, Special Report, 88-69; Health Studies, 89-371; insomnia, Special Report, 88-168; kidney transplantation, Special Report, 88-116; steroids, Special Report, 90-48. See also **Mental and Behavioral Disorders; Stress, Psychological.**

Psychotherapy: alcohol, Health Studies, 88-378; burns, Special Report, 90-225; depression, Special Report, 88-78; hyperactivity, Special Report, 89-194

Public health: AIDS, Special Report, 90-116; Health Professions, 88-363; People in Medicine, 89-340

Pulmonary function tests: asthma, Special Report, 90-190

Pupil: aging eyes, Special Report, 88-182

Q

Q fever: Legionnaires' disease, Special Report, 90-158

Quackery: health fraud, Special Report, 89-171
Quadriceps: knee, Special Report, 88-45

R

Radial keratotomy: eye and vision, 88-270
Radiation: breast cancer, Special Report, 90-32; Close-Up, 88-262; il., 89-279; skin cancer, Special Report, 89-29
Radiation sickness: radiation, Special Report, 88-143
Radiation therapy: skin cancer, Special Report, 89-37
Radiologist: radiation, Special Report, 88-147
Radium: radiation, Special Report, 88-147
Radon. See **Environmental Health.**
Rash: allergies and immunology, 88-223; Lyme disease, Special Report, 89-44
Raw fish: nutrition and food, 90-312
RDA's (Recommended Dietary Allowances): minerals, Special Report, 88-165; vegetarianism, Special Report, 90-106
Rebounding: migraine, Special Report, 89-23
Receptor cell: migraine, Special Report, 89-15
Recombigen HIV-I Latex Agglutination Test: AIDS, 90-232
Recombinant DNA technology. See **Genetic engineering.**
Recommended Dietary Allowances. See **RDA's.**
Reconstructive surgery: burns, Special Report, 90-224; cosmetic surgery, Special Report, 89-149
Rectal cancer: checkup, Special Report, 88-207; exercise and fitness, 88-267
Red blood cell: checkup, Special Report, 88-204; glands and hormones, 88-276
Registered nurse (RN): Health Professions, 88-353. See also **Health care facilities.**
Rehabilitation Institute of Chicago: Health Professions, 88-324
Rehabilitation nurse: Health Professions, 88-359
Relaxation: anxiety disorders, Special Report, 90-24; asthma, Special Report, 90-196; back problems, Special Report, 90-209; brain and nervous system, 90-253; diabetes, 90-264
Rems: radiation, Special Report, 88-144
Renal osteodystrophy: kidney, 89-307
Renin: kidney transplantation, Special Report, 88-112
Reproductive technology: books of health and medicine, 90-248; pregnancy and childbirth, 90-314
Respiratory distress syndrome: prenatal diagnosis, Special Report, 88-60

Respiratory infection: smoking, 88-310
Respiratory System, 90-316, 89-316, 88-300; allergies and immunology, 90-236, 89-238; asthma, Special Report, 90-189; Legionnaires' disease, Special Report, 90-155; tuberculosis, Special Report, 90-146
Respite services: caring for the aged, Special Report, 89-208
Restriction enzyme: genetics, 88-273
Retainer: orthodontics, Special Report, 88-93
Retina: aging eyes, Special Report, 88-183
Retinoblastoma: cancer, 88-241; genetics, 88-274
Retinopathy of prematurity: eye and vision, 89-282
Retrovirus: drugs, 88-254
Reverse transcriptase: drugs, 88-255
Rh disease: prenatal diagnosis, Special Report, 88-61
Rheumatic fever: Close-Up, 89-304
Rheumatoid arthritis (RA): arthritis and connective tissue disorders, 90-241, 88-224; bone disorders, 89-247; caring for the aged, Special Report, 89-204; left-handedness, Special Report, 89-168. See also **Arthritis and Connective Tissue Disorders.**
Rhinitis: Close-Up, 88-221
Rhinoplasty: cosmetic surgery, Special Report, 89-144
Ribonucleic acid. See **RNA.**
Rice bran: nutrition and food, 90-309
Rickets: minerals, Special Report, 88-162; vegetarianism, Special Report, 90-110
Rickettsia: Legionnaires' disease, Special Report, 90-158
Right to die: health policy, 88-279
Risk factors: coronary artery disease, Special Report, 89-75; osteoporosis, Special Report, 89-64
Ritalin: hyperactivity, Special Report, 89-193
RNA (ribonucleic acid): cancer, 88-241; drugs, 88-255; genetics, 89-289
'roid rage: steroids, Special Report, 90-48
Rotator cuff: arthritis and connective tissue disorders, 89-243
Roughage: dietary fiber, Special Report, 89-88
Running: arthritis and connective tissue disorders, 89-242; exercise and fitness, 89-281; glands and hormones, 88-277

S

Sabin, Albert B.: Health Studies, 90-368; polio, Special Report, 89-109
Safety, 90-318, 89-319, 88-302; fire safety, Special Report, 89-214; pediatric trauma, Special Report, 90-352
Salk, Jonas E.: Health Studies, 90-368; polio, Special Report, 89-109
Salmonella: infectious diseases, 88-288; safety, 88-304; Special Report, 89-131
Sanitariums: Soviet medicine, Special Report, 90-96; tuberculosis, Special Report, 90-142

Saturated fats: cholesterol, Special Report, 88-28
Scar tissue: burns, Special Report, 90-224; cosmetic surgery, Special Report, 89-148
Schizophrenia: genetics, 90-287; mental and behavioral disorders, 90-304, 89-309
School buses: safety, 89-319
Sciatica: back problems, Special Report, 90-203
Sclera: aging eyes, Special Report, 88-182
Scleral cryotherapy: eye and vision, 89-283
Scoliosis: Special Report, 88-124
Screening tests: cancer, 89-254. See also **Medical tests.**
Seasonal affective disorder (SAD): mental and behavioral disorders, 88-292
Seat belts. See **Safety.**
Selenium: minerals, Special Report, 88-158
Senile cataract: aging eyes, Special Report, 88-185
Senior center: caring for the aged, Special Report, 89-206
Sensorineural hearing loss: ear and hearing, 90-271
Sepsis: respiratory system, 88-301
Serotonin: mental and behavioral disorders, 88-293; weight control, 88-320
Serotype: salmonella, Special Report, 89-133
Set point: Health Studies, 89-380
Sex determinant: genetics, 89-288
Sex education: People in Medicine, 89-348
Sexual abuse of children: Special Report, 89-353
Sexually Transmitted Diseases, 90-324, 89-324, 88-306. See also **AIDS;** specific diseases.
Shell shock. See **Post-traumatic stress disorder.**
Shigella: arthritis and connective tissue disorders, 89-242
Shock: pediatric trauma, Special Report, 90-349; respiratory system, 88-301
Shoe: foot problems, Special Report, 89-128
Shyness: anxiety disorders, Special Report, 90-12; child development, 90-260, 89-259
"Sick headache": migraine, Special Report, 89-12
Sigmoidoscopy: checkup, Special Report, 88-208
Silent ischemia: coronary artery disease, Special Report, 89-74
Simian immunodeficiency virus (SIV): AIDS, 88-215
Skin, 90-326, 89-325, 88-308; allergies and immunology, 88-223; burns, Special Report, 90-215; foot problems, Special Report, 89-122; skin cancer, Special Report, 89-24
Skin cancer: cancer, 90-254, 89-259; Close-Up, 88-262; environmental health, 88-261; radiation, Special

Report, 88-143; Special Report, 89-24

Skin grafting: burns, Special Report, 90-221; cosmetic surgery, Special Report, 89-147

Skin test: tuberculosis, Special Report, 90-149

Sleep: back problems, Special Report, 90-206; brain and nervous system, 89-252; insomnia, Special Report, 88-166

Sleep apnea: insomnia, Special Report, 88-170

Slow virus: aging, 89-231

Smallpox vaccine: Health Studies, 90-370

Smoke detector: fire safety, Special Report, 89-220

Smokeless tobacco: cancer, 89-254, 88-239

Smoking, 90-328, 89-327, 88-310; cancer, 89-255, 88-239; Close-Up, 89-330; coronary artery disease, Special Report, 89-77; environmental health, 88-263; fire safety, Special Report, 89-218; Health Studies, 89-375; heart and blood vessels, 89-299; nutrition and food, 90-309, 88-297; People in Medicine, 89-348; respiratory system, 90-316, 89-318, 88-302; Soviet medicine, Special Report, 90-86; stroke, 88-312, Special Report, 90-65; ulcer, Special Report, 90-75

Snellen chart: eye and vision, 88-269

Snuff. See **Smokeless tobacco.**

Social phobia: anxiety disorders, Special Report, 90-12

Soft corn: foot problems, Special Report, 89-123

Soluble fiber: dietary fiber, Special Report, 89-89

Sore throat: mononucleosis, Special Report, 90-134

Soviet medicine: Special Report, 90-83

Spatial perception: left-handedness, Special Report, 89-160

Speech: left-handedness, Special Report, 89-161; stroke, Special Report, 90-58

Speech therapy: stroke, Special Report, 90-63

Speed limit. See **Safety.**

Spermicide: birth control, 88-227

SPF (sun protection factor): skin cancer, Special Report, 89-33

Sphygmomanometer: checkup, Special Report, 88-202

Spina bifida: prenatal diagnosis, Special Report, 88-57

Spinal fusion surgery: back problems, Special Report, 90-209; scoliosis, Special Report, 88-135

Spine: back problems, Special Report, 90-200; il., 89-60

Spirochete: Lyme disease, Special Report, 89-47

Spleen: mononucleosis, Special Report, 90-134

Spondylolisthesis: back problems, Special Report, 90-204

Sports: steroids, Special Report, 90-42

Sports medicine: knee, Special Report, 88-42

Sprinkler system: fire safety, Special Report, 89-221

Squamous cell carcinoma: nutrition, 88-296; skin cancer, Special Report, 89-26

Stanozolol: steroids, Special Report, 90-44

Staphylococcus aureus: salmonella, Special Report, 89-141

Steroids: Special Report, 90-42

Stimulant drugs: hyperactivity, Special Report, 89-193; steroids, Special Report, 90-53

Stomach acid: ulcer, Special Report, 90-73

Stomach stapling: Health Studies, 89-379

Strep throat: Close-Up, 89-304

Streptococcus mutans: dentistry, 89-263

Streptokinase: heart and blood vessels, 89-297

Stress, Psychological: asthma, Special Report, 90-189; books of health and medicine, 90-249; child development, 89-259; coronary artery disease, Special Report, 89-77; insomnia, Special Report, 88-170; mental and behavioral disorders, 89-310; migraine, Special Report, 89-21; ulcer, Special Report, 90-74

Stress fracture: knee, Special Report, 88-45

Stroke, 90-330, 89-330, 88-312; books of health and medicine, 90-248; cholesterol, Special Report, 88-29; smoking, 89-327; Special Report, 90-57

Structural disorders: foot problems, Special Report, 89-119; scoliosis, Special Report, 88-124

Subarachnoid hemorrhage: drugs, 90-270; stroke, Special Report, 90-58

Subliminal angioplasty: stroke, 90-331

Subunit vaccines: Health Studies, 90-376

Sudden death: exercise and fitness, 89-280

Suicide: alcohol and drug abuse, 88-218; depression, Special Report, 88-73; mental and behavioral disorders, 89-309, 88-291; Soviet medicine, Special Report, 90-95

Sun: skin, 89-325; skin cancer, Special Report, 89-26

Sunlight: depression, Special Report, 88-76

Sunscreen: skin cancer, Special Report, 89-33

Sun-tanning equipment: skin cancer, Special Report, 89-34

Surgeon general of the United States: People in Medicine, 89-340

Surgery: back problems, Special Report, 90-209; blood, 89-244; breast cancer, Special Report, 90-37; coronary artery disease, Special Report, 89-82; cosmetic surgery, Special Report, 89-144; Health Studies, 89-379; il., 89-253; Project Orbis, Special Report, 90-356; skin

cancer, Special Report, 89-37; Soviet medicine, Special Report, 90-84

Surgical implants: Close-Up, 88-237

Surrogate parenthood: health policy, 88-277

Symptomatic medication: migraine, Special Report, 89-22

Synthetic prostaglandins (PG's): digestive system, 88-253

Systemic desensitization: anxiety disorders, Special Report, 90-24

Systolic pressure: checkup, Special Report, 88-202

T

Tamoxifen: breast cancer, Special Report, 90-35

Tardive dyskinesia: mental and behavioral disorders, 90-305

Tarsal bone: foot problems, Special Report, 89-118

T cell: AIDS, Special Report, 88-13; allergies and immunology, 90-240, 89-240; Health Studies, 90-370

Teen-age suicide: mental and behavioral disorders, 88-291

Teeth, Crooked: orthodontics, Special Report, 88-82

Television: child development, 89-262

Temperature, Body: emergency medicine, 89-275; exercise and fitness, 88-264

Tendon: exercise and fitness, 88-265

Testicular cancer: cancer, 89-258

Testis determining factor: genetics, 89-289

Testosterone: glands and hormones, 90-290, 88-277; left-handedness, Special Report, 89-165

Tetanus: Health Studies, 90-378

Tetracycline: dentistry, 90-262

Tetrahydroaminoacridine (THA): aging, 90-228; Close-Up, 89-229

Thermometer: emergency medicine, 89-275

Three Mile Island: radiation, Special Report, 88-140

Thrombin: ear and hearing, 88-258

Thromboxane: Close-Up, 89-296

Thymus gland: left-handedness, Special Report, 89-168

Thyroid gland: glands and hormones, 89-292; minerals, Special Report, 88-159

Tibia: knee, Special Report, 88-43

Tick: Lyme disease, Special Report, 89-44

Ticlopidine: stroke, 90-330

Tissue expansion: cosmetic surgery, Special Report, 89-150

Toenail: foot problems, Special Report, 89-123

Tonometer: aging eyes, Special Report, 88-194

Tooth decay: dentistry, 89-263

Total parenteral nutrition (TPN): AIDS, Special Report, 90-122

Toxic chemicals: environmental health, 89-278

Toxic hepatitis: steroids, Special Report, 90-47

Toxin: brain and nervous system, 89-253; salmonella, Special Report, 89-141

Toxoid vaccines: Health Studies, 90-376

Toxoplasmosis: pregnancy and childbirth, 89-315

t-PA (tissue-type plasminogen activator): drugs, 89-272; heart and blood vessels, 89-298; stroke, Special Report, 90-62

Trabecular bone: osteoporosis, Special Report, 89-57

Tranquilizers: steroids, Special Report, 90-53

Transcutaneous electric nerve stimulation (TENS): back problems, Special Report, 90-207

Transducer: prenatal diagnosis, Special Report, 88-59

Transient insomnia: insomnia, Special Report, 88-168

Transient ischematic attack (TIA): stroke, Special Report, 90-58

Transplantation surgery: ils., 89-248, 268; respiratory system, 89-316

Transverse arch: foot problems, Special Report, 89-118

Trauma: anxiety disorders, Special Report, 90-12; mental and behavioral disorders, 89-309; pediatric trauma, Special Report, 90-342

Travel: Health Studies, 90-379

Tretinoin: skin, 89-325

Trichosanthin: AIDS, 90-231

Tricyclic antidepressant: anxiety disorders, Special Report, 90-20; depression, Special Report, 88-79

Trigger: asthma, Special Report, 90-189; migraine, Special Report, 89-16

Triglycerides: exercise and fitness, 90-279

Tuberculosis: Special Report, 90-141

Tumor: breast cancer, Special Report, 90-28; cancer, 90-254

Tumor infiltrating lymphocytes: cancer, 90-254; genetics, 90-286

Tumor necrosis factor: infectious diseases, 89-303

Type A personality: child development, 88-247

U

Ulcer: drugs, 90-269; sexually transmitted diseases, 89-324; Special Report, 90-71. See also **Digestive System.**

Ulcerative colitis: left-handedness, Special Report, 89-168

Ulcerative keratitis: eye and vision, 90-282

Ultrasonic humidifiers: Close-Up, 90-237

Ultrasound: arthritis and connective tissue disorders, 89-243; back problems, Special Report, 90-207; digestive system, 90-265; heart and blood vessels, 90-299; prenatal diagnosis, Special Report, 88-59; stroke, Special Report, 90-67; urology, 89-332

Ultraviolet (UV) radiation: Close-Up, 88-262; environmental health, 88-261; eye and vision, 90-284; skin cancer, Special Report, 89-29

Umbilical cord: pregnancy and childbirth, 88-299

Underbite: orthodontics, Special Report, 88-84

Uremia: kidney, 88-290

Urinalysis: checkup, Special Report, 88-204

Urology, 90-330, 89-332, 88-314

Ursodeoxycholic acid: digestive system, 90-265; drugs, 90-271

UV-A radiation: skin cancer, Special Report, 89-29

UV-B radiation: eye and vision, 90-283; skin cancer, Special Report, 89-29

V

Vaccines: AIDS, 90-233, 89-234, 88-214; birth control, 90-243; dentistry, 89-263; Health Studies, 90-368; polio, Special Report, 89-109; tuberculosis, Special Report, 90-151; veterinary medicine, 90-332, 88-318. See also by diseases.

Vaginal infection: sexually transmitted diseases, 88-307

Vaporizers: Close-Up, 90-237

Vasectomy: birth control, 88-226

Vasodilator drugs: heart and blood vessels, 88-280

Vegetarianism: Special Report, 90-99

Venereal disease. See **AIDS; Sexually Transmitted Diseases.**

Veterinary Medicine, 90-332, 89-333, 88-316; Lyme disease, Special Report, 89-48

Viralizer: allergies and immunology, 90-238

Virus: foot problems, Special Report, 89-124; Health Studies, 90-369; infectious diseases, 88-287; Lyme disease, Special Report, 89-44; mononucleosis, Special Report, 90-136; polio, Special Report, 89-104. See also **AIDS.**

Vision: aging eyes, Special Report, 88-181. See also **Eye and Vision.**

Vitamins: vegetarianism, Special Report, 90-110

W

Walking: Close-Up, 88-266

Wart: foot problems, Special Report, 89-124

Water pollution: environmental health, 88-261; lead poisoning, Special Report, 90-176

Watery eyes: aging eyes, Special Report, 88-193

Weight Control, 90-335, 89-336, 88-319; alcohol and drug abuse, 90-236; Close-Up, 88-266; exercise and fitness, 90-281; Health Studies, 89-368. See also **Obesity.**

Weight-loss products: health fraud, Special Report, 88-290

Wellness: books of health and medicine, 90-249

White blood cell: blood, 89-246; nutrition, 88-296. See also **Immune system.**

Withdrawal syndrome: alcohol, Health Studies, 88-377

Women: brain and nervous system, 90-250; breast cancer, Special Report, 90-26; cancer, 88-239; glands and hormones, 90-289; Health Professions, 88-357; smoking, 89-327, 88-311; stroke, 88-313; weight control, 90-337. See also **Pregnancy and Childbirth.**

Worker safety: AIDS, Special Report, 90-121; asthma, Special Report, 90-190; lead poisoning, Special Report, 90-171; safety, 90-323, 88-305

World Health Organization (WHO): AIDS, 88-214, Special Report, 88-20

Wrinkles: cosmetic surgery, Special Report, 89-152; skin, 89-325

X

X-linked lymphoproliferative syndrome: mononucleosis, Special Report, 90-137

X rays: arthritis and connective tissue disorders, 89-243; checkup, Special Report, 88-207; radiation, Special Report, 88-143; scoliosis, Special Report, 88-130; tuberculosis, Special Report, 90-149

Y

Yoyo dieting: Health Studies, 89-381

Yuppie flu: mononucleosis, Special Report, 90-137

Z

Zidovudine (AZT): AIDS, 90-230

Zinc: eye and vision, 89-283; lead poisoning, Special Report, 90-180; vegetarianism, Special Report, 90-108

Acknowledgments

The publishers of *The World Book Health & Medical Annual* gratefully acknowledge the courtesy of the following artists, photographers, publishers, institutions, agencies, and corporations for the illustrations in this volume. Credits should read from top to bottom, left to right, on their respective pages. All entries marked with an asterisk (*) denote illustrations created exclusively for *The World Book Health & Medical Annual*. All maps, charts, and diagrams were prepared by *The World Book Health & Medical Annual* staff unless otherwise noted.

4 Jeff Thompson*; © Ricki Rosen, Picture Group
5 Catherine Twomey*; © Leslie Jean-Bart; © David R. Frazier Photolibrary
8 Cary Henrie*; Donna Kae Nelson*; © Kevin Beebe, Custom Medical; TASS from Sovfoto; Jeff Thompson*
9 Terry Sirrell*
10-23 Jeff Thompson*
27 © SIU from Photo Researchers; Roberta Polfus*
29 Roberta Polfus*
30 JAK Graphics*
33 © Jon Riley, Medichrome
34 Art: Roberta Polfus*—photos: © Jon Riley, Medichrome
35 Photo: © Tom Tracy, Medichrome—art: Roberta Polfus*
38-39 Roberta Polfus*
42 John Figler*; Focus on Sports
45 SCALA/Art Resource; © *Time* Magazine
46 John Figler*
47 JAK Graphics*
49 John Figler*
50 UCLA Olympic Laboratories
51 Food and Drug Administration
53 John Figler*
56 Donna Kae Nelson*
59 JAK Graphics*
60 Donna Kae Nelson*; © Harry J. Przekop, Jr., Medichrome; Donna Kae Nelson*; © CNRI/Science Source from Photo Researchers
61 © Hank Morgan, Rainbow; © Hank Morgan, Science Source from Photo Researchers
64 © Larry Mulvehill, Photo Researchers
66 © Leonard Kansler, Medichrome; © John Lynch, Medichrome; © James Prince, Photo Researchers
67 © David York, Medichrome

68 JAK Graphics*
70-75 Terry Sirrell*
76 Evanston Hospital; University of Chicago Medical Center; University of Chicago Medical Center
78-80 Terry Sirrell*
82 TASS from Sovfoto
85 © Vlastimir Shone, Gamma/Liaison
86-87 TASS from Sovfoto
89-91 Sovfoto
95-96 Michael Woods*
98-109 Donna Kae Nelson*
112 Indre M. Lukas Design*
115 © Michael Grecco, Picture Group; © Tom Lyle, Medichrome
116 © Richard W. Shock, Black Star; © Liba Taylor, Select
119 © Ricki Rosen, Picture Group
120 © Michael Murphy, Medichrome; © Henry Martin, Custom Medical
122 © Linda Steinmark, Custom Medical
123 © Richard Lord, Black Star
126 Cary Henrie*
129 The Children's Hospital of Philadelphia
131-135 Cary Henrie*
136 © Harry J. Przekop, Jr., Medichrome
137 National Institutes of Health
138 © G. W. Willis, Ochsner Medical Institution from Biological Photo Service; © G. W. Willis, Ochsner Medical Institution from Biological Photo Service; © David York, Medichrome
140 American Lung Association
144 Granger Collection
145 Mary Evans Picture Library
147 American Lung Association
148 Ann Ronan Picture Library; American Lung Association; Ann Ronan Picture Library
150 Mary Evans Picture Library
151 © Hans Haberstadt, Photo Researchers
152 Trudy Rogers*; Trudy Rogers*; © Diane Rawson, Photo Researchers; © Mario Ruiz

154 Photos: UPI/Bettmann Newsphotos; AP/Wide World; UPI/Bettmann Newsphotos; Centers for Disease Control, Atlanta—art: Don Wilson*
159 American Legion; UPI/Bettmann Newsphotos; Don Wilson*
160 AP/Wide World; Don Wilson*; AP/Wide World
161 AP/Wide World
162 Don Wilson*; AP/Wide World
163 Hahnemann University Hospital; Don Wilson*
164 AP/Wide World; Don Wilson*; Don Wilson*; Centers for Disease Control, Atlanta
165 UPI/Bettmann Newsphotos
168-178 Robert Lawson*
182-191 Joe Rogers*
192 © Kevin Beebe, Custom Medical
194 John Frank*; © Richard Hutchings, Photo Researchers
198-210 Timothy S. Hooker*
212 Catherine Twomey*
215 Catherine Twomey*; © Alan Zuckerman, Sherman Oaks Community Hospital; Burns Institute of Shriners Hospitals for Crippled Children; Burns Institute of Shriners Hospitals for Crippled Children
217-218 Catherine Twomey*
220 Burns Institute of Shriners Hospitals for Crippled Children
223 AP/Wide World
226 University of Texas Southwestern Medical Center; Lawrence Berkeley Laboratory; Children's Hospital of San Diego
227 © Hank Morgan; Edward Mausner, NYT Pictures
228 Neurocom International, Inc.
230 © Sam C. Pierson, Jr., Photo Researchers

231 JAK Graphics*
232 © James D. Wilson, Woodfin Camp, Inc.
235 JAK Graphics*
236 © Beth Hansen
237 Ralph Brunke*
238 © Jacques Chenet, Woodfin Camp, Inc.
239 Ralph Brunke*
240 Stanford University Medical Center
241 Techmedica
243 © Vauthey, Sygma
244 Trudy Rogers*
245 Morris Simon, M.D., Beth Israel Hospital, Boston
246 University of Texas Southwestern Medical Center
247 Castblast, Inc.
249 WORLD BOOK photo
251 University of Colorado Health Sciences Center; JAK Graphics*
252 Smith-Kettlewell Eye Research Foundation; Peter Menzel
253 Pan-Asia Newspaper Alliance
254 Lawrence Berkeley Laboratory
255 Trudy Rogers*; National Cancer Institute
256 Laurie Jarvis, University of California at San Francisco
258 Catherine Best, Wesleyan University
259 Joseph Fagan, Case Western Reserve University
261 Washington University School of Medicine
262 University of Missouri at Kansas City
263 JAK Graphics*
264 Healthware Corporation
265 Barry J. Marshall, M.D.
266 THE FAR SIDE cartoon by Gary Larson is reprinted by permission of Chronicle Features, San Francisco, Calif.
267 Aprex Corporation
268 Ralph Brunke*
270 © Sidney Harris; *Time* Magazine
272 David R. Frazier Photolibrary
273 MEDphone Corporation
274 Igor Gamow
275 Dan Miller, NYT Pictures
278 © Chester Higgins Jr., Photo Researchers

279 JAK Graphics*
281 Joe Schwartz, Georgia Institute of Technology
282 ©Scott Arthur Masear
283 Denis G. Pelli, Syracuse University
287 Jean-Louis Cholet, The Institute for Dermatoglypics
288 Lawrence Berkeley Laboratory
290 © Donald Dietz, Stock, Boston
292 © Sudhir, Picture Group
293 Mayo Clinic; The Johns Hopkins University Medical Institutions
295 © Barbara Kinney, Gamma/Liaison; Chester Higgins, NYT Pictures
297 Patrick Dyson, University of Florida Health Science Center
298 Intermedics, Inc.
299 Cardiac Pacemakers, Inc.
300 Trudy Rogers*
301 © David York, Medichrome
302 Trudy Rogers*
303 George Tames, NYT Pictures
305 Children's Hospital of San Diego
306 Ralph Brunke*
308 © Will McIntyre, Photo Researchers
313 Michael Katz, M.D.
314 © Hank Morgan
315 © Ed Lettau, Photo Researchers
316 © Pierre Kopp, West Light
317 Trudy Rogers*
319 American Academy of Pediatrics
320 AP/Wide World
322 TRW, Inc.; © David Sears, Gamma/Liaison
323 Georgia Institute of Technology
327 AP/Wide World
328 AP/Wide World
329 JAK Graphics*; Lakeside Pharmaceutical
330 © J. H. Reeves
332 THE FAR SIDE cartoon by Gary Larson is reprinted by permission of Chronicle Features, San Francisco, Calif.
333 Edward Hausner, NYT Pictures

334 JAK Graphics*; Terence McCarthy, NYT Pictures
336 AP/Wide World
337 JAK Graphics*
338 © Barry Lewis, NETWORK; © Robert J. Bennett, Photri from Marilyn Gartman; © Jordan Coonrad
339 © Dennis Brack, Black Star; © Leslie Jean-Bart
340 Children's Hospital National Medical Center; © Andrea Krause, Photo Researchers; © Robert J. Bennett, Photri from Marilyn Gartman
341 © Leslie Jean-Bart
343 Children's Hospital National Medical Center
344-348 © Dennis Brack, Black Star
350 The Kennedy Institute, Baltimore
354 G. Robert Hampton, M.D., Project ORBIS
335 © Fred Ward, Black Star
358 David Loshak, Project ORBIS
359 © J. P. Laffont, Sygma
360-361 Art: JAK Graphics*—photos: © Barry Lewis, NETWORK; © Jordan Coonrad; © Jordan Coonrad
362 © Barry Lewis, NETWORK; © Jordan Coonrad
364 © Jordan Coonrad; © John Chiasson, Gamma/Liaison
366 Culver; Sygma; Merck Sharp & Dohme
367 Bettmann Archive; © David R. Frazier Photolibrary
368 Jason Weisfield, M.D. from The National Geographic Society
369 March of Dimes Birth Defects Foundation
371 JAK Graphics*
373 JAK Graphics*; Bettmann Archive
374 Culver
375 Merck Sharp & Dohme
377 JAK Graphics*
378 © SIU from Custom Medical; © David R. Frazier Photolibrary; Custom Medical
379 © Andrew Popper, Picture Group
381 Sygma
383 © James Pazarik, Gamma/Liaison; © Henry Martin, Custom Medical; The Skin Cancer Foundation
384 Copyright © The New York Times Company